Complaints, Controversies and Grievances in Medicine

Recent studies into the experiences and failures of healthcare services, along with the rapid development of patient advocacy, consumerism and pressure groups, have led historians and social scientists to engage with the issue of the medical complaint. As expressions of dissatisfaction, disquiet and failings in service provision, past complaints provide a vital antidote to progressive histories of healthcare. This book explores what has happened historically when medicine generated complaints.

This multidisciplinary collection comprises contributions from leading international scholars and uses new research to develop a sophisticated understanding of the development of medicine and the role of complaints and complaining in this story. It addresses how each aspect of the medical complaint – between sciences, professions, practitioners and sectors; within politics, ethics and regulatory bodies; from interested parties and patients – has manifested in modern medicine, and how it has been defined, dealt with and resolved.

Working from a critical and interdisciplinary humanities and social science perspective grounded in historical case studies of medicine and bioethics, this volume provides the first major and comprehensive historical, comparative and policy-based examination of the area. It will be of interest to historians, sociologists, legal specialists and ethicists interested in medicine, as well as those involved in healthcare policy, practice and management.

Jonathan Reinarz is Professor of the History of Medicine at the University of Birmingham, UK. His publications include *Healthcare in Birmingham: The Birmingham Teaching Hospitals, 1779–1939* (Woodbridge, 2009), and the edited collections *A Medical History of Skin* (with Kevin Siena; London, 2013), *Medicine and the Workhouse* (with Leonard Schwarz; Rochester, NY, 2013) and *Permeable Walls: Institutional Visiting in Historical Perspective* (with Graham Mooney; Amsterdam, 2009). He has also published on the history of the senses, including a special issue of the *Journal for Eighteenth-Century Studies* on 'The Enlightenment and the Senses' (edited with L. Schwarz, 2012) and *Past Scents: Historical Perspectives on Smell*

(Champaign, IL, 2014), and edited a special issue of the journal *Food and History* (forthcoming 2014) on the history of hospital food, which inevitably touches on the subject of complaining.

Rebecca Wynter is an Honorary Research Fellow in History and Visiting Lecturer in the History of Medicine Unit at the University of Birmingham, UK. As a Postdoctoral Researcher at Woodbrooke Quaker Study Centre, Birmingham, she is also co-curating a 2015 exhibition about Quakers in the Great War, to be mounted at Birmingham Museum and Art Gallery. Her current research centres on material culture, lunatic asylums and workhouses; neurodisabilities and epileptic colonies; focal sepsis theory in British psychiatry; and the Friends' Ambulance Unit, 1914–19. Her publications include '"Good in All Respects": Appearance and Dress at Staffordshire County Lunatic Asylum, 1818–54', *History of Psychiatry* (March 2011), and '"Horrible Dens of Deception": Thomas Bakewell, Thomas Mulock and Anti-Asylum Sentiments, *c.*1815–1860', in T. Knowles and S. Trowbridge (eds), *Insanity and the Lunatic Asylum in the Nineteenth Century* (London, 2014).

Routledge Studies in the Sociology of Health and Illness

Available titles include:

Dimensions of Pain
Humanities and social science perspectives
Edited by Lisa Folkmarson Käll

Caring and Well-being
A lifeworld approach
Kathleen Galvin and Les Todres

Aging Men, Masculinities and Modern Medicine
Edited by Antje Kampf, Barbara L. Marshall and Alan Petersen

Disclosure in Health and Illness
Mark Davis and Lenore Manderson

Complaints, Controversies and Grievances in Medicine
Historical and social science perspectives
Jonathan Reinarz and Rebecca Wynter

Forthcoming titles:

The Public Shaping of Medical Research
Patient associations, health movements and biomedicine
Edited by Peter Wehling and Willy Viehöver

Abuse, Mental Illness and Recovery in Everyday Lives
Beyond trauma
Nicole Moulding

Systems Theory and the Sociology of Health and Illness
Observing healthcare
Morten Knudsen and Werner Vogd

The Public Shaping of Medical Research
Patient associations, health movements and biomedicine
Peter Wehling, Willy Viehover and Sophia Koenen

Complaints, Controversies and Grievances in Medicine

Historical and social science perspectives

Edited by Jonathan Reinarz and Rebecca Wynter

Routledge
Taylor & Francis Group
LONDON AND NEW YORK

First published 2015
by Routledge
4 Park Square, Milton Park, Abingdon, Oxon OX14 4RN
605 Third Avenue, New York, NY 10017

Routledge is an imprint of the Taylor & Francis Group, an informa business

British Library Cataloguing-in-Publication Data
A catalogue record for this book is available from the British Library

Library of Congress Cataloging in Publication Data
Complaints, controversies and grievances in medicine : historical and social science perspectives / [edited by Jonathan Reinarz and Rebecca Wynter].
p. ; cm. – (Routledge studies in the sociology of health and illness)
Includes bibliographical references.
I. Reinarz, Jonathan, editor. II. Wynter, Rebecca, editor. III. Series: Routledge studies in the sociology of health and illness.
[DNLM: 1. Delivery of Health Care–history–Great Britain.
2. History, 19th Century–Great Britain. 3. History, 20th Century–Great Britain. 4. Patient Satisfaction–Great Britain. 5. Quality of Health Care–history–Great Britain. W 84 FA1]
RA394
362.1–dc23 2014022765

ISBN: 978-1-138-79490-0 (hbk)
ISBN: 978-1-315-75892-3 (ebk)

Typeset in Perpetua
by Wearset Ltd, Boldon, Tyne and Wear

For all those – physicians, nurses, surgeons, paramedics, care workers and whistleblowers – who are determined to continue Nye Bevan's fight for ideals in medicine, and for patients such as Violet Davies whose care fell far short.

Contents

Illustrations

Figures

Tables

Contributors

John Clarke is an Emeritus Professor in the Faculty of Social Sciences at the UK's Open University, where he worked for more than 30 years on the political and cultural struggles involved in remaking welfare, nations and states. His recent research has explored school inspection as a mode of governing and new sites of legal consciousness. Recent writing includes *Publics, Politics and Power* (with Janet Newman; London, 2009) and *Disputing Citizenship* (with Kathleen Coll, Evelina Dagnino and Catherine Neveu; Cambridge, 2014). A further collaboration (with Dave Bainton, Noémi Lendvai and Paul Stubbs) entitled *Making Policy Move: Towards a Politics of Translation and Assemblage* will be published by the Policy Press in 2015.

Hera Cook is a Senior Lecturer in Social Science and History in the Department of Public Health, University of Otago Wellington, in Wellington, New Zealand. Her previous research has examined the reasons behind societal commitment to sexual prudery and ignorance from the last third of the nineteenth century to the 1950s and the causal relationship between reproduction and English sexual culture. This has been published as a monograph, entitled *The Long Sexual Revolution: English Women, Sex and Contraception, 1800–1975* (Oxford, 2004), and in several articles. She is currently working on a history of the management of emotion in twentieth-century England. Recent publications include articles on romantic love and sexuality, on controlling emotion in mid-century England and on parental emotions and sex education.

Hilary Ingram is a PhD candidate in the Department of History at University College London. Her dissertation project, *A Complicated Calling: Female British Medical Missionaries and Professional Identity, 1874–1920*, explores female involvement in British Protestant medical missions over this period. Her research interests include the social history of the British Empire, missionary medicine, and women and medicine. She currently serves as a convenor for the Colonial/Postcolonial New Researchers' Workshop at the Institute of Historical Research.

June Jones is a Senior Lecturer in Biomedical Ethics at the University of Birmingham. Her publications include (with D. Willis) 'Specialist Palliative Care, Non-Cancer Conditions and Guilt: An Unholy Triad?' *International Journal of Palliative Nursing* (2014); (with A. Shanks) 'Laid Bare: Religious Intolerance within Online Commentary about "Bare Below the Elbows" Guidance in Professional Journals', *Health Care Analysis* (2013); and (with J. McHale) 'Privacy, Confidentiality and Abortion Statistics: A Question of Public Interest?' *Journal of Medical Ethics* (2011).

Steven King is Pro-Vice Chancellor and Head of the College of Social Science at the University of Leicester. His research interests span the histories of poverty, welfare, demography and medicine and run from the seventeenth century to the present. His most recent books have included *A Caring County: Social Welfare in Hertfordshire from 1600* (edited with G. Gear; Hatfield, 2013); *Migration, Settlement and Belonging in Europe, 1500s–1930s* (edited with A. Winter; Oxford, 2013); and *Networks of Knowledge in East-Central Europe* (edited with D. Sechel; special edition of the journal *East Central Europe*, 2014). His chapter for this volume draws on a wider project looking at the rights of patients and the duties of doctors between the eighteenth century and the twentieth.

Pilar León-Sanz is an Associate Professor of the History of Medicine and Medical Ethics at the University of Navarra, Portugal. Her research explores practices and healthcare professionals during the nineteenth and twentieth centuries. She has published 'Medical Assistance Provided by *La Conciliación*, a Pamplona Mutual Assistance Association (1902–84)', in B. Harris (ed.), *Welfare and Old Age in Europe and North America: The Development of Social Insurance* (London, 2012); *Health Institutions at the Origin of the Welfare Systems in Europe* (Pamplona, 2010); *La Tarantola Spagnola: Empirismo e tradizione nel XVIII secolo* (Lècce, 2008); *Vicente Ferrer Gorraiz Beaumont y Montesa (1718–1792), un polemista navarro de la ilustración* (with D. Barettino; Pamplona, 2007); and *La implantación de los derechos del paciente* (Pamplona, 2004). She is a member of the project 'Emotional Culture and Identity' at the Instituto de Cultura y Sociedad, University of Navarra.

Jean McHale is Professor of Healthcare Law and Director of the Centre for Health Law Science and Policy at Birmingham Law School, University of Birmingham. Her books include *Medical Confidentiality and Legal Privilege* (London, 1993); *Health Law and the European Union* (with T. K. Hervey; Cambridge, 2004); *Health Care Law Text and Materials* (with M. Fox; 2nd edn, London, 2007); edited collections include *Principles of Medical Law* (Oxford, 2010). Her new monograph, *European Health Law* (with T. K. Hervey; Cambridge), and edited collection, the *Routledge Handbook of Complementary and Alternative Medicine: Perspectives from Social Sciences and Law* (edited with N. Gale; London), will be published in 2015.

Alex Mold is a Lecturer in History at the Centre for History in Public Health, London School of Hygiene and Tropical Medicine. She is the author of *Heroin: The Treatment of Addiction in Twentieth Century Britain* (DeKalb, IL, 2008) and (with Virginia Berridge) *Voluntary Action and Illegal Drugs: Health and Society in Britain Since the 1960s* (Basingstoke, 2009). She has published a number of articles on the history of the patient as consumer, and her book on the topic will be published by Manchester University Press.

Matthew Newsom Kerr is an Assistant Professor of History at Santa Clara University in California. His recent publications include chapters on the visual culture of smallpox in *A Medical History of Skin* (London, 2013) and conditions at London infectious hospitals in *Residential Institutions in Britain, 1725–1970* (London, 2013). His article on the infectious possibilities of cabs, omnibuses and ambulances appeared in the *Journal of British History* (April 2010). He is currently completing a monograph on late-Victorian London isolation hospitals under the Metropolitan Asylums Board.

Kim Price is an Honorary Visiting Fellow at the University of Leicester, where he has also been a Wellcome Trust Postdoctoral Researcher. He has published articles about pre-NHS health policy and the history of medical negligence in the *Lancet* and the *Social History of Medicine*, and is the author of *Medical Negligence in Victorian Britain: The Crisis of Care under the English Poor Law, c.1834–1900* (London, 2014). He has also provided advice to public bodies and the media, including an appearance as lead contributor in a special broadcast of BBC Radio 4's *The Long View* on patient neglect in the NHS.

Jonathan Reinarz is a Professor of the History of Medicine at the University of Birmingham. His publications include *Healthcare in Birmingham: The Birmingham Teaching Hospitals, 1779–1939* (Woodbridge, 2009), and the edited collections *A Medical History of Skin* (with Kevin Siena; London, 2013) and *Medicine and the Workhouse* (with Leonard Schwarz; Rochester, NY, 2013) and *Permeable Walls: Institutional Visiting in Historical Perspective* (with Graham Mooney; Amsterdam, 2009). He has also published on the history of the senses, including a special issue of the *Journal for Eighteenth-Century Studies* on 'The Enlightenment and the Senses' (edited with L. Schwarz, 2012) and *Past Scents: Historical Perspectives on Smell* (Champaign, IL, 2014), and edited a special issue of the journal *Food and History* (forthcoming 2014) on the history of hospital food, which inevitably touches on the subject of complaining.

Andrew Scull is Distinguished Professor of Sociology and Science Studies at the University of California, San Diego. He has written extensively on the history of psychiatry. Recent books include *Madhouse* (New Haven, 2005); *The Insanity of Place/The Place of Insanity* (London, 2006); *Madness: A Very Short Introduction* (Oxford, 2009); and *Hysteria: The Disturbing History* (Oxford, 2011). His

Madness and Civilization will be published by Thames and Hudson and Princeton University Press in 2015.

Andrew Shanks is a Lecturer in Behavioural and Communication Sciences at the University of Birmingham. His research interests focus on language analysis in healthcare contexts and in particular on the nature of propositions in text. His analyses have contributed to publications on religious intolerance, discussing genetic conditions with children, and gaining opinions about care from people with learning disabilities. Most recently, he has written on the uses of language analysis with 'big data' for the *British Journal of General Practice* (2014).

Steven Thompson is a Senior Lecturer at the Department of History and Welsh History at Aberystwyth University. His publications include *Unemployment, Poverty and Health in Interwar South Wales* (Cardiff, 2006) and numerous articles and book chapters on various aspects of the provision of medical and health services in industrial south Wales in the nineteenth and twentieth centuries. He is currently engaged in a collaborative research project funded by the Wellcome Trust on disability and the British coal industry, and he is working on a monograph on medicine and health services in south Wales from 1780 to 1948.

Rosemary Wall is a Lecturer in Global History at the University of Hull and an Honorary Lecturer at the Florence Nightingale School of Nursing and Midwifery, King's College London. She is a historian of medicine, studying Britain and areas of British overseas settlement between 1880 and 1960. Her current project is an interdisciplinary book on British colonial nursing, co-authored with colleagues at King's College London. Her previous projects have investigated the use of bacteriology in hospitals, workplaces and local communities, and her book, *Bacteria in Britain, 1880–1939* (London), was published in 2013.

Rebecca Wynter is an Honorary Research Fellow in History and a Visiting Lecturer in the History of Medicine Unit at the University of Birmingham. As a Postdoctoral Researcher at Woodbrooke Quaker Study Centre, Birmingham, she is also co-curating a 2015 exhibition about Quakers in the Great War, to be mounted at Birmingham Museum and Art Gallery. Her current research centres on material culture, lunatic asylums and workhouses; neurodisabilities and epileptic colonies; focal sepsis theory in British psychiatry; and the Friends' Ambulance Unit, 1914–1919. Her publications include '"Good in All Respects": Appearance and Dress at Staffordshire County Lunatic Asylum, 1818–54', *History of Psychiatry* (March 2011), and '"Horrible Dens of Deception": Thomas Bakewell, Thomas Mulock and Anti-Asylum Sentiments, *c.*1815–1860', in T. Knowles and S. Trowbridge (eds), *Insanity and the Lunatic Asylum in the Nineteenth Century* (London, 2014).

Preface

This book had its origins in a two-day conference, entitled 'Complaining about Medicine', in November 2012, sponsored by the Institute of Advanced Studies at the University of Birmingham. It drew together scholars from across the University, and from Europe and North America, whose work directly engaged with some of the key themes identified in this volume's introduction. The opening keynote at the conference was delivered by Professor Andrew Scull, who has for this volume expanded on his original paper. The Afterword derives from our second keynote lecture, delivered at the conclusion of the event by Professor John Clarke. On that final day, his comments helped bridge chronological periods and regions and now offer a fitting conclusion to the subject as a whole, outlining both achievements in this area of research and some future challenges.

We wish to thank the conference sponsors, the Institute of Advanced Studies at Birmingham, and particularly Malcolm Press, Sue Gilligan and Sarah Myring, who continue to bring together academics from across the University of Birmingham's five colleges and encourage fruitful discussions and debates. We are especially grateful to the original members of the conference organising committee – Leonard Smith, Nicola Gale, Stuart Wildman and Jean McHale – for helping to identify participants and compile a stimulating programme. Leonard Smith and Cathy Hale, as well as many of the volume's contributors, were kind enough to cast their eyes over sections of the introduction and we are indebted to them for their help. Finally, we wish to thank the editorial team of Routledge's 'Health and Social Care' books, in particular Grace McInnes, James Watson and Louisa Vahtrick, as well as two anonymous reviewers, for their comments on an earlier draft of the book's chapters. They have not only made the entire publication process as painless as possible, but, ultimately, they leave us with no complaints.

The Editors
4 June 2014

Abbreviations

BMA	British Medical Association
BMJ	*British Medical Journal*
CEZMS	Church of England Zenana Missionary Society
CMS	Church Missionary Society
DDE	Doctrine of Double Effect
DSM	*Diagnostic and Statistical Manual*
GMC	General Medical Council
GP	General practitioner
LGB	Local Government Board
LSMW	London School of Medicine for Women
MAB	Metropolitan Asylums Board
MOH	Medical Officer of Health
NHS	National Health Service
PLB	Poor Law Board
SCTOC	South Croydon Typhoid Outbreak Committee
ZMC	Zenana Medical College

Introduction

Towards a history of complaining about medicine

Jonathan Reinarz and Rebecca Wynter

'I would be far from complaining about the treatment I have received in any English hospital, but I do know that it is a sound instinct that warns people to keep out of hospitals if possible, and especially out of the public wards.'

So wrote English novelist and journalist George Orwell, after recounting the 'horrors' of the medical care he experienced during his 1929 stay at Hôpital X in Paris.[1] The heritage of poor care is as much bound up in Orwell's haunted institutions as it is in inherited stories fossilised by the media. That great heroine of the hospital and reformer of nursing, Florence Nightingale, was not above publicising manipulated mortality figures in order to argue that medicine – as Hippocrates directed – should 'do the sick no harm'.[2] The municipal hospitals that emerged in England from workhouse infirmaries at exactly the same time as Orwell's stay in Hôpital X set off a new chain of events – one in which a host of official reports, again covered by the media, promoted a co-ordinated system in which inconsistencies might be eradicated. The 1948 National Health Service (NHS), in spite of the disgruntlement of many physicians, bloomed into a system in which the British people believed, and yet at the same time harboured those spectral superstitions of distress, discomfort, disease and death. In 1965, the press (in this case an open letter to the Editor of *The Times*) was used to confirm the worst fears of the public, fears which have only too recently re-emerged.

> Sir,
>
> We, the undersigned, have been shocked by the treatment of geriatric patients in certain mental hospitals, one of the evils being the practice of stripping them of their personal possessions. We have now sufficient evidence to suggest that this is widespread.
>
> The attitude of the Ministry of Health to complaints has merely reinforced our anxieties. In consequence, we have decided to collect evidence of ill-treatment of geriatric patients throughout the country, to demonstrate the need for a national investigation. We hope this will lead to the securing of

> effective and humane control over these hospitals by the Ministry, which seems at present to be lacking.
>
> We shall be grateful if those who have encountered malpractices in this sphere will supply us with detailed information, which would of course be treated as confidential.[3]

Among the 'yours faithfully' was Barbara Robb, associated with the pressure group Aid for the Elderly in Government Institutions (AEGIS), and editor of the influential 1967 critique *Sans Everything*, which drew on whistleblowers' letters received in response to the plea in *The Times*.[4] Another signatory was Brian Abel-Smith, a professor of social administration at the London School of Economics, a government policy advisor and a specialist in healthcare systems, who in his spare time 'unravelled' the myth of Florence Nightingale (1960),[5] and wrote *A History of the Nursing Profession* and *The Hospitals 1800–1948* (1964); the latter was published in the months prior to *The Times* letter of complaint.[6]

Those who research medical subjects, historical and contemporary, are well placed to contribute to discussions and debates about complaint and complaining culture; after all, the complaint is a reckoning with the past. Followers of recent events might also expect the British and American publics to be more than a little familiar with this general theme: not only given the storm surrounding phone hacking and the media, and the rumpus sparked by Obamacare, but also in light of the displacement of complaints about controversial NHS reforms with complaints about the NHS itself. These have centred on investigations at more than a dozen NHS Trusts following an inquiry into deaths at a hospital in Mid Staffordshire, England. In Britain, reporters have listened to complaints and revealed the details of individual scandals; they have also highlighted issues associated with those found in this volume, such as the agency of patient or pressure groups and voluntary organisations (including Cure the NHS and Action Against Medical Accidents) and of whistleblowers in generating reform, despite often being obstructed.[7] In order to challenge a so-called 'culture of fear' – which has been seen to have effectively silenced many healthcare workers, even if they were not subject to gagging orders – commentators and those in positions of authority are now emphasising a rediscovered 'duty of candour' required of all health service employees, from porters to chief executives, to ensure future transparency through speaking out about failures and mistakes. As part of this dramatic culture change, staff, rather than being legally bound to prevent the disclosure of 'unpleasant stories', have 'a duty to complain'.[8] Indeed, there had already been calls to recognise that 'complaining is good for medicine': it improved practice, maintained standards, reduced litigation, maintained trust, encouraged self-assessment, protected the public and reminded 'doctors of their legal and professional obligations'.[9]

Other countries have seen the emergence of similar trends, if not more aggressive manifestations of complaint cultures. In China, for example, grievance culture has reached new levels since the introduction of market reforms in the 1980s, with around 17,000 attacks on doctors being reported by the Ministry of Health in 2010 alone, some ending in the deaths of medical practitioners.[10] Much of the resentment stems from the escalating cost of treatment, but also from rumours of suspected corruption within the health services. As a result, following a recent attack and a subsequent online poll by a Chinese newspaper, it was reported that almost two-thirds of the more than 6,000 respondents said they were 'happy about the attack, since it was on a medical worker'.[11] When another doctor in Harbin in North-east China was stabbed, netizens similarly 'cheered for the murderer'. In response to this and similar stories, the English medical journal *The Lancet* declared in an editorial that 'China's doctors are in crisis', while others have described the country's hospitals as 'Battlegrounds of Discontent'.[12] More recently, doctors in India have staged strikes in protest at 'poor security after attacks from aggrieved relatives of patients they have treated'.[13] The extreme nature of such assaults will immediately remind some readers of attacks on American doctors who perform abortions,[14] only on a larger scale and, so far at least, without recourse to bombs or the full modern 'repertoire of contention', as sociologist and political scientist Charles Tilly has described the protestor's toolkit.[15]

At other times, complaining has been regarded as less political and so routine that it was hardly deemed worthy of serious examination. There are in fact few studies on the subject, historical or otherwise.[16] It is our assertion that the phenomenon of complaining, and its associated themes, is worthy of further investigation. This is, in essence, a complaint that complaining has not been listened to as intently as it should have been within the historiography – one that we hope will be the beginning of a wider and richer conversation. In medicine, as in many other areas of life, major advances and social reforms have started with a complaint. As noted elsewhere, 'complaint has a noble history. It has driven human society forward and led to the abolition of systematic injustice'.[17] That it is more commonly associated with inconsequential moans and is regarded as a pastime of the nostalgic is to be lamented; 'while moaning is the province of the disempowered, a complaint requires at the very least a hope that one might be heard. . . . A complaint is more than a moan; it is a call to action'.[18] Even so, the complaint takes on many guises. The *Oxford English Dictionary* variously defines complaint as 'outcry against or because of injury; representation of wrong suffered; utterance of grievance' and a 'statement of injury or grievance laid before a court of judicial authority for purposes of prosecution or of redress; a formal accusation or charge'.[19] A complaint is a serious, weighty charge and one that can be expressed in action, verbally or in writing; the success or otherwise of the method may be dependent on how reasonable the grievance or expression is considered to be, which in turn depends on its timing and on the temperament or acceptance of culpability by the point of contact with the complaint. Grievance may also be delivered in different theatres: on the street, in offices or branches of business, in parliaments, in courthouses, in the press, on the internet and in essays and books. With the space to write, analyse and assess, complaining takes on a specific form – the critique.

Complaining in the modern world may be considered as routine; it has also been formalised. As Julian Baggini states in one of the few scholarly studies to address the subject, 'complaint is doubly transitive'.[20] Most individuals complain *about* something, but also *to* someone. In his classic study, *Complaints against Doctors* (1973), Rudolf Klein outlined the two pathways available to British patients who were determined to complain about professional medical services: the law, or the relevant professional body.[21] The back of every Medical Card originally issued to users of the NHS directed the disgruntled to the Clerk of the Executive Council at a specified address. Clearly not all aggrieved patients took their remonstrations to this stage, for only 800 or 900 complaints were included in the statistics of the Department of Health and Social Security annually, just over half relating to community-based medical care. In 1970–71 alone, general practitioners (GPs) in London requested that 7,059 patients be removed from practice lists, so clearly relations between patients and practitioners were not harmonious.[22] With 200 to 250 million contacts between English patients and some 20,000 GPs each year, it became clear to Klein that recorded complaints were just the 'tip of the iceberg' in terms of dissatisfaction with British health-care, and the actual shape of that iceberg, let alone the specific types of complaints being made, was unknown.[23]

In some respects, Linda Mulcahy's work attempts to bring Klein's work up to date, but it simultaneously opens up many new avenues for examination. It also goes well beyond the identification of complaints, grumbles and frictions and considers the 'dynamics of disputes', such as the way in which both doctors and patients construct their accounts when such conflicts emerge.[24] Unlike Klein's, Mulcahy's work considers complaint handling within both general practice and hospital environments. Reviewed and revised by the Davies Committee report (1973), complaints procedures were recognised as being hampered by a lack of external involvement in handling grievances and as emphasising the rights of practitioners, rather than those of patients. Much else has changed in the three decades since the publication of Klein and the Davies report. For example, complaints processes have been more widely advertised in hospitals, while the Griffiths Report (1983) introduced general managers at regional, district and hospital levels, effectively triangulating the complaints issue and bringing new actors and considerations to grievance management. A new centralised complaints procedure, introduced in 1985 and examined in detail by Alex Mold in this volume, abolished separate hospital complaint mechanisms, but apparently left much else unchanged. Despite extensive reforms to official systems of complaining, including the new NHS complaints procedure inaugurated in 1996, Mulcahy has argued that doctors continue to exercise substantial control over procedures. Not only have hospital managers taken a minimalist approach to complaints handling post-1996, but often these complex issues have been handled at the local level and delegated to untrained or junior staff who rely primarily on clinicians' accounts of events.[25] Finally, the very act of making a complaint had not become any easier, the complexity of lodging formal complaints ensuring that the majority of the 'iceberg' remained submerged.

A visit to NHS Choices, the largest British healthcare website, reveals just how easy it has since become to register a complaint about medicine when – to echo the 1837 call to change of Scottish alienist W. A. F. Browne[26] – things are not as they ought to be. On arriving at this virtual 'front door' to the NHS, visitors are directed to one of three main sections, entitled 'You and the NHS'.[27] By clicking a link here, users are, in fact, directed to a page which advises 'How to complain'.[28] A brief passage clearly informs visitors to the website that 'Every NHS organisation has a complaints procedure', before this page runs through various related questions, including 'What are my rights?', 'Who should I complain to?' and 'When should I complain?' The homepage of the General Medical Council (GMC), the main regulator of the medical profession in the United Kingdom since the 1858 Medical Act, also features an obvious link on the main banner of its home page entitled 'Concerns about doctors'; when clicked, users are directed to three 'Featured sections', the first headed 'Making a complaint'.[29] *Inter alia*, this link will take visitors to a page containing further information, region-specific and in 10 different languages, including Welsh, Polish and Chinese. Indeed, the development of media has been further harnessed to propel the importance and impact of the complaint – evidenced as much by the number of website references in this 'Introduction' as by the suggestion that 'tweeting on the ward' will now help to circumvent closed and failing systems of complaint.[30] The issue also features prominently in this collection; after all, as the Parliamentary and Health Service Ombudsman argued in 2005, complainants were often left confused, isolated and exhausted by the NHS complaints system. Initially, all many had wanted was an apology, accountability and improvement in working practices; it was the complaints 'process itself [that made] them more likely to ask for financial redress ... [and] when compensation [was] offered, a small amount ... antagonise[d] them even further'.[31]

Yet private healthcare – a dominant global provider for all but the past few decades of history, as much for the UK and Europe as elsewhere in the world – 'has no standard complaints procedure',[32] with each supplier operating an in-house complaints system of varying approaches. Bupa, for example, an international healthcare group founded in 1950, operates as an insurance scheme. Their main online UK complaints page is indicative of the different frame in which they work: 'members' using subsidiary services are directed to splinter sites, 'Bupa care homes' or 'Bupa Home Healthcare', each with separate procedures and advice (the complaints procedure of the former follows instructions on sending 'comments, compliments and suggestions'; the latter consists of a 'Patient/customer feedback form'). Those remaining on the main page are advised of a helpline number, a customer relations email address, and an online form; if the complaint is not dealt with to complainants' satisfaction they are directed, not to the Parliamentary or Health Service Ombudsman, but to the Financial Ombudsman.

The overwhelming majority of UK private hospitals and clinics are committed to an umbrella organisation, the Independent Healthcare Advisory Services (IHAS). IHAS presents a standardised procedure for all but dental treatment sites, which have a separate complaints service. This standardised procedure is outlined in two online forms: 'Making a Complaint in the Independent Sector, A Guide for Patients' and 'Mumbles and Grumbles – A Complaints Guide for Children'. Not all vulnerable patients in private care are so lucky. In 2011, with the help of a previously ignored whistleblower, the BBC's *Panorama* programme secretly filmed the physical and emotional abuse inflicted on adults with autism or intellectual disabilities by staff at the private hospital Winterbourne View, owned and run by Castlebeck Care. Whistleblowers prompted 2012–13 official inspections of BMI Healthcare's Mount Alvernia private hospital in Surrey. A 'catalogue of chaotic and dangerous care' was facilitated by a culture of 'broke[n] rules and ignored critics' to which all patients were subject, but whose impact was especially significant for children and women.[33] Women were also subject to the fallout of a global medical manufacturing scandal in 2010–11. Private clinics in Europe, the US, Latin and South America installed the sub-standard cosmetic breast implants of French manufacturer Poly Implant Prothèse.[34] Without a formalised system of complaint and with the private sector refusing to replace faulty implants, women held protests and marched to secure compensation, often from the state.[35] The complaint therefore happens in the space before, or presages, indignant protest. Protest, an active manifestation of grievance, more often occurs if there is an ineffective structure to receive, handle and effectively address the complaint, or if there is no such structure. This study can, then – in the wake of twentieth-century controversies including eugenics, Tuskegee, thalidomide and 'mad cow disease', as well as those of the twenty-first century and the ongoing global issues surrounding AIDS – contribute to wider histories of protest and can inform how the personal is indeed the political. While some lesser-known or localised scandals reside within these pages, so too do grassroots complaints.

Although contemporary failures in something as seemingly straightforward as a complaint procedure might surprise some, perhaps more unexpected is that mechanisms for registering dissatisfaction with healthcare services have long existed in the United Kingdom and in many of its former colonies. We will begin by briefly outlining a couple of eighteenth- and nineteenth-century examples in order to demonstrate the way in which two of these early and very different grievance channels functioned; a third, more detailed case will help to introduce the development of frameworks of regulation and inspection, and the impact that service assessment can have on complainants, the gravity of complaints, and the views of frontline staff.

The first instance relates to general hospitals, which were founded in many British cities and towns in the early eighteenth century (many nineteenth-century institutions in North America followed this model). Despite having only a few dozen beds and consulting physicians and surgeons who attended patients weekly, their administration was fairly sophisticated and most, from the moment they opened their doors to patients, had formal complaints procedures in place. The process was run by the House Visitors, a select group of subscribers and governors of the hospital who took turns inspecting the building to ensure that patients were being routinely attended 'and that there was no neglect on the part of the medical and nursing staff'.[36] On completing their weekly tours of the hospital building, visitors entered the wards, staff vacated the area, and patients were required to stand beside their respective beds, 'so that the House Visitors might proceed upon their inspection unimpeded and be accessible for confidential communication and complaints'.[37] Occasionally, complaints stemmed from the visitors themselves, each having had very particular views about the proper and efficient running of a medical charity towards which they contributed financially. Their observations were recorded in a book provided for this purpose and findings were regularly presented to weekly board meetings, which visitors attended to justify any complaints made with the intention of seeing that matters were rectified. Evidence from hospital minute books reveals that cases were regularly and thoroughly investigated, some ending with the censure or, in extreme cases, discharge of a member of the medical staff, often a nurse, or even the punishment, expulsion and future exclusion of a patient, should the complaint have been unfounded or other misconduct come to light during the investigation.[38] As one might expect, many such complaints involved the quality of the food, but almost as regularly they document early cases of neglect, poor treatment and the unacceptable behaviour of medical staff. This localised system was not perfect, but it seems to have served to correct the worst abuses in a proto-medical service.

In contrast, at the medical schools which began to appear in various English provincial centres in the 1820s and 30s, formal systems to redress grievances and complaints do not seem to have existed. Many of these educational institutions were little more than businesses, where an affiliated group of local medical practitioners delivered lectures and collected fees from a dozen or more local youths who wished to attend their classes. Although officially recognised by the three medical royal colleges in London which then examined and licensed practitioners, these were often unrecognisable as schools. Not only were many unable to offer a full curriculum in order to prepare students for their professional examinations, but most were under-resourced and therefore possessed inadequate buildings, under-stocked libraries and museums, and almost certainly no facilities aimed at enhancing the student experience. Many undoubtedly appointed some good teachers, but the influence of local hierarchies on the appointment of 'professors' also ensured the election of some very poor lecturers. Many repeatedly cancelled scheduled teaching sessions if these conflicted with the demands of private practice, which led to a steady accumulation of gripes and grumbles in the years immediately following the establishment of these schools. Were one to scan the pages of provincial newspapers, little evidence of dissatisfaction is apparent, by contrast with the regularly reported anniversary dinners at which senior staff and governors endlessly toasted each other and the future of their educational enterprises. However, there is considerable evidence of annoyance should one look for alternative signs of malcontent. Occasionally, schools received actual letters of complaint from disgruntled parents; one might also reassess reports of unruly students who regularly disrupted lectures and destroyed school property.

One reason justifying such a reassessment is evidence from *The Lancet*, which, from its founding by surgeon Thomas Wakley in 1823 – in part to demystify medicine so that anyone might 'detect and expose the impositions of ignorant practitioners'[39] – became the mouthpiece of despondent and discontented pupils. Its pages are full of letters revealing the inadequacies of early medical educators, and its editors regularly took local teachers to task when the latter asked the journal to publish glowing accounts of festive occasions, annual dinners and their associated puffery, given the growing volume of correspondence the paper appears to have received. Provoked by endless toasting, the *Lancet* editors subjected the worst offenders to regular roasting. Besides advertising several cases of malpraxis at the leading London hospitals, Wakley and *The Lancet* presided over another key aspect of the history of complaining about medicine: the first recorded trial involving libel and medical negligence, following a lithotomy performed at Guy's Hospital, which ended fatally and featured in the journal's pages.[40] As later chapters in this volume suggest, legal recourse has had a central role in shaping medical treatment. However, as Phil Fennell has argued, for those traditionally unable to access the courts 'the legal substrata' of codes of practice and incremental common law have been of as much importance.[41]

Unlike voluntary hospitals and medical schools, the UK sites of psychiatric treatment have been some of the most regulated of the past two hundred years. Since the formation in 1763 of a Select Committee, scandal and serial instances of malpractice – something social scientists Ian Butler and Mark Drakeford have called 'scandal inflation',[42] a kind of outrage one-upmanship – have resulted in legislation and greater inspection. Provoked (admittedly rather slowly) by the 1763 hearings, in 1774 the state ordered local inspection of madhouses in England and Wales. Yet problems surrounding the care of lunatics continued to emerge and generated Select Committees in 1807 and 1815–16, the latter addressing particularly potent complaints. Fresh Select Committee investigations in 1827 addressed ongoing concerns about London's private asylums. From this, the first statutory authority and inspectorate for psychiatric sites emerged: the Metropolitan Commissioners in Lunacy. The 1834 'New' Poor Law put in place a national supervisory body for workhouses, which included the inspection of lunatic inmates. And in 1845, with state compulsion for local authorities to provide asylum places, and after their first nationwide assessment of facilities, the template provided by the Metropolitan Commissioners became that of the Commissioners in Lunacy for England and Wales. National inspection has since been undertaken by different agencies, including the 1913 Board of Control and NHS monitoring.

However, the system of complaint-handling and inspection in the UK has never quite been coherent, comprehensive or effective, a fact which historians have tended to suggest was largely due to pragmatic or toothless inspectorates,[43] and which provoked post-millennium concerns expressed by the Health Services Ombudsman.[44] Moreover, healthcare managers have often considered the complaint as part of the territory.

> Being worried one day with a discontented patient to the right of me, with worrying relatives of an inmate to the left of me, with a lazy and careless attendant behind me, and a nasty leak in a newly-made roof in front of me, the idea suddenly started from my irritated brain that I had never heard anyone declaim before an audience of sympathisers concerning the trials, the troubles, and grievances of an asylum superintendent.[45]

So began the 1894 speech of Dr Lionel A. Weatherly, proprietor of Bailbrook House private asylum, Bath, to an audience of fellow alienists. The sources of complaint did not stop there. Aside from local government and the Lunacy Commissioners, there was the general public: as Weatherly observed, '[do] your duty and hang public opinion may be very well theoretically, but, I fear, practically . . . "It don't wash"', noting also that the '*vox populi* when raised' could be 'a voice profoundly ignorant of what it is shouting about'[46] – something which has recently been felt in the British health services in conjunction with a media campaign against the management techniques used in end-of-life care.[47]

The routineness of complaint seemingly lent asylum doctors a specific attitude towards the complainant, who, according to Dr J. A. Campbell in 1881, was for the most part the aggrieved patient or, as Weatherly later put it, 'that *bête noir*',[48] some of whom published narratives on release (several of which are discussed in Chapter 1 of this volume).[49] Campbell, Superintendent of Garlands Asylum, Carlisle, delivered his paper 'Complaints of Insane Patients' to the Medico-Psychological Society at University College London. Anyone reading the address today might recognise that most widely deployed of feedback techniques: the poison sandwich. Bracketed by brief insistences of the grave importance and responsibility of listening to and handling patient complaints, particularly about abuse by staff – a matter of perpetual complaint in every branch of medicine and evident throughout this volume – Campbell's address proceeded to demolish the veracity of the grievances and their authors.[50] Illustrating with specific examples, Campbell asserted that habitual bruises and cracked ribs were due to all manner of self-harming behaviours and that many gripes were vexatious and rooted in 'ill-feeling to one attendant or official . . . [or] general ill-feeling to those looking after and detaining' inmates.[51] Moreover, 'many complaints [were] distinctly the result of delusions. . . . A female patient complain[ed] to me each morning that the female attendants [were] men in women's clothes, and that they "raped her" during the night'; improbable perhaps, but the reason why Campbell brushed this aside? 'She [was] over 60 years of age'.[52] This excerpt is indicative of another central aspect of the complaint, or more especially the response to it: that it is shaped by the milieu in which it is made.

Take, for instance, two investigations by psychiatric clinicians of local complaints against psychiatry and their resolution, which straddled the 1994 report of the Wilson Committee into NHS complaints procedures.[53] Drawing on two American studies,[54] Keith Ingram and Leena Roy gathered together grievances against psychiatrists made between 1988 and 1993 in the neighbouring populous Winchester and Basingstoke health districts of southern England. They discovered a grand total of 47 complaints, 79 per cent of which were made by relatives or other advocates after patients were released from hospital. These were dealt with within two months, and resolved by 'an explanatory letter'.[55] Iris Pitarka-Carcani, George Szmukler and Claire Henderson looked at complaints to South London and Maudsley Mental Health Trust in 1997. Over a single year, they found 325 written complaints recorded, with the majority of those examined made by patients, mostly about in-patient care;[56] '[all] complaints had been acknowledged with an apology within a month'.[57] In both of the two studies, the bulk of complaints 'concerned clinical aspects';[58] much of the dissatisfaction pertained to communication, essentially the explanations offered of diagnosis or treatment. However, in direct contrast to Weatherly's and Campbell's nineteenth-century beliefs, Pitarka-Carcani *et al.* found that there was little evidence to suggest that the complaint was due to psychosis or delusional states,[59] with potentially profound implications for how grievances are considered now and historically.

Unlike the example of early hospitals' official visitors, descriptions of some of the failings of the first provincial medical schools remind us that, where no formal complaint mechanisms exist, these will quickly appear. Students, like modern consumers, voted with their feet, and their collective criticisms quickly became very difficult for medical schools to ignore, especially when the numbers of institutions proliferated by mid-century. Like disgruntled medical students, aggrieved families and users of past mental health services, today's medical critics frequently use the press to begin their campaigns for change. While voting with their feet was (and is) not an option for the overwhelming majority of patients with mental illness, they were able to complain to management and, theoretically at least, to local inspectors and to the Lunacy Commissioners and their successors. Moreover, upon leaving, former inmates too used the press to air their grievances.[60] These examples should also demonstrate how quickly the parameters of this seemingly trivial issue – the act of complaining – rapidly expand and touch on important historical subjects which demand further theorising. When we first sat down to explore the role of the complaint in the history of medicine, we regarded the subject as a vital antidote to progressive histories of healthcare, but it revealed many other fertile seams for historical research. For example, it could tune into and amplify the voice of the patient, something the history of medicine has been trying to do since Roy Porter's clarion call in 1985.[61] In an age predating formal professional structures, the complaint could shed light on relations between medical practitioners, both orthodox and unorthodox, in what was a crowded and hugely competitive medical marketplace. Many related issues which have already been studied could also be taken forward into the twentieth century, and, at a time when the return of the medical marketplace is being discussed in Britain, perhaps even inform twenty-first-century healthcare.

As organisers of a conference that inspired this volume, we already recognised that Birmingham was an ideal, or at least an appropriate, location from which to 'complain' about medicine. In 1945, Thomas McKeown was appointed Professor of Social Medicine at the University of Birmingham; until his retirement in 1977, McKeown consistently critiqued medicine's role in bringing about recognised improvements in the population's health in the twentieth century. First, in articles written with R. G. Record and R. G. Brown, McKeown suggested that the decline in mortality from infectious diseases noted in the nineteenth century was due to social and economic factors, rather than clinical interventions.[62] These ideas were then expanded upon in McKeown's own books, such as his succinct *The Modern Rise of Population* (1976). He attributed the rapid population increases measured during the period of industrialisation not to the work of medical practitioners, but to improvements in the standard of living, hygiene and especially nutrition. He also suggested that the decline in virulence of the organisms that caused the killer infectious diseases of previous centuries had a greater impact on population growth than did medical interventions.

The timing of McKeown's critique was crucial to its impact. His commentary first appeared after a period of tremendous optimism about medicine. Penicillin had revolutionised the treatment of infections in the period following the Second World War, and other antibiotics were being introduced to civilian medical practice. Breakthroughs in chemo-therapeutics had significantly contributed to making the 1940s and 50s a veritable 'golden age' for medicine, 'unprecedented in any age'.[63] No surprise that Lord Horder, President of the British Medical Association, the professional and trade union, when asked where medicine was headed at the organisation's annual meeting in 1948, confidently stated 'straight ahead'.[64] Such optimism coloured many contemporary and historical discussions surrounding medicine in these years. At the same time, the 'Conquest of Disease' series was launched by publishers MacDonald and Company, with its first volume on penicillin appearing in 1946.[65] Medical practice was also being upgraded in America and Europe 'to a level appropriate for the age of penicillin and high technology'.[66] The language of 'conquest' and stories of medical 'victories' had been used in medical circles previously;[67] however, on this occasion, and a little more than a decade later, practitioners were not celebrating in the streets, but facing a crisis in confidence.

By the 1960s, people were increasingly beginning to question rising expenditure on medical technologies that seemed to offer diminishing returns in terms of quality of life; wellness was itself shifting in meaning, as evidenced by Barbara Baumann's 1961 essay.[68] The same year, hidden decay was becoming increasingly visible. In Britain, there had already been an examination by psychoanalyst Isabel E. P. Menzies which observed that in large organisations nurses disengaged from patients.[69] But in 1961, Enoch Powell – the now infamous Conservative Member of Parliament for Wolverhampton South West, a stone's throw from Birmingham – delivered 'The Water Tower Speech' to the annual conference of the National Association for Mental Health, a charity later renamed Mind. Chiming with the association's beliefs, Powell demanded the eradication of isolated Victorian asylums, yet did so with an eye on saving cash. On the other side of the Atlantic, the American Medical Association's LP *Ronald Reagan Speaks Out Against Socialized Medicine* was released. Reagan, then an actor and later Governor of California and US President, said:

> One of the traditional methods of imposing statism or socialism on a people has been by way of medicine. It's very easy to disguise a medical programme as a humanitarian project, most people are a little reluctant to oppose anything that suggests medical care for people who possibly can't afford it.[70]

From an alternative viewpoint, Vicente Navarro interpreted the crisis of medicine at this time as a crisis of capitalism and called for the better distribution of medicine in the name of 'democratization'.[71] He also described the state and medicine as agencies of control. The dangers of the increasing power of medical professionals over the lives of patients and ordinary people became common currency, and with accumulating examples of medical experiments running rampant, the public's attitude turned to one of cynicism, mistrust and therapeutic nihilism.

As historians L. Stephen Jacyna and Stephen T. Casper have noted,[72] this was not to be the last time that the polarised interests of Left and Right converged to produce a critique of medicine. In the late 1960s and the 1970s, the work of René Dubos, Michel Foucault, Thomas Szasz, Erving Goffman, R. D. Laing, Barbara Seaman, Barbara Ehrenreich and Ivan Illich, among others, began to challenge the 'medical model', which was revealed to be less objective than many had previously assumed. Emphasising the way in which pathologies were socially constructed, this body of literature stressed the way that medical narratives reinforced the Enlightenment discourses advanced by the rich and powerful, who 'located the domain of unreason among women, the mad, the poor, and the criminal classes'.[73] Inverting the orthodox position, social scientists instead proposed that the 'deviant' were the victims of labelling, stereotyping, and gendered, racial and economic injustices. In turn, the real villains were the doctors, psychiatrists and scientists who used their expert knowledge and authority to shore up the status quo and segregate, stigmatise and pathologise recalcitrant groups. Many physicians themselves, even if simply aiming to upgrade medical work in order to better achieve a commonly-held professional ideal, critiqued medicine's shortcomings and, in so doing, 'unwittingly opened the door for the latter-day critics who attacked not only [doctors'] priestly pretention but technical performance'.[74]

The above group of protesting scholars, it should be noted, was dominated by those working with mental illness and who helped to birth 'anti-psychiatry'. For the American psychiatrist Szasz, seventeenth-century witch-hunts had been reincarnated; this time 'they' were coming for the mentally ill. Yet his complaint went even further than that: mental illness, he declared, was a myth.[75] The British psychiatrist Laing concentrated on undermining established approaches to schizophrenia, a state that he felt was a different way of communicating or responding to the world, which was itself sick.[76] Perhaps in no other medical field has the wider literature impacted so profoundly than on psychiatry, traditionally criticised as being a specialism without a science. What Szasz, Laing and others did, stoked by controversial figures such as the London-based psychologist Hans Eysenck, was to create a vortex of dissent in Britain in the 1970s (as described by Irish psychiatrist Anthony Clare),[77] into which fell shifting policies, failing funding, controversial therapies, patient abuse and hospital scandal. None of these were new issues; nor was the unease about institutionalisation expressed by the Canadian-born sociologist Goffman.[78] Nevertheless, this time public perceptions of doctors rapidly transformed and metastasised, with many practitioners losing their saintly status and being reduced in the eyes of many to greedy monopolists, or businesspeople at the very least.

The Austrian philosopher, Catholic priest and social critic, Ivan Illich, added the concept of iatrogenic disease to the mix with his work *Medical Nemesis* in 1975.[79] Claiming that the cost of medical treatments was only rising, Illich also argued that doctors were anything but the life-savers they made themselves out to be. At the time, and in the United States, 7 per cent of those hospitalised were injured as a result of the procedures they endured; university hospitals, perhaps surprisingly, were also found to be more 'pathogenic', or 'sickening'.[80] As a result of what was described as negligence, error, callousness and incompetence, nearly 15,000 malpractice suits were lodged in US courts in 1971 alone.[81] Medical colonisation in many Western countries, according to Illich, had reached 'sickening proportions'.[82] Furthermore, medicalisation was interpreted as another aspect of state power, which expropriated the power of individuals to shape their environment and to heal themselves. Many others would pen biting studies of medicalisation, addressing, for example, hyperactivity, mental illness, child abuse and alcoholism, and would, in the process, transform the concept into a household word.[83]

Simultaneously, Thomas McKeown continued his penetrating assessment of medicine in *The Role of Medicine: Dream, Mirage or Nemesis* (1979). This critique of medicine extended to its organisation, with students in his opinion spending far too much time in prestigious university teaching hospitals – where high-tech services appeared to accumulate – treating acute accidents and illnesses (often very badly if one is to believe Illich), and not enough time developing preventive medicine and long-term care for the poor, elderly and mentally ill. According to McKeown, his and Illich's volumes were linked by the term 'nemesis' alone. In fact, he did as much as he could to distance himself from Illich, suggesting the books had little in common, 'except perhaps in the sense that the Bible and the Koran could be said to be identified by the fact that both are concerned with religious matters'.[84] This, however, was misleading, as both clearly addressed issues such as the poor distribution of doctors, who tended to 'deploy themselves as they like', gathering 'where the climate is healthy, where the water is clean, and where people work and can pay for their services'.[85] In *Psychiatry in Dissent* (1976), Anthony Clare described how profound were the implications for diagnosis and care. Clare quoted the 1975 UK government report on the regulation of the medical profession:

> [an] example is given of the doctor from abroad who interpreted the use of colloquialisms by the patient as a sign of confusion and disorientation.... Consequently, the ethical principles and cultural background peculiar to the United Kingdom also gave rise to a great deal of difficulty for doctors from different countries where values and principles are different.[86]

It is telling, then, that only in 2013 – and in consequence of unnecessary deaths – did the General Medical Council (the statutory regulator of doctors) acquire legal powers to check the standard of English for practitioners from the European Union working in the UK.[87]

Despite similar discussions about physician placement, McKeown's views crucially diverged from Illich's, primarily through his denial that medicine did more harm than good. He also rejected Illich's views on untreated pain and admitted that he would personally continue to seek medical treatment when ill, as in fact he did when diagnosed with cancer, dying in 1988. Even though Illich lived another 20 years following his own cancer diagnosis in 1983, the long-term influence of McKeown's critique has been impressive. It has also proved dangerous in times when politicians look for excuses to dismantle healthcare services. Much of its strength came from the fact that McKeown was an insider, a medical professional complaining about medicine. The terms 'dream' and 'mirage' in his 1979 subtitle tied him to studies by René Dubos and Macfarlane Burnet, two other renowned medical scientists, who, at the end of their careers, grew somewhat disillusioned with medicine's prospects, at the very least predicting slower progress than the public had seen in the first half of the twentieth century and anticipating not only disease resistance to antibiotics but also that non-infectious diseases such as cancer were here to stay.[88] Clare, on the other hand, was at the start of his career when his name, unlike those of other critics, would become widely known. In making sense of psychiatric controversy, Clare soberly portrayed a discipline in intellectual and even existential crisis and further complained of funding cuts, patients' relatives and the already failing care in the community ushered in by Powell; but for all of this, proving himself more on the side of McKeown, he fought for the good that psychiatry might do. McKeown was only one of a long line of medical critiques to arise from within the ranks of medicine. Though not made explicit in the subtitle of *The Role of Medicine*, his approach also linked him with other medical iconoclasts, such as Archie Cochrane, who launched a similar if not more influential criticism of medicine, *Efficiency and Effectiveness*, in 1972. In fact, McKeown engaged with Cochrane and made some effort to differentiate his approach from that of Cochrane in the book's introduction,[89] and only in the volume's penultimate chapter addressed Dubos, Burnet and others 'who have lost the faith in medicine'.[90] More recent research has regarded McKeown's thesis as more radical than Cochrane's, but also demonstrates McKeown's impact to have been greater in the social sciences, while Cochrane received a higher proportion of citations in medical journals.[91]

According to Illich, members of the public were already 'apprehensive about medicine' and only needed 'data to substantiate their misgivings'.[92] For example, in a section of his treatise entitled 'Useless Medical Treatment', Illich briefly addressed the way in which the medical profession created the 'dangerous delusion that contemporary medicine [was] highly effective'.[93] '[M]ost of the sky-rocketing medical expenditures' of the post-war period, he argued, were 'destined for diagnosis and treatment of no or of doubtful effectiveness'.[94] Rather than expand on this point, the lack of effectiveness of 'costly and high-risk medicine' was an issue which Illich declared himself unwilling to dwell upon further, and the subject was left to others, such as Dubos and Cochrane, to explore elsewhere.

Throughout his career and most famously in his published Carling Rock lectures, *Effectiveness and Efficiency*, Cochrane encouraged the more careful evaluation of medical procedures in order to remove bias from medical measurements. He himself was 'emotionally biased' in favour of a National Health Service, but had begun to view the NHS 'as one would a favourite child who is showing marked delinquent tendencies'.[95] More specifically, he believed that the all-encompassing pursuit of cure that he witnessed during his career had restricted the supply of care in the NHS. As a result, he encouraged the application of a cost/benefit approach to medical interventions. Moreover, his experiences in Greek and German prisoner-of-war camps during the Second World War and as a field epidemiologist studying defined communities convinced him that 'all medical administration would benefit from a scientific epidemiological training'.[96] However, before this could become a reality, two steps were essential. The first involved the wider implementation of measures such as the randomised controlled trial, which had greatly increased the ability to measure the effect of medical actions in altering the disease course.[97] It was in this way that Cochrane implied 'effectiveness' in his title. In terms of 'efficiency', Cochrane meant the optimum use of personnel and materials in achieving such clinical results. This was not restricted to the narrow issue of treatment either, but encompassed the activities of screening, diagnosis, the place and length of treatment, and rehabilitation.[98] In order to add some 'humanity' to his approach, Cochrane also added another 'e' to his conceptualisation, which was not included in his title: equality.[99]

During the period following our conference, we thought carefully about how best to organise the papers in this collection of essays. Taking a leaf from Cochrane's book, we too desired to make optimum use of the material presented to efficiently convey the human stories behind the multifaceted history and practice of complaining about medicine. At the same time, it was clear that we both wanted to disrupt the chronology; we wished instead to create themes around which our complaints and their mechanisms – or at least those present in the chapters – might coalesce. Between the Introduction and Afterword, we created four sections, Professionals, Politics, Patients and Public Relations, each of which comprises three chapters. However, the themes of the final and first papers in neighbouring sections are connected – so, Hilary Ingram and Steven Thompson both pick up on the negotiation of power at the periphery and the implantation of medicine; Kim Price and Steve King discuss the two partners (doctor and patient) of the medical encounter under the New Poor Law; and Rosemary Wall and Matthew Newsom Kerr consider oppositional relations in different areas of infectious disease policy. In this way, we hope that the sections are not rigid and defined but fluid and graduated.

The chapters in the first section – by Andrew Scull, Hera Cook and Hilary Ingram – centre on how complaints, grievances and critiques about and between different professional(ising) groups have shaped the credibility of medicine and its practitioners. Conflict arising from practitioner-inflicted pain, ineffective medicine and the inefficient organisation of healthcare and allocation of resources has always been a part of medical practice. In the very crowded medical marketplaces of the pre-modern period, for example, so-called quack doctors were regularly attacked as they encroached on the privileges of the medical colleges and companies when peddling what were depicted (rightly or otherwise) as their useless nostrums and harmful proprietary remedies. Though orthodox medicine up to the twentieth century was little more effective, a more fully-developed sacerdotal role appears to have been an effective antidote to complaints from patients.[100] Patients more often went to practitioners when seeking treatment for their medical complaints than to complain about their doctors' actual therapeutic impotence. Meanwhile, orthodox practitioners never missed an opportunity to complain about those whom they perceived to be quacks or who encroached on their most lucrative patients. The history of itinerant practice, unlike many other subjects in this volume, has been well researched and there was, consequently, little point in rehearsing further examples here.[101] The work that has emerged from this field, however, is crucial to the topic of complaining about medicine and informs other discussions concerning competition between medical people. For example, where competition or overlap with orthodox practice existed, even when perfectly legal, fierce battles were waged and complaints similarly proliferated. Eighteenth- and nineteenth-century accoucheurs, or obstetricians, for example, were quick to depict old 'granny' and Sarah Gamp midwives as ignorant and inept, despite their having managed normal births quite well.[102] While this subject has been thoroughly researched and has become a classic case in studies of medicalisation,[103] other examples of medical rivalry and the ever-increasing power of orthodox medicine are only beginning to be reconstituted by scholars. Of the three papers in the 'Professionals' section which do just so, all incorporate a similarly deep seam freighted with gender issues. Scull and Cook centre on what is perhaps the most consistently controversial area of modern practice: psychiatry and mental health. Yet, taken together with Ingram, the three also serve as a reminder that, even in the face of male-dominated medical and academic opposition, other voices could reverberate even more loudly, shifting fundamentally national and international attitudes, policy and law.

Indeed, from 1760s London to 1860s North America and Jamaica, back to 1890s England, it was often the complaints of women about poor care and wrongful confinement that generated change. The lunacy laws and the medical treatment under them were politically charged and bound up with women's rights and those of the free subject.[104] Yet mental health has also been politicised against complainers, whistleblowers and protesters, from 'sluggish schizophrenia' in post-1960 Soviet states to the present detention of political dissidents inside Chinese psychiatric hospitals.[105] Even within mainstream, Western, and seemingly apolitical psychiatry, protest has been considered as grounds for treatment.

While certain anxiety and personality disorders characterised by complaining remain firmly inserted in the American *Diagnostic and Statistical Manual* (*DSM*; the 'psychiatrists' bible'), one of the conditions which has previously been suggested, but failed to make it in, was 'Chronic Complaint Disorder', whose 'supposed sufferers' were mainly of Eastern European descent and 'revealed their malady when asked how things [were] going. "In those cases," the psychiatrists wrote, "the pathognomonic expression [became] 'Oy vey, don't ask'"'.[106]

The vernacular of complaint (and of diagnosis) is explored in Andrew Scull's chapter, which essentially traces the transatlantic 'culture of complaint' surrounding psychiatry. Scull charts the cultural embeddedness of critique across the past three centuries: by men and women, patients and psychiatrists, and social scientists; in fiction, through art and law, in film and the press – as well as through the vivid genre of ex-inmates' polemics and protests. Indeed, he describes the eighteenth- and nineteenth-century lineage of wrongful confinement, and places twentieth-century complaints about consent and concerning framing, reframing, expanding and inventing diagnosis as part of this transatlantic tradition, but one now laced with the drugs and money of Big Pharma. Scull considers the controversies surrounding the five incarnations of *DSM* from its first edition in 1952 to the latest, published in 2013, not only as part of this sustained and energetic castigation of psychiatry, but as recently having manifested in new and divergent ways.

Medical intervention in mental health, across the gamut from hospitalisation to leucotomy, has historically been predicated on forcible treatment or on the agreement of vulnerable people or people at their most vulnerable. To the great relief of some practitioners and perhaps many of the public, the ideas Sigmund Freud unleashed came to offer a new way: a way for mind managers to escape the asylum and treat based on consent. Shifting the emphasis from psychosis to neurosis also facilitated an active doctor–patient relationship and the expansion of treatment to middle-class consumers.[107] Conversely, office-based psychoanalysis and psychotherapy slammed into a new raft of complaints. Part of this has been the sexual, emotional or moral impositions of the practitioner on the therapeutic relationship and beyond. Until the 1970s, homosexuality was defined by psychiatry as a disorder. While this was overturned – again instigated by complaint – 'reparative', 'aversion' or 'conversion' therapy has continued to offer a controversial 'cure' for being gay.[108] Complaint and critique has come from groups as diverse as Stonewall and the British Medical Association, the latter in 2010 helping to pave the way for wider medical recognition by the Pan American and World Health Organisations that such therapy was 'a serious threat to the health and well-being – even the lives – of affected people'.[109]

The gender politics of therapy is included in Hera Cook's chapter. Rooted in 1950s criticism – largely emanating from the US, the home of psychotherapy after its Nazi eradication from Central Europe – Cook explores the past 60 years of shifting transatlantic therapy and complaints through discussion of the academics Philip Rieff, Christopher Lasch and Frank Furedi. Michel Foucault looms – as he so often does – over the key considerations of the chapter, which complicates understandings of complaint and of grievances against medicine. Dissatisfaction here seems not to stem from a personal encounter with medicine, medical intervention or professional boundaries, but centres on the cultural process of the medicalisation of society. The three men are not critiquing from a weakened position of sickness or recovery, or on behalf of the powerless; they are complaining about factors that have undermined their authority as wealthy, educated, white men. For them, the forces unleashed by psychoanalysis and the mass consumption of Freud have variously destroyed political engagement, social responsibility, the family, the home and privacy. Yet at the same time, and in the gendering of talking, tactile and group therapy by (almost solely male) critics, these complaints have been met with feminist reflection. Cook's chapter therefore evokes the possible wider mismatch of what men and women expect from medicine; for as much as they might belong to the same culture, the way they communicate may be as different as that between the foreign doctors and indigenous patients outlined by Anthony Clare, as suggested by recent studies gendering the complainant.[110]

This sense of tension surrounding gender, the foreign and the indigenous is also found in the broader history of the complaint in medicine. Just as the numbers of irregular popular healers proliferated in response to the low numbers and poor distribution of orthodox practitioners in European countries, nineteenth-century Protestant missionaries entered foreign climes where inhabitants appeared to have limited access to healthcare. Consequently, many missionaries used medicine as a tool to win over colonial communities and, in the process of healing its sick members, introduce them to the Gospel. Although offering medical services, and even operating on the sick and infirm, many missionaries were not actually qualified doctors and had received only limited medical training.[111] Some recent studies of missionary medicine have revealed the full scale of such non-state services, along with outsiders' regular conflicts with local healers, and have demonstrated that indigenous peoples were not passive recipients of missionary attention.[112] Hilary Ingram's chapter demonstrates the contempt with which medical missionary activities were held in the missionaries' home countries, and specifically among orthodox practitioners. Given the limited numbers of fully-qualified Western medics in the colonies, it was always recognised that a large proportion of individuals undertaking mission work would be only partially trained. Partial knowledge was therefore accepted by many missionary groups as better than none, but standards clearly varied, as did views concerning their medical competence. As Ingram highlights, much of this battle, like so many conflicts in medicine, was fought in the pages of the medical journals and lay periodicals. Ingram also demonstrates that race was at the heart of the debate and of negotiations of acceptable standards of care. Central too was gender, many women having forced the issue of full training so as to secure professional roles for themselves. This sense of an arena in which complaints were made and heard is, in Ingram's chapter, conceived at a transnational or global level (and in Scull's and Cook's chapters through transatlantic connections).

The second of the four sections, 'Politics', deals with the local arena, and continues the theme of pirouetting and colliding tensions between different groups found in Ingram's chapter. Here, Steven Thompson, Pilar León-Sanz and Kim Price explore not only how grievances have been negotiated, but also what they meant for patients and professionalising physicians in three national contexts. In Thompson's case, the setting is south Wales, more specifically the largest and most militant coalfield in Britain, where workers were particularly non-deferential towards doctors and were especially keen to hold medical practitioners accountable for the delivery of medical services to their mining communities. The chapter considers three workers' insurance schemes of three different communities between the late nineteenth century and the establishment of the NHS, and the complaints they dealt with. Employing Klein's categorisation of complaints, Thompson discusses the technical, organisational and stylistic aspects of complaints (involving doctors' professional knowledge, availability and manner respectively) and conveys dramatic evidence of the 'them' and 'us' mentality which challenged the autonomy of doctors in this region. Industrial relations helped establish a milieu which attracted only the 'flotsam and jetsam' of physicians, while the strains and isolation of practice in south Wales fuelled professional decline in others by way of insobriety. It also generated a militant patient body. As serious as grievances were, and although there was a high reported turnover of medical staff, Thompson also uncovers evidence of tremendous loyalty among patients, even in cases where doctors were clearly negligent. As importantly, he documents some of the only apologies appearing in this volume from practitioners who were willing to acknowledge their mistakes, or at least to recognise the emotionally-charged environment which shaped the doctor–patient relationship.

The role of emotion in the clinical encounter is further explored by León-Sanz. In Pamplona (the capital city of Navarra in northern Spain) between 1902 and 1936, insurance schemes and their governance, which proved so inflammatory in south Wales, were more pragmatic, undertaken by medical practitioners, employers and workers. As in Wales, León-Sanz identifies the three main reasons the thousand members of Pamplona's mutual insurance association complained about their scheme: failure of a doctor to attend promptly or at all when summoned, delays in delivering sick notes, and the payment of physicians' fees. Like Thompson's Welsh miners, the members of Pamplona's mutual aid society demonstrated considerable agency but appeared to lack sufficient power to deal with serious deficiencies in medical services. The dynamics of the doctor–patient relationship were altered because of location. Less isolated than their Welsh counterparts, Pamplona's doctors were prominent local figures; the potential for scandal that would be instigated by the dismissal of practitioners required workers to organise opposition more effectively and collectively. For León-Sanz, the complainants were an emotional community, and this is demonstrated in the way that mutual aid society members employed emotions to communicate their grievances to practitioners. Drawing on the society's rich files, León-Sanz examines the way in which members persuasively expressed their grief, distress and anger in their complaints. Although portraying themselves as vulnerable and helpless, worker-members communicated in a language that the society's management could not ignore. With the threat available for contributors to pull out of the scheme, complaints were negotiated and effected real change, evident in the types of assistance offered and even, perhaps, in the manipulation of attitudes by physicians.

In Kim Price's chapter, the framework fielding community desires and tensions was the New Poor Law. Although complaints about the poor law, especially following its reorganisation in 1834, have become the stuff of legend, very little attention has focused on the way in which doctors and patients dealt with sub-standard care, medical negligence – of which there was much – and iatrogenic harm, to use Illich's terminology. In fact, the medical work of the poor law has only recently begun to emerge in detailed regional studies.[113] Managing a service that was funded by local taxation, the Poor Law Guardians have been recognised as hard taskmasters. Eager to save ratepayers' money, guardians often saddled doctors with unmanageable workloads. Not surprisingly, although the poor often remained sick, each administrative area (or Union) generated a healthy number of complaints. In his chapter, Kim Price explores the long-recognised but neglected complaint and inquiry process under the New Poor Law. Price argues that today's headline statistics of litigation, and their interpretation as a barometer of complaints and the state of healthcare, obscure the truth of what is actually happening. Using the New Poor Law, he asserts that the layered meanings of the words 'negligence' and 'complaint' can only be understood if the administrative structure is explored. So, while he uncovers a rising number of complaints during the late nineteenth century made by paupers, doctors and government officials – and suggests that this might be only the tip of an 'iceberg' of dissatisfaction – he also finds that these complaints were evidence of short-sighted and swingeing cuts in funding by a central government intent on clipping the power of doctors. This is complicated still further by Price's exploration of the professional etiquette and pay structure for doctors who depended for income on private practice, but for reputation on the public employment provided by the New Poor Law. He asserts that the authorities' refusal to pay a fair wage or to honour payments while divesting responsibility for care to doctors meant that medical men were in a catch-22 situation; they were the scapegoats of scandal even though they were not its cause.

These voices are amplified in the third section of this collection: 'Patients'. While the history of mental health, for example, has long been strewn with advocacy and activist groups – including in Britain the Alleged Lunatics' Friend Society, the Lunacy Law Reform Association, Mind, the Mental Patients' Union and United Kingdom Advocacy Network, and in the US the more physician-informed National Committee for Mental Hygiene – the three chapters here offer different manifestations of self-help and patient assistance in three different settings. Steve King continues Price's strand of investigation into medical practice in the Victorian period in a chapter which focuses more overtly on patients' complaints under the English poor law. While many influential social critiques of medicine have claimed that health professionals in modern times accumulated power to an extent that destroyed the potential for ordinary people to deal with illness in personal and autonomous ways, patients are clearly not as defenceless as some have made out.[114] Medicine was not something that most ordinary patients, including the very destitute, such as the Victorian pauper, were subject to rather than actively shaped. From previous studies of childbirth, for example, it is clear that patients are not necessarily passive and could be active participants in the medical encounter, even in the process of medicalisation.[115] Drawing on a wide variety of records, including letters, diaries and newspaper accounts, King's chapter attempts to reconstruct the patient's voice and the nature of patient agency. Besides looking at when and to whom patients complained, King uses his rich sources to explore the way in which complaints were framed, rhetoricised and delivered – sometimes with physical force – by those ordinarily regarded as possessing very little influence. Not surprisingly, paupers often adopted the language of elevated social groups, and, in a pattern which will become familiar throughout this volume, used newspapers as highly effective mouthpieces. There was also a temporal element to delivering complaints; in other words, when it comes to complaining, timing is everything.

This sense of co-opting the language of authority discourse by patient groups is explored by Alex Mold. In her chapter, Mold charts the shift found in Britain and the US as the patient began to be reconceptualised as a consumer and to be given some consultative status through the market principles of consumer rights, and the impact this has had on complaining about medicine. She traces the UK development of the medical complaint as a distinct and managed entity from the 1962 establishment of the voluntary Patients Association in the UK. Statutory assistance was then to be provided by Community Health Councils from 1974, which overlapped with 1970s and 1980s patient consumer groups such as Which?. Finally, Conservative MP Michael McNair-Wilson, by way of a Parliamentary lottery, secured the 1985 Hospital Procedure Complaints Act. As elsewhere in this volume, Mold's discussions might be seen to echo what E. P. Thompson called 'moral economy'.[116] Mold interrogates the shaping of rights in health and medicine past traditional negotiations and more clearly from the collective since the 1940s to their framing by post-1960s governments emphasising the individual citizen, either in the guise of the whistleblower or, more usually, 'the patient'; the varying conceptions of the complainant (patient, consumer, citizen) sculpt what rights mean – from 'customs in common'[117] to the right to choose.

Both King and Mold offer windows into what sociologist Nick Crossley calls the 'culture of contention'; yet it is not only the 'vocabulary and common sense of history' that has shaped the actions of patients,[118] but also their politics, time, space and place. In Rosemary Wall's chapter, she explores this sense of shifting action and even resolution through outbreaks of typhoid in three different areas in Britain and at different points in the economic cycle of the 'Hungry Thirties'. One of these, the 1937 Croydon case, is exceptional in UK history in that it is an exemplar of a successful claim for compensation for damages sustained as the result of an epidemic. Using the local and national press, as well as local inquiry archives and official national reports, Wall anatomises the subtle politics of charitable assistance, local public health and healthcare, as well as the semantics of liability. In doing so, Wall indicates the role of class in the success of compensation claims; so too was proximity to London a factor, with NIMBYism (the cry of 'not in my backyard') perhaps accounting for the heightened response of the national press and the Ministry of Health (both situated in London) to the Croydon outbreak. Wall also underscores the vital, incremental role of law in establishing rights and complaints which took place before the formalisation discussed by Mold.

These themes – of politics and the shifting associations between medicine, medical authority and the law – also run through the final section of the volume: 'Public Relations'. Matthew Newsom Kerr's chapter explores what might be described as the 'self-serving complaint' in relation to the infectious disease hospitals established by London's Metropolitan Asylums Board (MAB) in the late Victorian period.[119] Rather than risk having such potentially weak cases dismissed, in the circumstances of those residing near the MAB hospitals erected in London between 1869 and 1885, protesters dressed up such self-interest to resemble a plea for justice; without the veneer of objective virtue, their complaints would not have elicited very much sympathy and were bound to fail. Instead, it is argued, despite the very real threats posed by infectious diseases to communities, opposition groups in the capital managed to disguise their NIMBYism (although less well than in Wall's case study) and organised protest movements involving mass demonstrations, petitions and press campaigns that convinced those in positions of power to regard the new hospitals as the greater threat facing the population.

Surveying the rhetoric of these public complaints in three metropolitan epicentres – Hampstead, Limehouse and Fulham – Newsom Kerr examines the way in which the location of a hospital was perceived to alter the lives of those resident in these districts. While it was one thing to open an hospital for the treatment of infectious disease in communities which were already regarded as unhygienic, it was an entirely different matter when the institution was located within a popular recreation area, such as Hampstead Heath, an archetypal 'high-class residential district'. Employing the contemporary language of foetid airs and miasmas, alongside the nascent theory of germs, residents of Hampstead emphasised the way in which hospitals concentrated poisons and infectious effluvia that would potentially seep into and infect the neighbourhood. Contrasting the way in which public health was debated and performed in the public sphere (once again in very emotional ways), Newsom Kerr highlights the class-specific and highly spatial nature of complaints. Besides exploring whose complaints are heard and whose dismissed, Newsom Kerr also demonstrates the way in which complaints shaped hospital practices, such as visiting, and even brought about the structural alteration of buildings, if not their periodic closure. Ultimately, the strength of these campaigns was influential in transforming 'infectious disease hospitals' into 'isolation hospitals' and in bringing about a modification of public health strategies in the English capital that was more than rhetorical in nature.

Communication is also at the heart of the chapters by June Jones and Andrew Shanks and by Jean McHale. In the former, the focus is less on emotions than on language concordancing, documenting the patterns in which words are used and how these change over time in order to reveal broader changes in social, or at least press, attitudes. In particular, these chapters share a focus on the prosecution of medical practitioners since the 1950s. Interestingly, at a time when the public was becoming more familiar with doctors who broke the law, it became increasingly common for conscientious bystanders to be punished for raising concerns about the quality of medicine.[120]

The chapters by Jones and Shanks and by McHale deal specifically with legal discourse (also alluded to in Newsom Kerr's chapter) and with its conveyance to the public, yet their wider themes link with chapters elsewhere in this collection. Jones and Shanks outline the doctrine of double effect and its centrality to the prosecution of doctors who were charged with killing their patients – the most serious complaint a practitioner might face. In their examination of the reportage of the sole five British cases of this nature (all involving drug overdose) in both *The Times* and *The Guardian* between 1957 and 2007, textual analysis reveals that familiar patterns of words emerged to describe the stories and their characters. In essence, Jones and Shanks uncover a media lexicon of medical complaint in the creation of myth, most notably in the trial of the Eastbourne physician Bodkin Adams, which became the touchstone for subsequent cases. Moreover, the authors demonstrate that, for the two most recent cases (in 1992 and 2007), reporters regularly emphasised compassionate reasons for ending a patient's life, steering readers' responses by referring to, for example, 'mercy killing' rather than 'murder'. Among other things, the outcomes of these latest cases suggest that even serious complaints might become part of accepted medical practice.

Additionally, though treated as a transcendent global ethical question, decisions about assisted dying are clearly linked to local and national contexts, as visible in the way in which cases are reported, recounted and discussed in individual jurisdictions and even newspapers.

Jean McHale considers the management of professional standards through the negotiation of precedent. Beginning again with 1957 – this time the Bolam Test, established in response to the unmodified use of electro-convulsive therapy (ECT) at a psychiatric hospital – and reflecting on the post-2001 fallout from the Bristol Royal Infirmary inquiry, McHale examines the impact of changing legal notions of informed consent on the ability and readiness of patients to complain. As one might expect, in the first years following the introduction of the NHS in Britain, there were few lawyers competent in medical litigation. Voluntary pressure groups, including those discussed by Mold and elsewhere in this Introduction, considerably improved the support available to patients; however, the costs and risks of litigation, not to mention the stressful and time-consuming nature of such cases, have discouraged large numbers of potential claimants from pursuing this route when faced with instances of presumed negligence and wrong-doing. Inadequate complaints procedures and an increase in the number of lawyers proficient in this field, on the other hand, eventually led greater numbers of complainants to try their luck in the courts.[121] Despite a steady increase in litigation against healthcare professionals in the last half century, the number of successful claims does not appear to have risen in recent decades. What McHale detects, on the other hand, is a noticeable decline in the deference shown by courts to doctors. Nevertheless, clinical judgement still holds considerable clout in the courtroom, possibly because the use of the law to complain about medicine largely involves attributing blame to individual medics and compensating particular patients for specific harms endured.[122] As this suggests, full investigation and the identification of systemic failures is less likely when the adversarial system of the courts is used to complain about medicine.

Outside the courtroom, on the other hand, the proliferation of clinical guidelines, from the medical colleges, pressure groups and the government, have more recently curbed clinical autonomy, though there is little evidence to suggest that clinical practice has changed much. There is, however, evidence that – as in the courtroom – public perceptions of medical practitioners have changed. McHale attributes much of this to inquiries into medical negligence since the 1990s, such as those following events at the Bristol Royal Infirmary and at Alder Hey Hospital in Liverpool. Not only have subsequent inquiries undermined the long-standing autonomy of medicine through efforts to allow patients genuine participation in their healthcare, but the 'club culture' that has for so long characterised medicine is gradually being replaced by a 'culture of candour' which many argue will better ensure respect and honesty in future medical encounters. While whistleblowers may continue to trigger further complaints, investigations and inquiries down the road, the threat is that reformers may no longer be on the lookout for a few bad apples, but are potentially tipping the entire cart in their efforts to reform a system that to some eyes appears rotten to the core. McHale claims that such extreme responses are unwarranted. Although inquiries appear to have allowed some parties to detach themselves from scandals and poor standards that are often made to appear the result of local circumstances, inquiry has brought considerable innovation and improvement. In the case of McHale's two chosen case studies, inquiries have introduced transparency in procedures and forums where errors may be discussed, and have led government and practitioners to implement stricter guidelines on staff training, among other remedies, and even radical mechanisms to ensure accountability. If inquiries are to bring about real and lasting change, the real challenge, according to McHale, is getting all of the groups involved – not only doctors and nurses but also ministers, managers and policy makers – to learn the associated lessons.

In his Afterword, John Clarke reflects on the complaint in the current round of NHS reforms. Rather than regarding complaints as endlessly recurring mishaps and evidence of systemic shortcomings which never get addressed, he emphasises that complaints have indeed driven change in medicine. Additionally, Clarke draws out four themes which he believes deserve further reflection and that centre on culture, power and authority. First, he alludes to an ambivalent relationship between patients and practitioners; the latter are treated with deference by the sick, and with scepticism should they fail to satisfy patients' expectations, often by simply communicating poorly. He considers what he prefers to call a 'hinterland of complaints' (to distinguish these expressions of disapproval from those that make up Klein's homogenous 'iceberg') and the way in which private gripes are transformed into public grievances, the moment when moans accumulate and make the transition into the formal complaint process. He then summarises and expands on the resources, techniques and technologies that are addressed by all of the contributors to this volume in their case studies of complaining, exploring the varied strategies, accepted repertoires, and languages used to register dissatisfaction, before considering where these experiences and emotional pleas take individuals, and who ultimately judges those who make their pleas public. Finally, he ends by reflecting on the politics of complaining, which has become part of institutional design, seemingly giving organisations greater control of the complaint, but often doing little to deal with these modest demands in any effectual manner. This is what Clarke describes as the 'micro-politics' of complaint, which many of the chapters of this volume reconstruct so vividly, and which healthcare institutions regularly and to the present day appear unable to manage effectively.

This collection is not, on the one hand, the pithy put-down contained in medical man Andrew Malleson's 1973 *Need Your Doctor Be So Useless?*,[123] nor is it as bounded as social scientist J. P. Martin's 1984 text, *Hospitals in Trouble*,[124] though, like them, this collection is a product of its social and political milieu. Indeed, while we have brought together chapters that illustrate a diversity of situations and scholars, we recognise that timing and place have inevitably shaped this volume. But we hope that it might be the beginning of a wider exploration of complaining about medicine and what it has meant in Eastern Europe, in Africa, in South America and elsewhere – the long lineage of whistleblowing and of vexatious complaints, though touched on in this volume, are clear areas for further research. Our intent is not to become part of any ideological war against medicine, but to demonstrate how powerful the complaint has been and the important ways in which it can inform wider historical and contemporary discussions. That so many of the chapters here implicate the centrality of notions of the consumer at the same point as a lack of investment or the privileging of profit implies that there is yet time for further scandal. We suggest that the complaint – and most pointedly the complaint as a fundamental part of regular negotiations and normal relations, now and historically – can be harnessed as a positive agent of public healthcare development and not simply act as a by-product of 'the market' and privatisation.

Notes

1 G. Orwell, 'How the Poor Die', *Decline of the English Murder and Other Essays* (Harmondsworth, 1946/1978), pp. 32–44, p. 39 and p. 43.
2 J. Woodward, *To Do the Sick No Harm: A Study of the British Voluntary Hospital System to 1875* (London, 1974), pp. 124–125.
3 Strabolgi, Beaumont, Heytesbury, B. Abel-Smith, E. Ardizzone, A. Harvey, J. Hewetson, B. Robb, B. Sargent, D. Woolgar, and O. P., 'Old People in Mental Hospitals', *The Times* (10 November 1965), p. 13.
4 B. Robb (ed.), *Sans Everything: A Case to Answer* (Edinburgh, 1967).
5 P. Townsend, 'Obituary: Professor Brian Abel-Smith', *The Independent* (9 April 1996), www.independent.co.uk/news/obituaries/obituary-professor-brian-abelsmith-1303950.html, accessed 12 March 2013.
6 B. Abel-Smith, *A History of the Nursing Profession in Great Britain* (London, 1960); B. Abel-Smith with R. Pinker, *The Hospitals 1800–1948: A Study in Social Administration in England and Wales* (London, 1964).
7 www.bbc.co.uk/news/health-21455723, accessed 14 February 2013; www.itv.com/news/central/story/2013–02–14/ex-nhs-chief-break-gagging-order/, accessed 14 February 2013; www.guardian.co.uk/uk/2013/feb/14/nhs-whistleblower-quit-gagged, accessed 14 February 2013.
8 http://blogs.bmj.com/bmj/2012/02/15/richard-smith-you-have-a-duty-to-complain/, accessed 14 February 2013.
9 M. Walton, 'Why Complaining is Good for Medicine', *Internal Medicine Journal*, 31, 2 (2001), pp. 75–76.
10 T. Hesketh, D. Wu, L. Mao and N. Na, 'Violence against Doctors in China', *British Medical Journal*, 345, e57307 (September 2012); 'Heartless Attacks: Medical Staff are Fearful as Anger against their Profession Grows', *The Economist* (21 July 2012), www.economist.com/node/21559377, accessed 13 May 2014.

11 'Heartless Attacks'.
12 L. Jie, 'New Generations of Doctors Face Crisis', *Lancet*, 379, 9829 (19 May 2012), p. 1878; www.nytimes.com/2010/08/12/world/asia/12hospital.html?_r=0, accessed 14 February 2013.
13 'Maharastra Government is Told to End Doctors' Strikes over Poor Security in Hospitals', *British Medical Journal*, 346 (2013), f742, www.bmj.com/content/346/bmj.f742, accessed 18 April 2013.
14 M. Wilson and J. Lynxwiler, 'Abortion Clinic Violence as Terrorism', *Terrorism*, 11, 4 (1988), pp. 263–273.
15 C. Tilly, *Regimes and Repertoires* (Chicago, 2006).
16 See J. Baggini, *Complaint: From Minor Moans to Principled Protests* (London, 2008); R. M. Kowalski, 'Complaints and Complaining: Functions, Antecedents and Consequences', *Psychological Bulletin*, 119, 2 (1996); R. Klein, *Complaints against Doctors: A Study in Professional Accountability* (London, 1973); C. F. Hanna, 'Complaint as a Form of Association', *Qualitative Sociology*, 4, 4 (1981), pp. 298–311; L. Mulcahy, *Disputing Doctors: The Socio-legal Dynamics of Complaints about Medical Care* (Maidenhead, 2003); J. Weeks, *Unpopular Culture: The Ritual of Complaint in an English Bank* (Chicago, 2004); T. V. Hitchcock, *Richard Hutton's Complaint Book: The Notebook of the Steward of the Quaker Workhouse at Clerkenwell, 1711–1737* (London, 1987); R. Gregory and P. Giddings, *The Ombudsman, the Citizen and Parliament: A History of the Office of the Parliamentary Commissioners for Administration and Health Service Commissioners* (London, 2002).
17 Baggini, *Complaint*, p. 3.
18 C. Allen, 'Why Some Complaints Pack a Greater Punch than Others', *Guardian: Society Guardian* (4 March 2009), p. 6.
19 'Complaint', *Oxford English Dictionary*, www.oed.com/view/Entry/37620?redirectedFrom=complaint&, accessed 8 May 2013.
20 Baggini, *Complaint*, p. 2.
21 Klein, *Complaints against Doctors*, p. 16.
22 Ibid., p. 19.
23 Ibid., pp. 16–17, 34.
24 Mulcahy, *Disputing Doctors*, p. 3.
25 Ibid., p. 126.
26 W. A. F. Brown, *What Asylums Were, Are and Ought to Be* (Edinburgh, 1837).
27 www.nhs.uk/Pages/HomePage.aspx, accessed 13 February 2013.
28 www.nhs.uk/choiceintheNHS/Rightsandpledges/complaints/Pages/NHScomplaints.aspx, accessed 13 February 2013. Similar sites have been created by the UK Financial Ombudsman, and, at the time of writing this introduction, it had been announced that record numbers of complaints had been filed against British banks in 2013: www.financial-ombudsman.org.uk/consumer/complaints.htm, accessed 8 March 2013.
29 www.gmc-uk.org/concerns/index.asp, accessed 13 February 2013.
30 Dr P. Hodgkin (founder and Chief Executive of the UK independent feedback site Patient Opinion), speaking on 'The Shelagh Fogarty Show', BBC Radio 5 Live, 6 February 2013.
31 Parliamentary and Health Service Ombudsman, *Making Things Better: A Report on the Reform of the NHS Complaints Procedure in England* (London, 2005), p. 10.
32 http://news.bbc.co.uk/1/hi/health/6999307.stm, accessed 8 May 2013.
33 S. Boseley, 'Surgeons at Mount Alvernia Private Hospital "broke rules and ignored critics"', *Guardian* (3 May 2013), p. 20.

34 www.english.rfi.fr/americas/20111230-french-breast-implant-fraud-boss-tries-start-new-company, accessed 8 May 2013; www.thelocal.fr/20111227/2128, accessed 8 May 2013.

35 D. Orr, 'The Breast Implants Scandal is Bringing Out the Worst Kinds of Private Sector Attitudes', *Guardian* (14 January 2012), p. 47. For protests see, for example, www.bbc.co.uk/news/world-latin-america-22619407, accessed 30 May 2013; www.manchestereveningnews.co.uk/news/greater-manchester-news/fix-our-breasts-pip-implant-women-680457, accessed 30 May 2013; www.guardian.co.uk/world/2012/jan/14/pip-implants-scandal-march-replacements, accessed 30 May 2013.

36 W. B. Howie, 'The Administration of an Eighteenth-century Hospital', *Medical History* (1961), p. 44; J. Reinarz, 'Receiving the Rich, Rejecting the Poor: Towards a History of Hospital Visiting in Nineteenth-Century Provincial England', in G. Mooney and J. Reinarz (eds), *Permeable Walls: Historical Perspectives on Hospital and Asylum Visiting* (Amsterdam, Rodopi, 2009), pp. 31–54, p. 33.

37 Reinarz, 'Receiving the Rich', p. 33.

38 For some examples, see J. Reinarz, 'Investigating the "Deserving" Poor: Charity and the Voluntary Hospitals in Nineteenth-century Birmingham', in A. Borsay and P. Shapely (eds), *Medicine, Charity and Mutual Aid: The Consumption of Health and Welfare in Britain,* c.*1550–1950* (Aldershot, 2007), pp. 111–134, pp. 113–116.

39 Preface, *The Lancet*, 1, 1 (5 October 1823), p. 2.

40 T. Wakley, *A Report of the Trial of Cooper* v. *Wakley, for an Alleged Libel, Taken by Short-hand Writers Employed Expressly for the Occasion; with an Engraving of the Instruments, and the Position of the Patient, together with Mr. B. Cooper's 'Prefatory Remarks' on the Evidence, and Copious Explanatory Appendix* (London, 1829). See also S. Squire Sprigge, *The Life and Times of Thomas Wakley* (Huntington, NY, 1974), pp. 130–155.

41 P. Fennell, *Treatment Without Consent: Law, Psychiatry and the Treatment of Mentally Dis-ordered People since 1845* (London and New York, 1996), p. 278.

42 I. Butler and M. Drakeford, *Scandal, Social Policy and Social Welfare*, revised second edition (Bristol, 2003/2005).

43 N. Bethell Hervey, *The Lunacy Commission 1845–63, with Special Reference to the Implementation of Policy in Kent and Surrey* (University of Bristol, 1987). See also N. Hervey, 'A Slavish Bowing Down: the Lunacy Commission and the Psychiatric Profession, 1845–60', in W. F. Bynum, R. Porter and M. Shepherd (eds), *The Anatomy of Madness: Essays in the History of Psychiatry*, volume II: *Institutions and Society* (London and New York, 1988), pp. 98–131; P. Bartlett, *The Poor Law of Lunacy: The Administration of Pauper Lunatics in Mid-nineteenth-century England* (London and Washington, 1999), pp. 197–277; D. J. Mellett, 'Bureaucracy and Mental Illness: The Commissioners in Lunacy, 1845–90', *Medical History*, 25, 3 (July 1981), pp. 221–250; E. Murphy, 'The Lunacy Commissioners and the East London Guardians, 1845–1867', *Medical History*, 46, 4 (October 2002), pp. 495–524. Recent research has, however, begun to challenge Hervey's characterisation of inspection for the years 1745–1828 (R. Wynter, '"Good in All Respects"': Appearance and Dress at Staffordshire County Lunatic Asylum, 1818–54', *History of Psychiatry*, 22, 1 (March 2011), pp. 40–57, p. 42).

44 Health Service Ombudsman for England, *Making Things Better? A Report on Reform of the NHS Complaints Procedure in England* (London, 2005).

45 L. A. Weatherly, 'The Trials and Troubles and Grievances of a Private Asylum Superintendent', *Journal of Mental Science*, 40, 170 (July 1894), pp. 345–354, p. 345.

46 Weatherly, 'The Trials and Troubles', p. 345.
47 See article and responses to www.bmj.com/content/345/bmj.e7316, accessed 22 March 2013.
48 Weatherly, 'The Trials and Troubles', p. 347.
49 For more examples, see anthologies including R. Hunter and I. MacAlpine (eds), *Three Hundred Years of Psychiatry, 1535–1860: A History Presented in Selected English Texts* (London, 1963); A. Ingram (ed.), *Patterns of Madness in the Eighteenth Century: A Reader* (Liverpool, 1998); R. Porter (ed.), *The Faber Book of Madness* (London, 1991).
50 J. A. Campbell, 'Complaints by Insane Patients', *Journal of Mental Science*, 27, 119 (October 1881), pp. 342–352.
51 Campbell, 'Complaints by Insane Patients', p. 351.
52 Ibid., pp. 347–348.
53 For more on the Wilson Committee (and indeed the Health Ombudsman and its forerunners), see Gregory and Giddings, *The Ombudsman*, pp. 614–621 (and throughout).
54 P. F. G. Slawson and F. G. Guggenheim, 'Psychiatric Malpractice: A Review of the National Loss Experience', *American Journal of Psychiatry*, 141, 8 (1984), pp. 979–981; J. J. Bradley, 'Malpractice in Psychiatry', *Medico-legal Journal*, 57, 3 (1989), pp. 164–173.
55 K. Ingram and L. Roy, 'Complaints against Psychiatrists: A Five Year Study', *Psychiatric Bulletin*, 19, 10 (1995), pp. 620–622, p. 621.
56 I. Pitarka-Cacani, G. Szmukler and C. Henderson, 'Complaints about Care in a Mental Health Trust', *Psychiatric Bulletin*, 24, 10 (2000), pp. 372–376, p. 372.
57 Pitarka-Cacani, Szmukler and Henderson, 'Complaints about Care', p. 376.
58 Ibid., p. 372.
59 Ibid., pp. 373–374.
60 R. Wynter, '"Horrible Dens of Deception": Thomas Bakewell, Thomas Mulock and Anti-Asylum Sentiments, *c.*1815–1858', in T. Knowles and S. Trowbridge (eds), *Insanity and the Lunatic Asylum in the Nineteenth Century* (London, 2014).
61 R. Porter, 'The Patient's View: Doing Medical History from Below', *Theory and Society*, 14, 2 (1985), pp. 175–198.
62 T. McKeown and R. G. Brown, 'Medical Evidence Related to English Population Changes in the Eighteenth Century', *Population Studies*, 9, 2 (1955), pp. 119–141; T. McKeown, R. G. Brown and R. G. Record, 'An Interpretation of the Modern Rise of Population in Europe', *Population Studies*, 26, 3 (1972), pp. 345–382.
63 J. C. Burnham, 'American Medicine's Golden Age: What Happened to It?', *Science*, 215 (19 March 1982), p. 1474.
64 Lord Horder, 'Whither Medicine', *British Medical Journal*, 1 (1949), pp. 557–560, p. 558.
65 G. Bankoff, *The Conquest of Disease: The Story of Penicillin* (London, 1946).
66 Burnham, 'American Medicine's Golden Age', p. 1475.
67 See, for example, the surgeon's conquest of the body, which ushered in the 'Century of the Surgeon'; see J. Duffin, *History of Medicine: A Scandalously Short Introduction* (Toronto, 2010), p. 266.
68 B. Baumann, 'Diversities in Conceptions of Health and Physical Fitness', *Journal of Health and Human Behavior* 2, 1 (1961), pp. 39–46.
69 I. E. P. Menzies, 'A Case-study in the Functioning of Social Systems as a Defence Against Anxiety: A Report on a Study of the Nursing Service of a General Hospital', *Human Relations*, 13, 2 (1960), pp. 95–121.

70 www.youtube.com/watch?v=fRdLpem-AAs, accessed 14 February 2013.
71 V. Navarro, *Crisis, Health, and Medicine: A Social Critique* (New York, 1986), p. 11.
72 L. S. Jacyna and S. T. Casper, 'Introduction', in L. S. Jacyna and S. T. Casper (eds), *The Neurological Patient in History* (Rochester, NY, 2012), pp. 1–21, p. 3.
73 R. A. Nye, 'The Evolution of the Concept of Medicalization in the Late Twentieth Century', *Journal of the History of the Behavioral Sciences*, 39, 2 (2003), pp. 115–129, p. 116.
74 Burnham, 'American Medicine's Golden Age', p. 1479.
75 T. S. Szasz, *The Myth of Mental Illness: Foundations of a Theory of Personal Conduct* (New York, 1961).
76 R. D. Laing, *The Divided Self: An Existential Study in Sanity and Madness* (London, 1960).
77 A. Clare, *Psychiatry in Dissent: Controversial Issues in Thought and Practice*, second edition, Foreword by M. Shepherd (London, 1976/1980).
78 E. Goffman, *Asylums: Essays on the Social Situation of Mental Patients and other Inmates* (New York, 1961).
79 I. Illich, *Medical Nemesis: The Expropriation of Health* (London, 1975), p. 22.
80 Ibid., p. 25.
81 Ibid., p. 25.
82 Ibid., p. 11.
83 P. Conrad, 'The Discovery of Hyperkinesis: Notes on the Medicalization of Deviant Behaviour', *Social Problems*, 23, 1 (1975), pp. 12–21; A. T. Scull, 'From Madness to Mental Illness: Medical Men as Moral Entrepreneurs', *European Journal of Sociology*, 16, 2 (1975), pp. 218–261; S. J. Pfohl, 'The "Discovery" of Child Abuse', *Social Problems*, 24, 3 (1977), pp. 310–323; J. W. Schneider, 'Deviant Drinking as a Disease: Deviant Drinking as a Social Accomplishment', *Social Problems*, 25, 4 (1978), pp. 361–372.
84 McKeown, *The Role of Medicine: Dream, Mirage or Nemesis* (Oxford, 1979), p. vii.
85 Illich, *Medical Nemesis*, p. 19.
86 Clare, *Psychiatry in Dissent*, pp. 401–409, quote from p. 408.
87 www.bmj.com/content/346/bmj.f1297, accessed 1 March 2013.
88 R. Dubos, *The Mirage of Health* (London, 1960); M. Burnet, *Genes, Dreams and Realities* (Aylesbury, Bucks, 1971).
89 McKeown, *The Role of Medicine*, pp. xiv–xv.
90 Ibid., pp. 178–179.
91 C. Alvarez-Dardet and M. T. Ruiz, 'Thomas McKeown and Archibald Cochrane: A Journey through the Diffusion of their Ideas', *British Medical Journal*, 306 (8 May 1993), p. 1252.
92 Illich, *Medical Nemesis*, p. 11.
93 Ibid., p. 19.
94 Ibid., p. 19.
95 A. Cochrane, *Effectiveness and Efficiency: Random Reflections on Health Services* (London, 1972), p. 4.
96 Ibid., p. 6.
97 Ibid., p. 2.
98 Ibid., p. 2.
99 Ibid., p. 3.
100 Burnham, 'American Medicine's Golden Age', pp. 1476–1477.
101 See, for example, J. H. Young, *The Toadstool Millionaires: A Social History of Patent*

Medicines in America before Federal Regulation (Princeton, 1961); J. H. Young, *The Medical Messiahs: A Social History of Health Quackery in Twentieth Century America* (Princeton, 1967); W. F. Bynum and R. Porter (eds), *Medical Fringe and Medical Orthodoxy, 1750–1850* (London, 1987); M. Ramsey, *Professional and Popular Medicine in France, 1770–1830* (Cambridge, 1988); R. Porter, *Health for Sale: Quackery in England, 1660–1850* (Manchester, 1989); M. Sax (ed.), *Alternative Medicine in Britain* (Oxford, 1992); R. Porter, *Quacks: Fakers and Charlatans in English Medicine* (Stroud, Gloucestershire, 2000); R. Bivins, *Alternative Medicine? A History* (Oxford, 2007).

102 J. Donnison, *Midwives and Medical Men: A History of Inter-Professional Rivalries and Women's Rights* (London, 1977).

103 A. Oakley, *The Captured Womb* (New York, 1984).

104 See, for example, Parliamentary Papers, *A Report from the Committee, Appointed (upon the 27th Day of January, 1763) to Enquire into the State of the Private Madhouses in This Kingdom. With the Proceedings of the House thereupon* (London, 1774); B. Sapinsley, *The Private War of Mrs. Packard* (New York, 1991); L. V. Carlisle, *Elizabeth Packard: A Noble Fight* (Champaign, IL, 2010); M. Jones, 'The Most Cruel and Revolting Crimes: The Treatment of the Mentally Ill in Mid-nineteenth-century Jamaica', *Journal of Caribbean History*, 42 (2), 2008, pp. 290–309; L. D. Smith, *Insanity, Race and Colonialism* (London, forthcoming), Chapter 3; R. S. Porter, H. Nicholson and B. Bennett, *Women, Madness and Spiritualism: Georgina Weldon and Louisa Lowe* (London, 2003); A. Owen, *The Darkened Room: Women, Power and Spiritualism in Late Victorian England* (Chicago, 1984/2004). For 1860s England, see, for instance, V. Blain, 'Rosina Bulwer Lytton and the Rage of the Unheard', *Huntington Library Quarterly*, 53, 3 (summer 1990), pp. 210–236.

105 See, for example: G. Wilkinson, 'Political dissent and "sluggish" schizophrenia in the Soviet Union', *British Medical Journal (Clinical Research Edition)*, 293, 6548 (13 September 1986), pp. 641–642; R. van Voren, 'Political Abuse of Psychiatry: An Historical Overview', *Schizophrenia Bulletin*, 36, 1 (January 2010), pp. 33–35; R. Munro, *Dangerous Minds: Political Psychiatry in China Today and its Origins in the Mao Era* (Geneva, 2002); C. MacLeod, 'Chinese Citizens Sent to Mental Hospitals to Quiet Dissent', *USA Today* (29 December 2011), http://usatoday30.usatoday.com/news/world/story/2011–12–28/china-mental-hospitals/52260592/1, accessed 28 January 2013.

106 R. Grossman, 'Psychiatric Manual's Update Needs Openness, not Secrecy, Critics Say', *Chicago Tribune* (27 December 2008), www.christopherlane.org/DSM5Tribune.html, accessed 05/06/2014.

107 E. Shorter, *A History of Psychiatry: From the Era of the Asylum to the Age of Prozac* (New York, 1997), pp. 145–153.

108 J. N. Katz, *Gay American History: Lesbians and Gay Men in the U.S.A.* (New York, 1978), p. 296.

109 Pan American Health Organization, '"Therapies" to Change Sexual Orientation Lack Medical Justification and Threaten Health', press release (17 May 2012), http://new.paho.org/hq/index.php?option=com_content&view=article&id=6803&Itemid=1926, accessed 14 February 2013.

110 See, for example, E. C. Halperin, 'Grievances against Physicians', *Western Journal of Medicine*, 173, 4 (October 2000), pp. 235–238; G. Lester, B. Wilson, L. Griffin and P. E. Mullen, 'Unusually Persistent Complainants', *British Journal of Psychiatry*, 184, 4 (April 2004), pp. 352–356.

111 D. Hardiman, *Missionaries and their Medicine: A Christian Modernity for Tribal India* (Manchester, 2008), p. 1.

112 D. Arnold, 'Introduction: Disease, Medicine and Empire', in D. Arnold (ed.), *Imperial Medicine and Indigenous Societies* (Manchester, 1988), p. 2.
113 J. Reinarz and L. D. Schwarz (eds), *Medicine and the Workhouse* (Rochester, NY, 2013).
114 Illich, *Medical Nemesis*, pp. 25–26.
115 P. Conrad, 'Medicalization and Social Control', *Annual Review of Sociology* (18 August 1992), pp. 209–232, p. 219.
116 E. P. Thompson, 'The Moral Economy of the English Crowd in the Eighteenth Century', *Past & Present*, 50 (1971), pp. 76–136.
117 E. P. Thompson, *Customs in Common* (London, 1993).
118 N. Crossley, *Contesting Psychiatry: Social Movements in Mental Health* (London and New York, 2006), p. 29.
119 Baggini, *Complaint*, pp. 45–49.
120 For further reading on the subject, see G. Hunt (ed.), *Whistleblowing in the Health Service: Accountability, Law and Professional Practice* (London, 1995).
121 M. Stacey, 'Medical Accountability', in G. Hunt (ed.), *Whistleblowing in the Health Service: Accountability, Law and Professional Practice* (London, 1995), pp. 40–41.
122 L. Mulcahy, 'Mediation of Medical Negligence Actions: An Option for the Future?', in M. M. Rosenthal, L. Mulcahy and S. Lloyd-Bostock (eds), *Medical Mishaps: Pieces of the Puzzle* (Buckingham, 1999), 154–167, p. 154.
123 A. Malleson, *Need your Doctor be So Useless?* (London, 1973).
124 J. Martin, with D. Evans, *Hospitals in Trouble* (Oxford, 1984).

Part I

Professionals

1 A culture of complaint

Psychiatry and its critics

Andrew Scull

I venture to suggest that few branches of the medical profession have been as subject to complaints as psychiatrists. The mad (or some of them) were vocal critics of their doctors long before there was such a thing as psychiatry – or at least an organised profession that went by that name. For psychiatry as a term of art only came into broad usage in the English-speaking world a century or so ago. Before the early twentieth century, those purporting to minister to diseased minds called themselves (or were referred to by others) asylum superintendents, medical psychologists, or alienists. Earlier still, in the eighteenth century and through the first part of the nineteenth, they answered to the name 'mad-doctor', a label that nicely captures the ambivalence with which society at large always seems to regard those who lay claim to expertise in the treatment of the mentally ill. (As Hilary Ingram reminds us elsewhere in this volume, defining and defending a profession often brings questions of semantics to the foreground.) Complaints about psychiatry continue to the present, as the introduction to this volume similarly makes clear. Indeed, as I shall show in the concluding section of this chapter, in the last half century, the voices of the patients have been amplified by other powerful complainers – by social scientists who have suggested that the psychiatric emperor has no clothes; and, more disturbingly still, by critics from within the profession of psychiatry itself, and not just renegades like Thomas Szasz and Ronald Laing, but mainstream psychiatrists as well.

Complaints have frequently functioned as a motor of change in this arena, as in other fields of medicine. Complaints about the horrors of the *ancien régime* madhouse and about the confinement of the sane amidst the lunatic played a vital role in generating the moral outrage that fuelled the Victorian lunacy reform movement, and in successive revisions of commitment laws – though it has to be added that the law of unintended consequences operated with particular force in these arenas. The asylums that were one generation's solution to the problems of serious psychosis became the object of complaints and agitation for a later generation seduced by the siren song of 'community psychiatry'; and the hedging about of the psychiatric commitments process with legal entanglements likewise became a late-twentieth-century *bête noir*. But complaints have also been directed against particular forms of psychiatric treatment and have played an important role in creating greater circumspection among psychiatrists about the use of treatments such as lobotomy and the shock therapies, and more recently even in raising concerns about the contemporary reliance on psychopharmacology as the sheet anchor of current psychiatric practice.[1] Though, of course, and as Hera Cook has described elsewhere in this collection, a transatlantic swell was created by critiques of psychoanalysis and US therapy culture – complaining about talking therapies and their rationale also punctuated the late twentieth century.

Most recently of all, as I shall discuss in the concluding sections of this chapter, complaints from the very centre of the psychiatric enterprise – the authors of the two editions of the psychiatric 'bible', the *Diagnostic and Statistical Manual of the American Psychiatric Association*, immediately preceding the one issued in May 2013; and the head of the US National Institute of Mental Health, Thomas Insel, who presides over the vital federal presence in basic mental health research, dispensing billions of dollars – have threatened to destabilise the psychiatric enterprise in its entirety. *DSM 5*, as it is called, has been labelled a useless, anti-scientific document, a hindrance to progress. Perhaps worse, Insel has complained openly about the mythical status of such 'diseases' as schizophrenia and depression.[2] Complaining about psychiatry scarcely gets more dangerous and delegitimising for the psychiatric profession than that.

Though medical speculations about the origins of madness have an ancient lineage, the emergence of what ultimately became the modern profession of psychiatry – that is, the routine engagement of some medics in the management of the mad – cannot really be traced back much further than the eighteenth century. As the nineteenth-century term 'asylum superintendent' suggests, the emergence of what ultimately became a community of practitioners specialising in mental illness was intimately bound up with the parallel creation of a new social space – the madhouse or the asylum. It was in and through the management of these establishments that doctors developed some claims to skill in the management of the depressed, the demented and the deranged, and it was their control over the rapidly expanding network of such places in the Victorian era that ultimately helped to constitute and consolidate their position as an organised, well-defined, but still suspect profession.

The eighteenth-century 'trade in lunacy' was produced by and responded to the opportunities created by the growth of a consumer society, the emergence of a market for all sorts of goods and services that had traditionally been supplied on a subsistence basis, if they were supplied at all. It must be understood, as the late historian Roy Porter suggested, as part of the same developments that saw the rise of dancing masters, fencing instructors, hairdressers, pottery manufacturers, and other novel service occupations.[3] Those practising the trade in lunacy took over the burdens of coping with some initially small fraction of those whose disturbed emotions, cognitions and behaviours rendered them inconvenient if not positively impossible to live with – rather as undertakers now began to emerge to handle the comparatively unpleasant and stigmatising task of dealing with and disposing of corpses. The mad had traditionally been a liability that fell primarily on the shoulders of their families. The disruptions they visited on the texture of daily life – the uncertainties, the threat, the terror they might provoke – were ones their relations bore primary responsibility for dealing with. In the entrepreneurial culture that prevailed in eighteenth-century England, those who could afford it might for the first time relinquish these problems to others, and where poor lunatics were judged sufficiently threatening and disruptive, the creaky mechanism of the Old Poor Law might occasionally pay to confine pauper lunatics in these new-fangled madhouses.

By no means was the new trade in lunacy a medical monopoly. To the contrary, in its early years, the madhouse business attracted all manner of entrepreneurs willing to speculate in, and earn a living from, trafficking in this particular form of misery. The keepers of madhouses were a heterogeneous lot, for there were no barriers to entry, and no oversight of the industry. And though traditional humoral medicine could readily stretch its explanatory schema to account for mania and melancholia, and its bleedings, vomits, purges and dietary regimens could be easily rationalised as remedies for the excesses of bile and blood that supposedly produced mental turmoil, there was no compelling reason, so far as many potential customers were concerned, to prefer those who professed some sort of medical expertise to others who offered similar services: respite from the travails madness brought in its train, and the shutting up of a source of social shame and embarrassment out of public view. To be sure, the growing numbers of madhouses, and the experience of attempting to control and manage the mentally disturbed day after day, meant that those running these places perforce developed techniques and some measure of skill in the handling of such awkward customers. The very variety of establishments and operators led to experiments with different approaches, and since claims to provide cure as well as care could provide a comparative advantage when it came to securing clients, many were not slow to advance them; some rather bizarre pieces of apparatus – swinging chairs, devices to mimic the experience of drowning, chairs to immobilise the patient and cut him or her off from sources of sensory stimulation – were invented to assist in the task.[4]

One of the key benefits madhouses could potentially offer families was the capacity to draw a veil of silence over the existence of a mad relation in their midst. But this shutting up of the mad in what purported to be a therapeutic isolation could easily be cast in a more sinister light. Drawing boundaries between the mad and the sane is scarcely a simple task. At the margin, ambiguities abound. Madhouses, with their barred windows, high perimeter walls, isolation from the community at large, and enforced secrecy, inevitably invited gothic imaginings about what transpired hidden from view, and such stories almost immediately began to circulate.

Some were fictional. Pulp fiction was another innovation of the emerging consumer society, and Grub Street hastened to produce melodramas with a madhouse setting. One of the most successful of these, first published in 1726 and passing through myriad editions, staying in print for more than three-quarters of a century, was Eliza Haywood's novella, *The Distress'd Orphan*. As was customary in such gothic productions, the confinement that structured the story arose from familial conflict over a romantic liaison and the control of a personal estate: Annilia, the daughter of an eminent city merchant, who had lost both parents at a young age and was heiress to a substantial fortune, finds herself nefariously confined as insane by her uncle and guardian, Giraldo, after falling in love with a foreigner, Colonel Marathon. Her uncle is determined that she should marry his own son, Horatio, thus ensuring the passage of her estate as her dowry. The confinement (mimicking what was often the case in reality) was initiated in her own home by the uncle ordering her door locked and 'one of the Footmen to bring a Smith, that her Windows may be barr'd', under the pretence of protecting Annilia from her own mischievous and suicidal propensities: 'for 'tis not Improbable but when she finds she is restrain'd in her Humour she may offer to throw herself out'.[5]

Annilia, however, is not to be so easily intimidated, and her uncle ratchets up the pressure by arranging for her to be carted off to a madhouse, secretly and in the dead of night, her screams silenced by 'stopping her mouth'.[6] Here, she finds herself at the mercy of 'inhuman Creatures', 'Ruffians', 'pityless [*sic*] Monsters' and 'ill-looked fellows', wedded to the terrific mode of instilling 'awe' and dread in their patients via lashings, mechanical restraint and neglect.[7] Heywood's melodrama plays up the symbolic homology between the constraints of the madhouse – its bolts, bars, and chains – and the tyranny of life as a lady, bereft of any semblance of legal and social equality. Only the intervention of her lover, Colonel Marathon, who surreptitiously enters the madhouse and then heroically scales its wall with his 'trembling' sweetheart draped across his broad shoulders, allows her to escape back to 'freedom' after three months of confinement.[8] Then the evil are punished, and virtue is rewarded, and the titillating story comes to a satisfying close.

Haywood's portrait of the mad-business as corrupt and cruel, unconcerned with the mental status of those it confined, struck deep chords with an audience prone to believe the worst about what happened in the madhouse. Nor were such complaints confined to the realm of fiction. Mrs Clerke's case came before the courts in 1718, and the testimony at the trial made plain that women with fortunes (in this case, a rich widow) were genuinely vulnerable to incarceration as mad in just the ways that were exploited in these literary narratives – all the more so, given the hazy boundaries of those disorders of mind and body being constituted by doctors and owned by sufferers as vapours, spleen and nerves.[9] Research by the Cambridge historian Elizabeth Foyster into the records of the King's Bench court has shown that Mrs Clerke's case was scarcely unique. Women were, indeed, especially liable to false confinement in madhouses, locked away by husbands eager to enforce their authority over the property of wives and to sanction their 'reasonable' restraint and correction.[10]

Whereas emotionally and socially susceptible females predominated as the victims and complainants in this partly literary and partly literal construction of the madhouse, there were also a fair number of actual and fictional male equivalents suffering similar fates. A particularly noisy example was the obsessive–compulsive printer and proof-reader, and author of a *Concordance to the Holy Bible* (1737) that remains in print to this day, Alexander Cruden. The very obsessiveness that allowed Cruden to compile his monumental work in his garret after work each day translated less well into his picaresque daily life. When he lost his job in 1729 as reader in French to the Earl of Derby (it turned out that he had never heard spoken French, learning the language through his work as a proof-reader, and attempting a Scots-inflected phonetic pronunciation of the text put before him) he rushed off to learn French at the hands of a family of Huguenot refugees, and then rode to Lancashire, nearly killing his horse in the process, to demand his job back – to no avail. But when in 1739 he obsessively stalked ladies above his station, informing them that God had chosen each of them for his spouse, he was imprisoned in a madhouse, as he was later in 1753 when he fought with a group of drunken youths who were swearing and blaspheming in the London streets.

Escaping on the first occasion by sawing through the bed leg and gathering up the chain that had bound him to it, he hobbled through the streets of London one foot shod in a slipper, the other bare, till he reached the Lord Mayor's house. There followed a lawsuit for £10,000 in damages, which he lost, and then a series of pamphlets, in which he pronounced himself a 'London citizen exceedingly injured' by a form of 'British Inquisition'.[11] James Monro, the mad-doctor who had treated him, was denounced as a Jacobite and an adulterer. James' son, John Monro, was called in to treat him on the occasion of his confinement for the fight, but he was at least spared from being the target of Cruden's second unsuccessful lawsuit, though lampooned in the next round of pamphlets Cruden wrote to protest his confinement.

James Newton (*c.*1670–1750), the proprietor of a madhouse in Islington, was one of few to be convicted (and the many to be lambasted) for a false confinement, or, as an anonymous 1715 pamphlet put it, for 'violently keeping and misusing' William Rogers at the behest of his wife.[12] But many another was suspected of following suit. Calling upon a growing common knowledge and concern about such abuses, the novelist Tobias Smollett arranged for his mock-heroic English

Don Quixote, *Sir Launcelot Greaves* (1762), to be seized and carried off to a madhouse run by Bernard Shackle, an occasion for a warning that

> in England, the most innocent person upon earth is liable to be immured for life under the pretext of lunacy, sequestered from his wife, children, and friends, robbed of his fortune, deprived even of necessaries, and subjected to brutal treatment from a low-bred barbarian, who raises an ample fortune on the misery of his fellow-creatures, and may, during his whole life, practice this horrid oppression, without question or control.[13]

Daniel Defoe had earlier raised similar fears,[14] which by the 1730s had become sufficiently universal to become the subject of an opera-burlesque.[15] Before the century's end, in the wake of further critiques and protests by pamphleteers and disaffected former patients,[16] the image of these 'mansions of misery' could scarcely have been less salubrious.

The mid-eighteenth century thus saw a torrent of criticism of the unregulated state of private madhouses, fed by scandalous tales of alleged false confinement and intermittent, but influential, appeals for legislative intervention – all of which were met initially with official indifference. Eventually, however, the rising tide of complaints of corruption, cruelty and malfeasance in the mad trade forced a reluctant House of Commons to launch a half-hearted inquiry into the mad-business in 1763; the limited testimony it took proved damning. All the instances of false confinement that came to light involved women who had allegedly been falsely confined by their husbands and other family members. Witnesses stressed the use of ruses and trickery to initiate and perpetuate these confinements, and the obstruction of contact with the outside world, in particular through being locked up and mechanically restrained night and day, having visitors refused and correspondence barred, and being 'treated with Severity' by keepers. The women themselves complained that they received no medicines or medical treatment whatsoever, and were never even attended by a medical practitioner, or not, at least, until a *habeas corpus* was affected.

Complaints notwithstanding, it was another 11 years before an Act for Regulating Madhouses (14 George III *c*.49) was finally passed. Porter has suggested that the prolonged delay in enacting legislation should be seen as a function of the opposition of the College of Physicians, some of whose members 'had a large financial stake in metropolitan madhouses'.[17] Yet Parliament handed over the power to license and inspect madhouses in the metropolis to the College, who proved as indolent at the task as the magistrates who were charged with these tasks in the provinces. In every respect, the legislation seems to have been little more than a token gesture.

Patient protest against their mad-doctors became even fiercer in the nineteenth century, as lunacy reformers secured legislation compelling the tax-supported construction of mental hospitals, and thousands upon thousands of patients flooded into the expanding empire of asylumdom. Perhaps the most socially prominent contributor to this literature was John Perceval, son of the last British Prime Minister to be assassinated, Spencer Perceval. The younger Perceval patronised a prostitute while a student at Oxford. A pious Evangelical Christian, he feared he had contracted syphilis, dosed himself with mercury, and soon lapsed into a delusory religious state, which led his family to lock him up, first in Edward Long Fox's madhouse near Bristol, Brislington House, and then in what became the favourite asylum for the English upper classes, Ticehurst House in Sussex. Elaborate as these establishments were, they could not provide accommodations that matched Perceval's expectations. He complained of violence from his attendants and of their failure to display sufficient deference to their distinguished, gentlemanly patient. Shortly after his transfer to Ticehurst in 1832, he considered himself cured. Yet his confinement continued. The angrier he became, the more the Newingtons, in whose establishment he was now confined, insisted that he was still unfit for release – another of Kim Price's (after Joseph Heller) catch-22 crucibles of complaint (see Chapter 6 in this volume). Deprived of his privacy and his dignity, Perceval was furious. Released in October 1833 (though his doctors were still not sure of his sanity), he subsequently penned an anonymous account of his captivity, savaging both Fox and the Newingtons; when that volume failed to attract much attention, he issued a revised and enlarged version under his own name, something that permanently alienated him from many of his family.[18]

Finding his complaints were still largely ignored, Perceval subsequently was one of the founders in 1845 of that wonderfully named Victorian organisation, The Alleged Lunatics' Friend Society (ALFS) – a forerunner to the twentieth-century advocacy movement shadowed by Alex Mold's chapter in this volume. Perceval and his cohorts (who included Luke Hansard, whose family published the parliamentary proceedings and who had two mad sisters confined in asylums; Captain Richard Saumarez, two of whose brothers were locked up as lunatics; and Richard Paternoster, a discharged lunatic who claimed he had always been sane) now made usually fruitless efforts to secure the release of patients whom they claimed were improperly confined. The *Medical Times* spoke scornfully of their activities:

> The members of this Society are apt to see things through a hazy and distorted medium. . . . They have wandered about the country, prepared to lend an ear to the idle story of every lunatic they could meet with; they have pestered the Home Secretary, and ever and anon obtruded their opinions and schemes upon such members of the Upper and Lower House as would listen to them.

Others had a pithier put-down: they called them 'The Lunatics' Society'.[19]

Most of those whose cases the society took up were men, but the most famous complainer of the late 1840s was a woman, Miss Louisa Nottidge, whose suit against her brothers for kidnapping and false imprisonment in a madhouse produced a string of newspaper reports that titillated literate Englishmen, and a proclamation from the judge who heard the case which cast scorn upon the pretensions of the alienists who had confined her. Louisa was a maiden lady of a certain age, one of several unmarried sisters upon whom their father had settled considerable sums and who subsequently became devotees of a defrocked Anglican clergyman, a certain Mr Prince, who set up a commune in the West of England he called Agapemone or the Abode of Love. Prince preached that the Day of Judgment had come, and that only his followers would be saved. Later, he appeared to announce (his preaching was convoluted and confusing) that he was the Holy Ghost made flesh. And flesh was something the Abode of Love appeared to worship: there were rumours that female recruits had to present themselves naked, or risk damnation. Three of Louisa's sisters had already married members of the sect, turning over their fortunes to them, and when Louisa seemed likely to follow suit, her brother and brother-in-law descended at night and abducted her, locking her up in Dr Arthur Moorcroft's asylum, Moorcroft House in Hillingdon, Middlesex. Learning of where she was confined, her co-religionists brought a writ of *habeas corpus* and secured her release. Hence the lawsuit, which was decided in her favour (though damages were assessed at a mere £50), and a scathing statement from the judge that mad-doctors were a danger to the liberty of free-born Englishmen, and that 'no lunatic should be confined in an asylum unless a danger to himself or others'. (Louisa, incidentally, had fled back to the Abode of Love, and handed over all her money to Prince. She would remain there till her death in 1858.)[20]

And other women were far more audible if not the most famous complainers during the second half of the nineteenth century. They stand in contrast to the predominantly male complainers about medicine – Szasz, McKeown and Illich – discussed in the introduction to this volume, and their distinctive set of utterances deserves serious attention of its own. The novelist and politician, Sir Edward Bulwer Lytton (he of the infamous 'It was a dark and stormy night' opening line), had a sharp-tongued and spendthrift wife, Lady Rosina, of whom he eventually tired. His novels proving hugely successful, he set up a stable of mistresses. The married couple's domestic bliss was by now gone. Bulwer Lytton on occasion beat Rosina, and perhaps sodomised her. They officially separated in 1836, nine years after their marriage. Then Lady Lytton began her own career as a writer, much of what she wrote being barely veiled criticism of her estranged husband, and full of her sense of rage and betrayal.[21] He threatened to ruin her if she kept it up. An affair in Dublin cost her custody of her children, and the whole sorry business of a broken Victorian marriage took a further turn for the worse when Lady Lytton discovered that her daughter, dying of typhoid, had been exiled to a down-at-heel boarding house.

Lady Rosina now began to bombard her well-connected husband and his powerful friends with letters filled with obscenities and libels, and eventually, in 1858, when Bulwer Lytton stood for re-election at Hertford, she showed up and denounced him before the electors, haranguing them for nearly an hour. The response from her angry spouse was immediate: he cut off her allowance (which in any event he had paid only intermittently and with great reluctance) and he cut off her contact with their son. But then he took a further step, which he would live to regret: obtaining the legally required lunacy certificates from two compliant doctors, he had Rosina confined in a madhouse run by Robert Gardiner Hill.

Shutting up Lady Rosina was intended to silence her: it had the opposite effect. Bulwer Lytton evidently relied for impunity on his many connections – his close friendship with one of the Lunacy Commissioners, John Forster, for example, and with the editor of *The Times* (who indeed tried to protect him by suppressing all mention of the scandal). But *The Times*' great rival, the *Daily Telegraph* (whose very existence, ironically enough, owed much to Bulwer Lytton's efforts to reduce the stamp tax newspapers had to pay), took great delight in pursuing the salacious scandal. Within weeks, Bulwer Lytton, facing an avalanche of bad publicity, had capitulated, releasing his wife on condition that she relocate abroad – something she briefly did, only to return and spend the rest of her life blackening his name, not desisting even after his death from complications following ear surgery.[22]

The enormous suspicion with which many regarded those running asylums intensified in the aftermath of a series of other cases calling into question the motives and competence of even the most prominent alienists of the age. John Conolly, previously superintendent of the first public asylum for London at Hanwell, and famous for his role in abolishing mechanical restraint in his asylum, was held liable for major damages in the case of a Mr Ruck, whose certificates he had signed at the instigation of his wife. It turned out that the proprietor of the madhouse to which the alcoholic Ruck had been consigned paid Conolly fees for the referral, not to mention a further £60 a year for so long as Ruck remained in his hands.[23] Forbes Winslow, who in 1848 had founded the first English journal on the science and treatment of mental illness, the *Quarterly Journal of Psychological Medicine*, had a different problem: he testified at the lunacy inquisition held in the case of the immensely wealthy William Windham that the gentleman was mad: he openly masturbated; ate voraciously at dinner parties, then vomited at table so he could eat yet more; impersonated a train guard and nearly caused a train crash; wore servant's clothes; contracted syphilis and then married a prostitute. But, for whatever reason, many of his colleagues, Conolly prominent among them, insisted that Windham was eccentric, not mad. The jury agreed. At a staggering cost of some £20,000, Windham had secured his freedom.[24] He drank, spent, and fornicated his way to oblivion in the space of scarce two years, dying at only 25. The jury's verdict in this extraordinary case had been just one more sign of how deeply suspicious of the madhouses and those running them the British public remained, and it was a mistrust that would be nurtured and fed by yet more scandal and evidence of financial corruption on the part of alienists in the remaining years of the nineteenth century.

The cases of Ruck and Windham remind us that a great many of the Victorian *causes celèbres* revolved around the improper confinement of men, not women – though, like the Nottidge affair and the case of Lady Rosina, the newspaper attention to these cases was often intensified by lurid tales of sexual impropriety (Ruck had fathered two children in a long-running affair with his sister-in-law, and Windham's sexual escapades were legion). Still, perhaps the most determined and in some ways the most effective complainers about psychiatry were two women: Louisa Lowe and Georgina Weldon, both spiritualists, and both major sources of trouble for those claiming expertise in mental medicine.[25]

Beliefs in automatic writing and in communing with spirits in the other world might be enough for some of us to conclude that persons holding such views had a tenuous hold on reality, but in the Victorian era, such notions were seen as plausible even by many highly educated folk – Lunacy Commissioners and alienists included.[26] But the content of the messages Louisa Lowe received from the netherworld had its own complications: her automatic writing included much that was obscene and upsetting, not least the allegation that her husband, the Reverend Lowe, was engaged in an incestuous relationship with his seven-year-old daughter and was a serial adulterer besides. (No other evidence existed to support either accusation.) And Georgina Weldon was a real-life Mrs Jellyby, persuading her husband to lease the grand Tavistock House and then turning it into a slum: her pet dogs leaving their excrement everywhere; her children running wild, dressed in rags and living in filth; adopted 'orphan' children brought in randomly and given singing lessons and put up to public performances conducted by the estimable Mrs W. All sorts of dubious adults – the French opera composer Gounod and his mistress, a con-man and his common-law ex-prostitute wife – added to the mix, till the household grew so unbearable that poor Mr Weldon moved out, though he continued to pay the bills.[27]

The gentlemen who had made the mistake of marrying these formidable ladies sought to shake themselves loose from the domestic horrors that enveloped them by arranging for their wives to be certified and sent to a madhouse: Brislington House and then Lawn House, Hanwell, for Mrs Lowe (John Conolly's old madhouse now run by his misanthropic and misogynist son-in-law Henry Maudsley); and Lyttleton Forbes Winslow's Sussex House Asylum in Hammersmith for Mrs Lowe. Foreseeing the fate that awaited her, Mrs Lowe escaped from her would-be captors, waited for her certificates to expire, got a clean bill of health from her own choice of doctors, and then launched a whole series of lawsuits against all comers that occupied and entertained British courtroom onlookers for much of the 1880s.

As with Bulwer Lytton and Lady Rosina, Messrs Winslow and Lowe badly miscalculated. Louisa Lowe wrote harrowing accounts of her captivity and spent nearly two decades attacking the motives and competence of the alienists with whom she had come into contact, most notably in the best-selling critique *The Bastilles of England, or The Lunacy Laws at Work* (1883). Georgina Weldon proved even more resourceful. She launched a string of lawsuits (17 in 1884 alone), and these delivered her endless publicity and not a few damage awards. Juries and judges seem to have shared her low opinion of the mad-doctors and their diagnoses, and to have sympathised with the notion that it was odious to lock up the eccentric and the unconventional in asylums. It became her life's work to humiliate her husband and the medics he had employed to try to bring her to heel. 'May God give me the means, give me the allies, to ruin them', she wrote in her diary. And God duly obliged, or Mrs Weldon acted nobly in his place.[28] Reputational ruin was her goal, and her accomplishment – as also was a change in the lunacy laws. In 1890, a new Lunacy Act required the involvement of a magistrate in all certification of lunatics, and certificates were made valid for only a year at a time. In practice, such legal changes served only to ossify still further the empire of asylumdom.

Louisa Lowe and Georgina Weldon's complaints were far from a uniquely English phenomenon. Indeed, in the United States a clergyman's wife, Elizabeth Packard, had anticipated their arguments about the dangers of women being railroaded into asylums by husbands anxious to shut them up. Packard had been sent to the Illinois State Asylum by her clergyman husband in 1860, by her account because she argued with him on points of theology, by his, because she heard voices and believed she was talking to God. (Mrs Packard, not unusually for the age, was a spiritualist). Illinois commitment laws at the time generally required medical certificates before someone was confined as a lunatic, but they made an exception for married women and children, who could be sent to the asylum simply on the husband or father's representations. Like Lowe and Weldon, Packard would not be silenced. She brought a *habeas corpus* lawsuit, and three years after she had been locked up, notwithstanding some embarrassing revelations about the crush she had developed on the asylum's superintendent, she was declared sane and freed. She spent much of the rest of her life publishing and republishing denunciations of the involuntary commitment laws,[29] and campaigning to require a jury trial before any patient accused of being mad could be locked up against his or her will. Illinois, then Michigan, Iowa, Massachusetts and Pennsylvania enacted at least some of the changes she sought during the 1870s and 1880s.

Neither these American nor these British legal changes sufficed to choke off the culture of complaint. Consider just the examples of Virginia Woolf, Janet Frame and Sylvia Plath. Sir William Bradshaw in *Mrs. Dalloway* (1925) is a brutal fictionalised rendition of Woolf's own disastrous encounter with Sir George

Savage, whose psychiatric practice centred on the chattering classes. Sylvia Plath's roman-à-clef *The Bell Jar* (1963), a novel that became a feminist classic in the aftermath of its author's suicide, casts mid-twentieth-century psychiatry, and particularly its resort to shock treatments, in a distinctly unflattering light. From the late 1940s onwards, the New Zealand novelist Janet Frame spent years of her life in a series of dire mental hospitals, where, like many of her contemporaries, she endured life-threatening insulin comas, not to mention more than 200 electroshocks, all for naught. At one point, she came within weeks of being lobotomised, only to have her brain and her talents spared when she won a major literary prize, the Hubert Church Memorial Award, in 1951. These encounters with the horrors of institutional psychiatry are the dominant theme of her novels and her three-volume autobiography,[30] which was made into an award winning film, *An Angel at My Table* (1990).

And, as in the nineteenth century, complaints came from pens of men as well. Ken Kesey's *One Flew Over the Cuckoo's Nest* (1962) was based on its author's experiences in a California mental hospital. Adapted by Milòs Foreman, the film version featured Jack Nicholson in the role of a lifetime, as the rebel Randle P. McMurphy. Fairly or unfairly, it cemented psychiatry's reputation in many quarters as an instrument of repression, with the irrepressible McMurphy reduced to a vegetable by a lobotomy.[31]

As this volume's introduction and Cook's chapter suggest, among social scientists, the period between the late 1950s and the 1970s saw the development of a steadily more elaborate set of complaints about psychiatry and its pretensions. A series of increasingly critical ethnographies of the mental hospital in particular culminated in Erving Goffman's searing 1961 critique of them as 'total institutions'.[32] Their nearest analogues, he suggested, were such things as prisons and concentration camps. So far from being places of treatment and cure, they were engines of degradation, misery and oppression that worsened, even created, the symptoms of chronic mental illness. Within five years, the California sociologist Thomas Scheff had advanced a more audacious hypothesis yet: mental illness, he alleged in his *Being Mentally Ill* (1966), was not a medical disease at all, but a matter of labels, an intervention discussed in this book's introduction. Scheff's arguments were seriously flawed, conceptually and empirically, and over the years he steadily retracted his more extreme statements. But the fact that they were granted credence in some quarters is a measure of how much damage the culture of complaint had done to psychiatry's public standing.

Besides, in those same years, equally fierce complaints were being launched from within psychiatry. Scottish psychiatrist R. D. Laing was voicing the heretical (and in my view absurd) claim that schizophrenia was a voyage of discovery that should be indulged and encouraged, and was temporarily receiving a respectful hearing among intellectuals. Across the Atlantic, Thomas Szasz published the best-selling *The Myth of Mental Illness* (1960), which was followed by a host of derivative publications that repeated the theme that mental illness was nothing more than a bad metaphor, with no legitimate status as an object of medical science. His fellow psychiatrists, he proclaimed, systematically violated their patients' rights and trust, acting as gaolers and agents of social control on behalf of society at large, not as therapists.

Szasz's assaults on his profession were legitimised in part by accumulating evidence of its inability to distinguish the mad from the sane. Throughout the 1960s and 1970s, a series of careful studies had demonstrated that psychiatrists, when confronted with a patient, could not be relied upon to reach a reliable conclusion about his or her mental state.[33] A meticulous cross-national comparison had shown that depression was diagnosed five times as often in Britain as in the United States, the mirror image of the situation with respect to schizophrenia.[34] In the courtroom or the clinic, psychiatrists cast doubt on their collective clinical competence by routinely failing to agree about what was wrong with a given patient, or whether anything was wrong at all.[35] This embarrassing state of affairs was made far worse in 1973 when *Science* published a paper by the Stanford psychologist David Rosenhan, 'On Being Sane in Insane Places', that purported to show how readily psychiatrists were deceived when confronted with sham patients.[36]

Though American psychiatry had published two previous editions (1952, 1968) of a manual that purported to list a variety of types of mental disorder, most psychiatrists paid them little mind, and in any event they proved useless as practical guides to diagnosis.[37] But amidst the rising tide of complaints, the unreliability of the diagnostic process had become a major liability for the profession, a threat to its very legitimacy that was far greater than the long-standing culture of complaint among patients, whose grumblings were always vulnerable to the counter-allegation that they came from those of dubious mental competence.[38] Stung into action, mainstream psychiatry urgently sought to address the problem. The upshot, in 1980, was the publication of the third edition of the *Diagnostic and Statistical Manual of the American Psychiatric Association*, *DSM III* for short. Because of the linkages which quickly emerged between the new *DSM* categories and developments in psychopharmacology, with efforts made to link particular drugs to particular kinds of mental pathology, as defined in the manual, its influence soon extended far beyond the United States, and successive editions of the *DSM* became a global phenomenon.

What *DSM III* and its successors represent, however, is not an effort to cut nature at the joints, but a cynical effort to maximise inter-rater reliability among psychiatrists. Unable even at this late date to demonstrate convincing chains of causation for any major form of mental disorder, the task force that produced the manual abandoned any pretence at doing so. Instead, they concentrated on maximising inter-rater reliability, developing lists of symptoms that allegedly characterised different forms of mental disturbance, and matching those to a 'tick the boxes' approach to diagnosis. Faced with a new patient, psychiatrists would record the presence or absence of a given set of symptoms, and once a threshold number of these had been reached, the person they were examining was given a particular diagnostic label, with 'co-morbidity' invoked to explain away situations where more than one 'illness' could be diagnosed. Disputes about what belonged in the manual were resolved by committee votes, as was the arbitrary decision about where to situate cut-off points: i.e. how many of the laundry list of symptoms a patient had to exhibit before they were declared to be suffering from a particular form of illness. Questions of validity – whether the new classificatory system was really cutting nature at the joints, so that the listed 'diseases' corresponded in some sense with distinctions that made etiological sense – were simply set to one side. If diagnoses could be rendered mechanical and predictable, consistent and replicable, that would suffice.[39]

In the years that have followed, the successive editions of the *DSM* have grown like the Yellow Pages of the old-fashioned telephone directory on steroids. Definitions have been broadened, ever-newer forms of pathology have been 'discovered' (most neatly helping to create markets for new versions of psychoactive drugs), and more and more of the range of normal human experience has been drawn into psychiatry's net.[40] Bipolar disorder, once rare, has become epidemic, and psychiatrists have 'discovered' for the first time its presence in children. Depression is now widely called the common cold of psychiatry, so broad is its remit and so frequent the diagnosis. The decision in 2013 to treat grief as a mental illness will amplify that trend. There has been a massive expansion of children diagnosed with autism and with Attention Deficit Hyperactivity Disorder, not to mention things like school phobia.

One might expect this expansion of the psychiatric imperium to encounter some push-back – and so it has in some quarters. In Oregon as early as 1970, complaining patients formed the short-lived Mental Patients Liberation Front. In California, angry patients formed NAPA in 1974 (named after California's largest remaining traditional mental hospital – the initials stand for Network Against Psychiatric Assault). In 1988, patients who now called themselves consumer-survivors created Support Coalition International, later renamed MindFreedom International: each of these organisations is reflective of the disability and patients rights movement that Mold writes of in this collection. But there have also been some paradoxical developments. NAMI, the National Alliance on Mental Illness, was formed in 1979, primarily by the families of mental patients, and has acted largely to defend contemporary, somatically-orientated psychiatry, and to promulgate the notion that mental illness is purely biological, simply brain disease – a notion so congenial to Big Pharma that they have secretly underwritten NAMI's operations with large sums of money.[41] And efforts by some to tighten the wording of diagnoses such as autism – loosened with devastating effect in *DSM IV* in 1994 – have encountered huge push-back from parents who want the diagnosis and the state assistance it brings in managing their children.[42]

But perhaps the most striking thing about the debates that erupted over the latest, fifth edition of the American Psychiatric Association's diagnostic manual was their source. For the most vocal critics of the document that for more than three decades has taken its place at the very heart of contemporary psychiatric practice, and that must be used in the United States if the mental health provider expects to receive reimbursement from the medical insurance industry, have turned out to be psychiatrists themselves, and not just any psychiatrists, but the editors of the third and fourth editions of the manual, Robert Spitzer and Allen Frances.[43] Relentlessly, these two men attacked the science (or lack of science) that lay behind the proposed revisions, and raised warnings that the revisions would further extend psychiatry's tendency to pathologise normal human behaviours. For orthodox psychiatrists, it was a deeply embarrassing spectacle. It is one thing to be attacked by Tom Cruise and the Scientologists (a group easy to dismiss as a cult), quite another to come under withering assault from one's own. (The medical enterprise more broadly suffered similar internal critiques from people like McKeown, Dubos and Burnet in the 1960s, an episode alluded to in this book's introduction). Wounded, the leaders of American psychiatry struck back with *ad hominem* attacks, alleging that Spitzer and Frances were clinging to past glories, and going so far as to suggest that the latter, by far the more energetic of the two, was motivated by the potential loss of $10,000 a year in royalties he still collected from *DSM IV*.[44] (Left unmentioned was how dependent their professional association had become on the multi-millions in royalties a new edition promised to provide). The prolonged controversy forced a delay in the issuance of the new manual, but seems to have done little to alter its basic structure and contents.

It has sufficed, however, to undermine, perhaps fatally, the legitimacy of the new *DSM 5*, and possibly the psychiatric profession's standing more broadly. On 6 May 2013, just two weeks before *DSM 5* was due to hit the marketplace, came an announcement from Thomas Insel, the director of the National Institute of Mental Health. The manual, he proclaimed, suffered from a scientific 'lack of validity. . . . As long as the research community takes the D.S.M. to be a bible, we'll never make progress. People think everything has to match D.S.M. criteria, but you know what? Biology never read that book.' NIMH, he said, would be 'reorienting its research away from D.S.M. categories [because] mental patients deserve better.' In the spirit of piling on, one of his predecessors as director of the Institute, Steven Hyman, added his assessment of the whole enterprise. It was, he opined,

> totally wrong in a way [its authors] couldn't have imagined . . . what in fact they produced was an absolute scientific nightmare. Many people who get one diagnosis get five diagnoses, but they don't have five diseases – they have one underlying condition.[45]

Just what that condition might be remains startlingly unclear. A few months before his savage dismissal of *DSM 5*, Thomas Insel had gone even further, expressing incredulity that most of his psychiatric colleagues

> actually believe [that the diseases they diagnose using the *DSM*] are real. But there's no reality. These are just constructs. There is no reality to schizophrenia or depression . . . we might have to stop using terms like depression and schizophrenia, because they are getting in our way, confusing things.[46]

Some might argue that to hear the head of NIMH saying such things might itself be construed as being a trifle confusing, or even more than a little destabilising. Surely if someone in his position keeps uttering such unpalatable truths, he threatens the very legitimacy of the psychiatric enterprise. A century ago, it was the inmates in the asylum who were complaining about psychiatry. Now the psychiatric piñata is being whacked by the mad-doctors themselves. An extraordinary development to be sure. Whatever else these developments portend, one thing is certain: the old tradition of complaining about mental medicine shows no sign of withering away, though complaining about psychiatry in its latest incarnation has assumed some newly surprising forms.

Notes

1 See, for example, D. Healy, *Mania: A short History of Bipolar Disorder* (Baltimore, 2008); D. Healy, *Pharmageddon* (Berkeley, 2012); E. Shorter, *Before Prozac: The Troubled History of Mood Disorders in Psychiatry* (Oxford, 2008).

2 www.nimh.nih.gov/about/director/2013/transforming-diagnosis.shtml, accessed 8 May 2014.

3 R. Porter, *Mind Forg'd Manacles: A History of Madness in England from the Restoration to the Regency* (Harmondsworth, 1990; 1987), pp. 164–165.

4 See A. Scull, *The Most Solitary of Afflictions: Madness and Society in Britain, 1700–1900* (London, 1993).

5 *The Distress'd Orphan, or Love in a Mad-house* (London, 1726, 2nd edition), p. 35. The book appears anonymously, but was advertised as by, and clearly is by, the prolific Eliza Haywood, novelist, actress, and editor of *The Female Spectator*, 4 volumes (London, 1744–1746). One of her later novels was *The History of Miss Betsy Thoughtless*, 4 volumes (Dublin, 1751), a reworking of the story of Betty Careless, a dissolute brothel keeper, whose name Hogarth had depicted scratched on the banister rails of his Bedlam scene in *The Rake's Progress*. For a recent biography, see K. King, *A Political Biography of Eliza Haywood* (London, 2012). Other late-eighteenth-century novels with madhouse themes written by women include Mary Wollstonecraft's *Maria: or, the Wrongs of Women* (1798) and Charlotte Smith's *The Young Philosopher* (1798). My account here of the scandals and complaints that swirled around the trade in lunacy in the eighteenth century draws heavily upon my earlier researches published in *The Most Solitary of Afflictions: Madness and Society in Britain, 1700–1900*; and, more particularly, my book written with Jonathan Andrews, *Undertaker of the Mind: John Monro and Mad-Doctoring in Eighteenth Century England* (Berkeley, 2001).

6 Haywood, *The Distress'd Orphan*, pp. 39–40.
7 Ibid., p. 42.
8 Ibid., pp. 50, 52, 58, 59.
9 See J. Andrews, '"In her Vapours [or] Indeed in her Madness"? Mrs Clerke's Case: An Early Eighteenth-century Psychiatric Controversy', *History of Psychiatry*, 1 (1990), pp. 125–143.
10 See E. Foyster, 'Wrongful Confinement in Eighteenth-century England: A Question of Gender?', unpublished paper delivered at the conference 'Social and Medical Representations of the Links between Insanity and Sexuality', University of Wales, Bangor, July 1999. I am greatly indebted to Dr Foyster for permitting me to quote from this paper.
11 A. Cruden, *The London Citizen Exceedingly Injured, or a British Inquisition Display'd* (London, 1739); A. Cruden, *The Adventures of Alexander the Corrector, with an Account of the Chelsea Academies, or the Private Places for the Confinement of Such as are Supposed to Be Deprived of the Use of their Reason* ((London, 1754).
12 *A Full and True Account of the Whole Tryal, Examination, and Conviction of Dr. James Newton, who Keeps the Mad House at Islinstton [sic], for Violently Keeping and Misusing of William Rogers, . . . by his Wife's Orders* (London, 1715).
13 T. Smollett, *The Adventures of Launcelot Greaves* (London, 1762). Smollett borrowed heavily from John Monro's *Remarks on Dr. Battie's Treatise on Madness* (London, 1758) in constructing his images of treatment in a madhouse.
14 D. Defoe, *Augusta Triumphans* (London, 1728).
15 R. Baker, *A Rehearsal of a New Ballad-opera Burlesqu'd, Call'd The Mad-house. After the Manner of Pasquin. As it is now Acting at the Theatre-Royal in Lincoln's-Inn-Fields. By a Gentleman of the Inner-Temple* (London, 1737).
16 Cf. Allan Ingram (ed.), *Voices of Madness* (Stroud, Gloucestershire, 1997); *Proposals for Redressing Some Grievances Which Greatly Affect the Whole Nation* (London, 1740); 'A Case Humbly Offered to the Consideration of Parliament', *Gentleman's Magazine*, 33 (1763), pp. 25–26.
17 R. Porter, *Mind Forg'd Manacles*, pp. 151–152.
18 J. T. Perceval, *A Narrative of the Treatment Received by a Gentleman During a State of Mental Derangement*, 2 volumes (London, 1838 and 1840).
19 Cf. N. Hervey, 'Advocacy or Folly: The Alleged Lunatics' Friend Society', *Medical History*, 30 (1986), pp. 254–275.
20 See the discussions of this case (and the Ruck case which follows) in A. Scull, *Social Order/Mental Disorder* (Berkeley, 1989), pp. 201–204; and with much more circumstantial detail in S. Wise, *Inconvenient People: Lunacy, Liberty, and the Mad-Doctors in Victorian England* (London, 2012), pp. 94–129, 267–277. Also very useful for the Ruck case is Akihito Suzuki's splendid *Madness at Home: The Psychiatrist, the Patient, and the Family in England, 1820–1860* (Berkeley, 2006), pp. 144–146.
21 See V. Blain, 'Rosina Bulwer Lytton and the Rage of the Unheard', *Huntington Library Quarterly*, 53 (1990), pp. 210–236.
22 See R. Bulwer Lytton, *A Blighted Life: A True Story* (London, 1880), for her polemical account of her travails, and Wise, *Inconvenient People*, pp. 208–251, for a more balanced assessment of the case.
23 For contemporary commentary from the psychiatric perspective, see 'Report on the Ruck Case', *Journal of Mental Science*, 4 (1858), p. 131.
24 For a contemporary report on this inquisition in lunacy, as it was called, see *The Times* (17 December 1861).

25 In addition to Wise's work, see R. Porter, H. Nicholson, and B. Bennett (eds), *Women, Madness and Spirtualism* (London, 2003), for examples of Lowe's and Weldon's complaints.

26 On this phenomenon, see A. Winter, *Mesmerized: Powers of Mind in Victorian Britain* (Chicago, 1998); and A. Owen, *The Darkened Room: Women, Power, and Spiritualism in Late Victorian England* (Chicago, 2004).

27 The overlap between Georgina Weldon and Mrs Jellyby of Dickens' *Bleak House* is extraordinary, whether one looks to her marital relations, her treatment of her children, her obsession with 'philanthropy', or the squalor in which she lives. But there is a further historical connection which is distinctly odd: the leasehold of Tavistock House, Weldon's home during her campaigns, had been purchased and the house extensively renovated by Charles Dickens in 1851, and he had planned to live there for the rest of his life, before changing his mind and selling the place in 1860 in the aftermath of the breakup of his marriage. And the first novel Dickens wrote on moving in was *Bleak House*.

28 Wise, *Inconvenient People*.

29 See, for example, E. Packard, *Modern Persecution, or Insane Asylums Unveiled* (Hartford, CT, 1873); E. Packard, *Great Disclosures of Spiritual Wickedness!! In High Places, with an Appeal to the Government to Protect the Inalienable Rights of Married Women* (Boston, 1865).

30 J. Frame, *To the Is-Land* (New York, 1982); J. Frame, *An Angel at My Table* (New York, 1984); J. Frame, *The Envoy from Mirror City* (Auckland, 1989).

31 For further discussion, see K. Gabbard and G. Gabbard, *Psychiatry and the Cinema* (Chicago, 1987); and A. Scull, *Madness and Civilization* (London, forthcoming), Chapters 11 and 12.

32 I. Belknap, *Human Problems of a State Mental Hospital* (New York, 1956); H. W. Dunham and S. K. Weinberg, *The Culture of the State Mental Hospital* (Detroit, 1960); E. Goffman, *Asylums* (New York, 1961).

33 See, for example, A. T. Beck, 'The Reliability of Psychiatric Diagnoses: A Critique of Systematic Studies', *American Journal of Psychiatry*, 119 (1962), pp. 210–216; and A. T. Beck, C. H. Ward, M. Mendelson, J. Mock and J. K. Erbaugh, 'Reliability of Psychiatric Diagnoses: A Study of Consistency of Clinical Judgments and Ratings', *American Journal of Psychiatry*, 119 (1962), pp. 351–357.

34 J. E. Cooper, R. E. Kendell and B. J. Gurland, *Psychiatric Diagnosis in New York and London: A Comparative Study of Mental Hospital Admissions* (London, 1972).

35 Scornfully, lawyers dismissed psychiatric claims to expertise, pointing out that their diagnostic competence was essentially non-existent: B. Ennis and T. Litwack, 'Psychiatry and the Presumption of Expertise: Flipping Coins in the Courtroom', *California Law Review*, 62 (1974), pp. 693–752.

36 D. Rosenhan, 'On Being Sane in Insane Places', *Science*, 179, 19 (January 1974), pp. 250–258.

37 Cf. R. Spitzer and J. Fleiss, 'A Re-Analysis of the Reliability of Psychiatric Diagnosis', *British Journal of Psychiatry*, 125 (1974), pp. 341–347.

38 Linda Mulcahy has, of course, argued that many medical complainants are similarly labelled as 'sick', which challenges the validity of their complaints. See L. Mulcahy, *Disputing Doctors: The Socio-legal Dynamics of Complaints about Medical Care* (Maidenhead, 2003), p. 112.

39 H. Kutchins and S. A. Kirk, *Making Us Crazy: The Psychiatric Bible and the Creation of Mental Disorders* (New York, 1997).

40 A. V. Horwitz and J. C. Wakefield, *All We Have to Fear: Psychiatry's Transformation of Natural Anxiety into Mental Disorder* (Oxford, 2012); D. Healy, *Mania: A Short History of Bipolar Disorder* (Baltimore, 2008).

41 A. Johnson, 'Under Criticism, Drug Maker Lilly Discloses Funding', *Wall Street Journal* (1 May 2007), http://online.wsj.com/news/articles/SB117798677706987755, accessed 28 February 2014.

42 B. Carey, 'New Definition of Autism will Exclude Many, Study Suggests', *New York Times* (19 January 2012), www.nytimes.com/2012/01/20/health/research/new-autism-definition-would-exclude-many-study-suggests.html?pagewanted=all&_r=0, accessed 28 February 2014; B. Carey, 'Psychiatry Manual Drafters Back Down on Diagnoses', *New York Times* (8 May 2012), www.nytimes.com/2012/05/09/health/dsm-panel-backs-down-on-diagnoses.html, accessed 28 February 2014.

43 Cf. A. Frances, 'DSM-V Badly Off Track', *Psychiatric Times*, 26 (26 June 2009), www.psychiatrictimes.com/articles/dsm-v-badly-track, accessed 28 February 2014; R. Spitzer, 'APA and DSM-V: Empty Promises', *Psychiatric Times*, 26 (2 July 2009), www.psychiatrictimes.com/articles/apa-and-dsm-v-empty-promises, accessed 28 February 2014.

44 A. F. Schatzberg, J. H. Scully, D. J. Kupfer and D. A. Regler, 'Setting the Record Straight: A Response to Frances [*sic*] Commentary on DSM-V', *Psychiatric Times*, 26 (1 July 2009), www.psychiatrictimes.com/dsm-5–0/setting-record-straight-response-frances-commentary-dsm-v, accessed 28 February 2014.

45 Both quoted in P. Bellick and B. Carey, 'Psychiatry's Guide is Out of Touch with Science, Experts Say', *New York Times* (6 May 2013), www.nytimes.com/2013/05/07/health/psychiatrys-new-guide-falls-short-experts-say.html?pagewanted=all, accessed 28 February 2014.

46 Quoted in G. Greenberg, *The Book of Woe: The DSM and the Unmaking of Psychiatry* (New York, 2013).

2 Complaining about therapy culture

Hera Cook

In contrast to much of the rest of this volume, this chapter is about complaints from the privileged rather than from the sick and the vulnerable. From the late 1950s, socially conservative academics began to complain that there had come into existence a therapeutic culture stretching across Western society and creating a supposed obsession with the self. This is a form of medicalisation, but these complainants have no interest in radical critiques concerned with those labelled as mad, bad, poor or deviant. They are protesting the undermining of the order and authority on which their privilege is based. This chapter discusses two major figures in this influential conservative discourse, Philip Rieff and Christopher Lasch, and a recent British example, Frank Furedi, whose work shows the development of these complaints. Rieff and Lasch assume that therapy has been integrated into the wider culture and produced major negative changes in many aspects of everyday life from political engagement to intimate relations. Evidence about the prevalence, or experience, of actual therapy or counselling practices is not treated as relevant to the complaints; therapy is rather a form of societal governance about which statements can be made.

The French philosopher-historian Michel Foucault's ambivalent attitude to psychoanalysis and the powerful cultural pessimism that shaped his early work on madness and prisons has reinforced this narrative of cultural decline, though he did not share these authors' social conservatism.[1] The gendered nature of the complaints about therapy was unexpected at the outset of this research project.[2] Occasional brief criticisms about therapy from women have surfaced during this research, but women do not appear to have produced any sustained socially conservative complaints about therapy of the type described in this chapter. There were a striking number of prominent female psychoanalysts, and occupations into which counselling was integrated, such as social work, were among those with a high proportion of women, creating an alignment of counselling with female occupations.[3] Traditional femininity is also associated with emotional labour, and complaining about therapeutic culture may have been experienced by women as devaluing an ethic of care relevant to both traditional femininity and women in the workplace.

Psychoanalysis and counselling

Psychoanalysis is an approach created by Sigmund Freud in the late nineteenth and early twentieth century to healing those suffering from mental distress, and was founded upon his theory of human development and culture. Classic Freudian analysis involved hourly sessions five days a week during which the patient free-associated – that is, the client was instructed to discuss anything that crossed his or her mind – while the analyst listened and provided interpretations, usually infrequently, of what he heard. The majority of the counselling procedures and analytical therapies that have emerged since then share the basic feature of Freud's method; they are 'talking cures'.[4] Those who provide them include psychiatrists, lay and medical psychotherapists, psychoanalysts and clinical psychologists, social workers, probation officers, GPs and a wide range of counsellors.[5] Paul Halmos, who categorised all those who provided talking cures as counsellors, estimated in 1965 that there were under 6,000 in Britain, and, in 1960, only 400 were psychotherapists; this can be compared to nearly 280,000 medical personnel in the 1951 census.[6] These numbers already suggest that the reach of therapeutic culture in the UK was insufficient to achieve the changes claimed in the complaints of social conservatives.

Attempts to assess the cultural impact of Freud in the UK reinforce this. In early twentieth-century Britain, psychoanalysis met with strong resistance, especially from within medicine.[7] Those who promoted Freud to the public prior to the later 1930s were largely sex reformers and other radical thinkers who took an oppositional stance to mainstream culture.[8] Success with treating shell shock during the Great War led to the slow adoption of the method as a practical, therapeutic method of achieving emotional control.[9] The initial resistance to psychoanalysis was weaker in the USA and, by the 1930s, psychoanalysts were required to obtain a medical qualification, thus ensuring they became part of the medical establishment. Though adherents continued to cluster in the major cities, disciplines, such as child guidance, that embraced Freud were far better funded and more influential in the USA, and images of psychoanalysis became part of popular culture.

Philip Rieff: Freud and authority

The first major contribution to the discourse on the negative impact of therapy on Western culture emerged in the late 1950s. Philip Rieff (see Figure 2.1) was born in Chicago in 1922, the son of Jewish working-class refugees from the Ukraine. He served in the forces during the Second World War, then obtained a BA from the University of Chicago in 1946, an MA in 1947, and in 1954 his PhD, on the topic of Sigmund Freud's contribution to political philosophy. This became his first book, *Freud: The Mind of the Moralist* (1959). He was offered a lecturing post

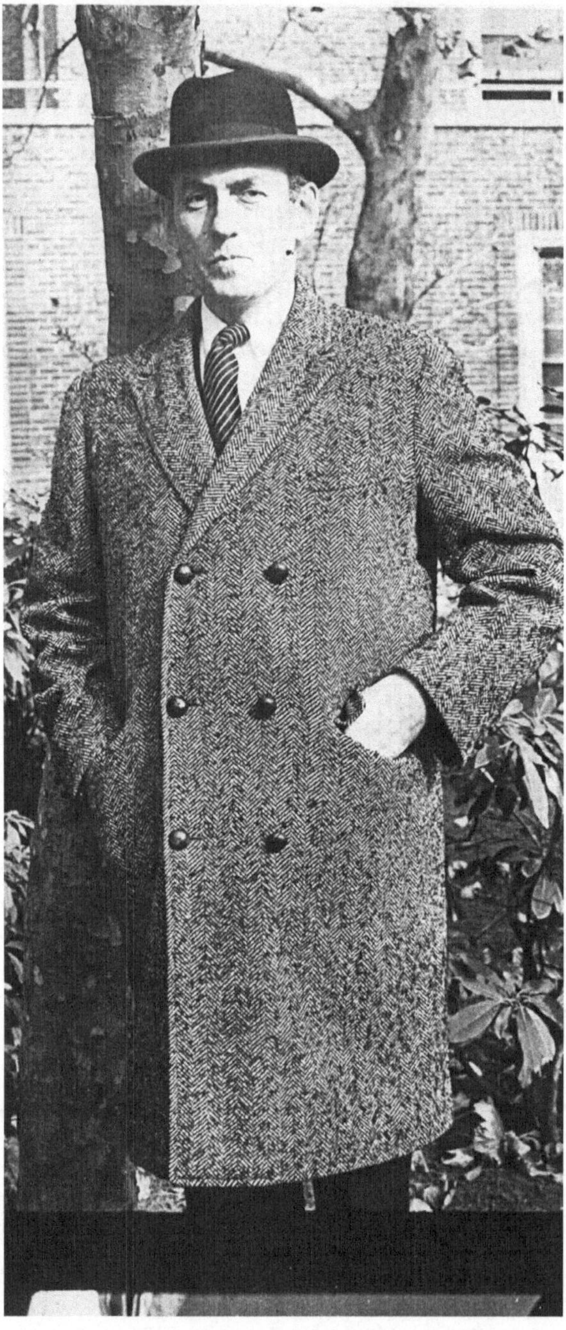

Figure 2.1 Philip Rieff; from *The 1968 Record* (undergraduate yearbook, University of Pennsylvania, Philadelphia), page 119 (courtesy of the University of Pennsylvania Archives).

at Chicago before completing his BA and taught in universities for the rest of his working life. By the mid-twentieth century in the USA, psychoanalysis was a widely influential professional therapy requiring formal qualifications in psychiatry.[10] Academic disciplines such as anthropology and sociology had developed psychoanalysis as a cultural theory and it was widely used as a critical method by literary scholars.[11] As a sociologist, Rieff's interest lay in psychoanalysis as a cultural theory.

Rieff told an interviewer in 1999 that his interest stemmed from his perception in the 1940s that 'Freudianism, in some form or another appeared to become the dominant form of ideation among American intellectuals . . . whether they knew it or not.'[12] According to Rieff, 'a new cultural ideology [had emerged] in which political, economic, or religious modes of explanation [were] . . . superseded by psychological ones'.[13] Freud's aim, he claimed, was to produce 'a personality type unknown to history thus far, the psychological man – man emancipated by rational analysis from commitments to the prototypical past'.[14] Rieff believed this Freudian 'psychological man' was the dominant moral personality of the twentieth century. In his second book, *The Triumph of the Therapeutic: Uses of Faith After Freud* (1966), Rieff defined what had taken place as a shift from a 'creedal', or religious culture, to an analytic attitude, in relation to which Freud was the formative figure. Out of this analytic attitude emerged a therapeutic culture that Rieff fiercely rejected. Notwithstanding this, as Paul Robinson suggests, for Rieff, Freud was 'the great moral intelligence of the century and the virtual creator of the modern conception of the self'.[15]

Rieff's Freud was, however, deeply pessimistic; Freud 'assures us of nothing except perhaps that, having learned from him, the burden of misery we must find strength to carry will be somewhat lighter'.[16] This pessimism was central to Freud's conception of development, Rieff argued, because the possibility and extent of positive change is limited by the presence within the unconscious of immutable, instinctive desires or libidinal energies, as well as mechanisms, primarily the Oedipus complex, created by culture, for deflecting libidinal energy toward fulfilling the demands of society. Freud, according to Rieff, believes the conflict between social and antisocial impulses is situated within the unconscious. Internal conflict and ambivalence is thus biological and unavoidable. This means that neurotic symptoms, that is to say illness, arise from the structure of instinct and that there can be no such thing as 'simple animal expressivity'.[17] Thus, Rieff rejected the concept that psychoanalytic theory promoted sexual revolution and greater expression of instinct; rather Freud believed that the social repression of the instincts was necessary and inevitable.[18] In Rieff's reading, Freud supported a conservative vision of humanity with limited potential for change.

Rieff's hostility to 'psychological man' arose not from the social theory implicit in psychoanalysis, but from the outcomes of Freud's therapeutic practice. He argued that Freud had an ambivalent attitude to authority. It was inevitable and necessary in the form of the unconscious controls that were a precondition for normal psychic and social life, but identification with authority figures was also the cause of neurosis. According to Rieff, in the process of analysis, psychological man learns that to cease being ill he has to become an autonomous individual. He must cease to identify unconsciously with traditional figures of authority. This takes place through the process of transference, which is the displacement onto a new object of unresolved conflicts and emotions, frequently those from the child's relations with their parents. The analyst used the transference to attach the patient to the therapy; 'love', Freud said, 'was the great educator'. The analyst then pointed out to the patient at every step that the emotions he felt (love, anger, frustration, envy and so on) arose from the transference of early childhood experiences, in order finally to free the patient from his unconscious acceptance of authority. It was this freeing of the patient from the transference to which Rieff objected. Once freed from the unconscious transference to the authority figures learned in early childhood, the individual's own independent rational powers of judgment became his or her highest authority. From a conservative perspective, undermining the acceptance of authority challenges the foundations of duty and belief that enable society to endure.

For Rieff's generation, psychoanalysis interpreted duty, self-sacrifice and other altruistic feelings and aspirations reductively as redirected libido. Religious belief was obsessional neurosis, parental love was re-interpreted as narcissism, while children's love and respect for their parents became deeply conflicted oedipal desires, and political passion was merely emotional identification.[19] In Freudian terms, to be rational was to question altruism, public commitments and religious belief and to reject feelings of guilt about personal failure to live up to higher societal ideals.[20] In Christianity repressing higher, moral feelings produced shame and guilt, but in analysis patients were taught that guilt resulted from the repression of lower instinctual desires. Thus, Rieff argued, indulgence and acceptance of the self was promoted at the expense of traditional cultural authority and purposes.

Rieff believed that the authority of the sacred gave people's lives direction and meaning, and that without this they are lost in panic and emptiness. He argued, sacred culture survives according to:

> The power of its institutions to bind and loose men in the conduct of their affairs with reasons which sink so deep into the self that they become commonly and implicitly understood – with that understanding of which explicit belief and precise knowledge of externals would show outwardly like the tip of an iceberg.[21]

This belief that the unspoken acceptance of institutions and authority is central to the health of a culture is fundamental to conservatism. The concept of tacit, or implicit, knowledge becomes conservative when the knowledge so constructed is treated as common-sense and natural and placed in opposition to claims concerning the value of conscious knowledge and autonomy.[22] It is this belief about the nature of culture that enabled Rieff to claim that the despoiling of authority could reach from American intellectuals who were influenced by Freud 'whether they knew it or not', through to the 'ignorants of a culture' binding them all into the 'great chain of meaning' within which every person had their place.[23] It was this embeddedness in sacred culture that, Rieff complained, 'psychological man' had lost.

Rieff's emphasis on limits and moderation was central to the conservative tradition that stretched back to the eighteenth-century Irish statesman and political theorist Edmund Burke. He greatly admired the imagined high culture of 'Old England' and styled himself as a man of prudence and tradition, dressing in dapper suits and taking on an 'Oxfordish' accent.[24] This affiliation may have replaced religious belief for Rieff, as, despite his claim that Christianity was crucial to the maintenance of Western civilisation, he was unable to give the Church his personal support; 'I have not the slightest affection for the dead church civilization of the West. I am a Jew. No Jew in his right mind can long for some variant of that civilization.'[25] Corey Robin, a historian of conservative thought, shows in an analysis of conservatism that even Rieff's ambivalence about past creedal cultures and his absorption of fundamental aspects of Freudian thought are central to the 'reactionary imperative'. This imperative, says Robin, pushes 'first to a critique and reconfiguration of the old regime; and second to an absorption of the ideas and tactics of the very revolution or reform it opposes'.[26] Rieff could venerate Freud in part because, though Freudian thought had been a radical innovation only half a century earlier, by the 1950s classic psychoanalytic theory had become an integral component of socially conservative understandings of the personality and a new extreme had emerged in a variety of therapuetic forms, including neo-Freudian analysis.

Neo-Freudian and radical Freudian optimism

Neo-Freudian thought emerged primarily among the more than two hundred European analysts who immigrated to the USA in the 1930s and 40s. Together Karen Horney, Erich Fromm and an American, Harry Stack Sullivan, created the new school of thought known as neo-Freudian. Rieff put Horney and Fromm, together with Alfred Adler and John Dewey among others, in the single category of 'liberal revisors of Freud'.[27] Rieff's inclusion of John Dewey, an influential American philosopher, psychologist and educational reformer, increased the range of societal changes he critiqued.

Dewey believed that the purpose of education was not the acquisition of a set of skills and passing of exams, but the realisation of the child's full potential and their ability to contribute to the greater good. He had a major influence on the development of progressive education, which reshaped education in the mid-twentieth century and has been a particular target of conservatives. Dewey believed that conflict can be used to create psychic growth and that by adaptation we can fulfil our needs and desires. Rieff argued that Freud's concept of sublimation served the same role as Dewey's adaptation but, while both concepts involved a given instinct changing in response to repressive social process, sublimation involved a cost to the individual whereas Dewey's adaptation did not. Freud emphasised that humans had a limited capacity for enduring sublimation as the instincts will not easily tolerate substitutes for the real gratifications of life. Dewey, however, located the conflict between society and the person instead of within the unconscious. This was the foundation for his rejection of Freud's pessimism and his optimistic view of human beings' potential for change.[28]

The neo-Freudian analysts Horney, Fromm and Stack Sullivan also rejected Freud's emphasis on biological instincts and the argument that there are dichotomous social and antisocial impulses or instincts situated within the unconscious.[29] They conceived of the individual's desires as a striving for growth and the forces inhibiting realisation of them as the cultural precepts that protect the interests of society. Thus, as with Dewey, for them the conflict was between the person and society. Rather than an internal, immutable struggle within the human psyche, the neo-Freudians believed that the central focus of psychoanalytic theory should be the individual's search for identity, for loving relations with others, and for fulfilling, secure engagement in work and the broader society. This led them to break away from both classical Freudian theory and the increasingly medically oriented American psychoanalytic establishment.

Historian Neil McLaughlin points out that, by the 1990s, the neo-Freudians' conception of the psyche dominated Freudian thought.[30] Even more importantly, their ideas, and those of other breakaway psychoanalysts such as Otto Rank and Alfred Adler, influenced the development of humanistic psychology and counselling, which reached a far larger number of people than classic psychoanalysis. Carl R. Rogers introduced what he described as a client-centered or non-directive approach to counselling in the early 1940s. This was enormously influential across the range of counselling professions, from probation officers to marriage guidance counsellors. Rogers believed that the individual had 'the capacity . . . to reorganize himself and his relationship to life in . . . such a way as to bring a greater degree of internal comfort'.[31] This optimism was the opposite of the pessimism that Rieff so admired in Freud, and Rieff warned his readers not to accept this optimistic view of the possibilities of human growth.[32]

A key aspect of both neo-Freudian psychotherapy and Roger's non-directive counselling was an emphasis on the expression of feelings. Horney argued that 'in therapy only that counts which is felt and experienced'.[33] This emphasis had not been present in orthodox Freudian theory.[34] In a transcript of non-directive counselling sessions published in 1943, William Snyder, a former student of Rogers, explained that 'one of the principal aims of the non-directive counselor is to recognize the feeling (rather than the intellectual content) expressed by the client'.[35] Jessie Taft, an American social worker who was the most important single influence on Rogers, translated the work of Otto Rank, an Austrian psychoanalyst who had been one of Freud's earliest colleagues and came to the USA after being expelled by Freud from his inner circle.[36] Rank commented in 1930 that 'the emotional life develops from the sexual sphere, therefore [Freud's] sexualization in reality means emotionalization'.[37] Emotion was defined by Freud primarily as energy released in abreaction, that is to say the discharge of emotion following the recall and reliving of painful memories or as libido. It was the unconscious ideas and instincts that Freud believed were important; the emotions attached to them were a byproduct of the processes of the mind.[38] Thus, this new emphasis on emotional expression reflected an important shift away from classic Freudian psychoanalysis.

Other influential social theorists opposed the neo-Freudian conception of Freud from the left. Herbert Marcuse and Norman O. Brown were an important influence on the counterculture by the 1960s. Like Rieff, they rejected the neo-Freudian conception of the instincts. Marcuse argued that the revisionists erased the threatening and unnerving elements in the psyche, such as life and death instincts, aggression and repression.[39] They insisted that the essential libidinous conflicts are within the person, not between them and the social order, but they also rejected the classic psychoanalysis championed by Rieff. Brown believed that society could be altered through the liberation of Eros (sexuality) from oppressive cultural structures and that this would result in the freeing of individuals from ascetic moral imperatives. Orthodox psychoanalysis had, Brown argued, recreated the soul–body dualism in the form of the ego 'defence mechanisms' that fought against the possibilities for pleasure offered by the body or id (instincts). This closed off the potential for more open and less repressed personal relations.[40] Rieff loathed the counterculture and in his second book, *The Triumph of the Therapeutic*, he argued against these 'utopian fantasies' of cultural liberation, suggesting that a hollow 'gospel of self-fulfilment' was being produced as a result of urbanisation and modernity.[41]

By the mid-1960s, the neo-Freudian ideas about the importance of the expression of feelings and the individual's potential for change had combined with the ideas of utopian Freudian social theorists to form the foundation for a wide range of new optimistic and fast therapies. Many of these therapies took place in groups and involved touching, crying, moving – they broke away from the model of therapy with doctor and patient alone in a private room.[42] These therapies aroused critics to heights of anxiety, contempt and complaint similar to responses to psychoanalysis in the early decades of the century. A young journalist, Richard D. Rosen, complained about what he labelled 'the cult of candour' in a 1975 book, entitled *Psychobabble*: 'Everything must now be spoken. . . . It is as if the full bladder of civilization's squeamishness had burst. The sexual revolution, this therapeutic age, has culminated in one profuse steady stream of self-revelation.'[43] This metaphor reveals the strength of belief in a negative inner life that was disgusting and should be concealed. Rosen suggested that Rieff's 'Psychological Man' had 'regressed in the 1970s to an adolescent . . . the victim of interminable introspection'.[44] The complaint that a person who thought and talked about their feelings to others was adolescent reveals how psychotherapy conflicted with expectations of emotional control and restraint, especially from adult men.

Rosen linked the new therapies with sexuality:

> It is not uncommon these days to hear people speak about their homosexuality as a 'preferred' form of sexual life or defend their three divorces on the grounds that 'marriage simply doesn't work for me anymore' . . . as if understanding one's childhood experiences is irrelevant, just a quaint Freudian ploy to undermine one's will, one's ability to do and be exactly what one wants.[45]

In this comment, Rosen implies that new sexual mores are self-indulgent and an avoidance of the demands of reality according to which we cannot do or be what we want. He produces a popularised version of Reiff's Freud, who insists on the inevitability of repression and acceptance of the limitations that society placed upon us. Rosen's complaints were limited to examination of actual therapy, but such contempt for these new therapies and the young radicals who were experimenting with them provided the conservative social context in which the cultural historian Christopher Lasch developed his complaints about narcissism and society.

Christopher Lasch and the invention of the narcissistic culture

In *The Culture of Narcissism* (1979), Lasch complained that 'the contemporary climate is therapeutic': America had become a society of narcissists who lived in the present, expected instant gratification, lacked moral and ethical capacity, and were inner-directed and sexually permissive.[46] Freud had originally conceived of narcissism as a dynamic in the formation of healthy subjectivity, but Lasch turned to pathological forms for his definition of the modern self. The book was on the *New York Times* best-seller list for seven weeks and President Jimmy Carter referred to Lasch's conception of USA society in a major speech on 15 July 1979.[47] The concept has also continued to attract popular and academic attention in succeeding decades.[48]

Lasch was born in Nebraska in 1932 to progressive, secular parents. His mother was a social worker and feminist and his father a prominent newspaper editor. After obtaining his first degree from Harvard, he went to Columbia to undertake graduate research and became a historian of nineteenth- and twentieth-century American culture. Lasch was a Marxist, but his approach to subjectivity and personal life sets him firmly down among social conservatives.[49] Rieff's discussion of Freud and the concept of 'psychological man' influenced Lasch, who understood the human psyche in Freudian terms. The ideas of Michel Foucault also fascinated Lasch, and this influence is evident in his focus on government and official intrusion into the family, although he did not adopt a Foucauldian methodology. His analysis continued to be located at the level of the individual in the context of society, rather than at that of discourses.[50]

In the first chapter of *The Culture of Narcissism*, Lasch attacks the 'Awareness Movement' and the young radicals, generalising from, for example, the experience of social activist and American anti-war leader Jerry Rubin, a remarkable and atypical individual. Such carelessness with evidence is apparent throughout the book. Sociologist Richard Kilminster has pointed out that there was a substantial problem with the evidence Lasch used to support his complaints about the rise of narcissism in contemporary culture.[51] Lasch introduced clinical psychoanalytic studies of extreme narcissistic disorders, suggesting these 'depict a type of personality that ought to be immediately recognizable, in a more subdued form, to observers of the contemporary cultural scene'.[52] The clinicians who produced these studies had explicitly stated that the apparent rise in number of these cases resulted from the increased research interest and not from developments in the psychological make-up of the American population.[53] Kilminster commented that Lasch 'has to cover himself against the obvious accusation that it is not legitimate to generalize from clinical, psychoanalytic studies of pathological personalities to an empirical psychological trend which is spreading across the population at large'.[54] Lasch does so by equivocating at key points, asserting, for example, that the narcissistic 'type of personality "ought" to be immediately recognizable to observers of contemporary society', thus evading the important issue of the prevalence of the personality type that his book is complaining about.[55] Given that Lasch's argument was, and continues to be, influential, the extent to which this type actually existed should be an important question; however, the growth of narcissism rapidly came to be seen as a common-sense notion, concerning which evidence was irrelevant.

A nostalgic vision of the past and the claim that the current generation had been transformed informed Lasch's social theory even more powerfully than was the case with Rieff. Lasch claimed that:

> to live for the moment is the prevailing passion – to live for yourself, not for your predecessors or for posterity. We are fast losing any sense of historical continuity, the sense of belonging to a succession of generations originating in the past and stretching into the future.[56]

He explained that he saw

> the past as a political and psychological treasury from which we draw the reserves . . . that we need to cope with the future. Our culture's indifference to the past – which easily shades over into active hostility and rejection – furnishes the most telling proof of that culture's bankruptcy.[57]

Lasch's earlier historical research created a vision of a past in which the domination of the ruling class over subordinate groups, including that of men over women and children, was acceptable because the rulers were shaped by chivalry and civility and a principled commitment to public honour. Thus for Lasch respecting the past meant accepting the existing relations of authority. He argued, however, that from the later nineteenth century advanced capitalism had undermined patriarchal authority, as government in the form of professional experts invaded the family claiming to be improving family relationships and childrearing. The 'possibility of genuine privacy' was receding and, as a result, the 'common life' was being undermined.[58] The sector of contemporary society that Lasch valued was the lower-middle class whom he saw as still maintaining an appropriate and necessary insistence on the necessity for limits and resistance to change in family forms or sexual mores.[59] Lasch contrasted them with the narcissistic personality that he claimed was now emerging.

By the end of the 1970s, the emergence of Women's Liberation had produced a major shift in the cultural context. Rieff did not use the word feminism in his first two books (except in relation to Wilhelm Reich). During the 1950s, when Rieff was completing his doctoral thesis and turning it into his first book, he was married to Susan Sontag, the cultural critic. Scholar Daniel Horowitz, who has compared Rieff's thesis with the book that emerged from it, believes that Sontag had some influence on Rieff's thesis and played a major part in writing the book on Freud. Their archives have led him to believe that it was as part of their divorce settlement that the book appeared as authored by Rieff alone.[60] Certainly, there is an unexpected insistence on Freud's 'misogyny' and domination in the book. Kenneth Piver points out that in *Fellow Teachers* (1975), Rieff's tone has changed to one of misogynist dismissal of women's intellectual pretentions.[61] It seems possible that in the 1950s, Freud's attitude to women did not seem very important to Rieff, whereas, by the 1970s, following his divorce and the resurgence of feminism, the threat that women posed to the stable and hierarchical social order Rieff prized had become all too obvious.[62]

In contrast to the early Rieff, Lasch pays considerable attention to female protest as he saw it. Bernice Fisher, a feminist scholar, who published a review in 1979, thought that the book 'concerns the rise of a new class of women and their participation in the assault on the American family'.[63] Lasch argues, she writes, that:

> 'Woman' seeks expression in the public world because she is 'disappointed' with her family life. 'Family life' . . . seems to mean her relationship with her husband . . . Lasch suggests a close link between contemporary women's struggles and the inability of modern husbands to fulfil their wives 'demands' for 'sexual satisfaction and tenderness'.[64]

The implied complaint that women's political demands have made their husbands impotent and that wives' demands are unreasonable was a commonplace response to feminism in this decade. Similarly, the concept of narcissism is the only novelty in Lasch's claim that 'the black power movement grew out of a need, on the part of black men, to assert their masculinity against the suffocating feminine narcissistic culture of the ghetto'.[65] In a study of the impact of Lasch's narcissism, Imogen Tyler has argued that:

> The attribution of narcissism to stereotyped figures – sexually liberated women, feminists, career women, African-Americans, queers, etc. – enabled white heterosexual masculine subjects and patriarchal forms of sociality to be defined in contrast as legitimate, authoritative, ethical and loving. At the same time, the increasing cultural and political visibility of minorities is interpreted as 'evidence' of their narcissistic claims for 'special attention'.[66]

Such complaints about narcissism have purchase because, from a socially conservative perspective, women, African-Americans, the young and other subordinate groups have no legitimate claim to attention. Therefore, any claim they make can be denigrated as narcissism, whether it be in the political form of demands for equality and an end to discrimination, or merely by virtue of the increasing visibility that is the result of greater equality. Tyler's focus was on the emergence and development of the Freudian concept of narcissism as a basis on which to undermine the legitimacy of the demands being made by groups, such as women and people of colour, whom she identifies as those who have gained from identity politics. Her analysis of the use of narcissism as a political tool contributes understanding of what is taking place in the critiques of therapy. Psychotherapy in all its variations, from classical psychoanalysis to the most radical and challenging groups, is frequently described, and dismissed, in terms that reveal engaging in therapy to be an exemplary instance of narcissism.

Frank Furedi: therapy and common sense

There are fewer substantial British complaints about therapy, probably due to the lesser acceptability of therapy or discussion of emotions in British culture. Sociologist Frank Furedi's criticisms reveal however, that the conception of the therapeutic society has been welded into an enduring socially conservative discourse, presented as self-evidently correct and readily available for the elaboration of further complaints. Born in Hungary in 1947, Furedi emigrated to Canada with his family in 1956 after the Prague Spring. After completing his MA and PhD at the School of African and Asian Studies in London, Furedi settled in Britain. He was involved in founding the British Revolutionary Communist Party in the 1970s, and is now an extreme libertarian.[67] Both Rieff and Lasch also had allegiances to left-wing politics in their youth. The apparent conflict between these seemingly radical political convictions and their later support for traditional relations of power in intimate and public life has aroused confusion among commentators, as does Furedi's political trajectory. This suggests that the crucial issue of how those who hold power and authority operationalise their power has not been fully attended to in our politics and our society. Rieff himself argued that the revolutionary ideology of our time was not communism but psychoanalysis.[68] Communism rejected sacral or religious structure, but accepted a social order that embodied enduring hierarchically-structured authority at all levels of society. Furedi's libertarianism is not the reverse of his communism, but another means of complaining about challenges to the social order he wishes to protect.

Unlike Rieff and Lasch, Furedi does not attempt to address subjectivity and he is not a Freudian thinker. His grievances are less original than were those of Reiff and Lasch. Furedi describes therapy as 'constructing a form of personhood whose defining feature is its vulnerability. Terms like depression, addiction and trauma are routinely designated to describe people's encounters with the problems of everyday life.'[69] Furedi has no interest as to whether people are actually suffering distress and to what extent therapy might or might not address their difficulties. He repeatedly implies that emotional problems are manufactured through discourse and explicitly complains that in the past, prior to the creation of the therapeutic discourses, people managed such problems more effectively:

> The provision of counselling advice – no matter how sound and commonsensical – further diminishes the capacity of people to negotiate the problems they encounter. The problem is not that professional people are always misguided, but that it short-circuits the process through which people can learn how to deal with problems through their own experience. Intuition and insight gained from personal experience is continually compromised by professional knowledge.[70]

Here Furedi is attacking the whole concept of expertise, or knowledge, as it can be taught, or offered by trained persons, to others in intimate and domestic life. The claim that counselling diminishes the capacity of people to manage their own distress is vaguely credible, perhaps because it is evocative of concepts such as medicalisation, or Foucault's biopower. But Furedi compares this supposed compromise with a past in which 'notions of stoicism, understatement, the stiff upper lip and of fortitude . . . helped frame the interpretation of everyday life', and so he claims, made counselling unnecessary.[71] Similarly to Lasch, Furedi is offering 'an ideological description of what he intensely dislikes about society written in such a way as to try to convince readers to see it as he does'.[72]

Furedi shares Rieff and Lasch's commitment to privacy as central to the maintenance of social order:

> victimologists have been in the forefront of a clamour to allow more public scrutiny of private life. . . . Many feminists argue that in the private sphere women are rendered invisible, their work becomes unrecognised and therefore devalued and their lives become subject to male violence.[73]

By collapsing feminists and 'victimologists' into the same category, and conflating the threat of violence and the lack of recognition for women's work in the home, Furedi trivialises these concerns. Privacy, on the other hand, is presented as a threatened moral value: 'contemporary culture still retains a resilient strain of respect for privacy and family life'.[74]

Feminist history and ideas are misrepresented by Furedi: 'This development which is symbolised by the motto "the personal is political", has as its premise the conviction that the solutions to both individual and social problems have an important therapeutic dimension.'[75] The argument made by the Women's Liberation movement that 'the personal is political' was, rather, a claim that the events and practices that took place in intimate relationships and in the home involved power and authority and could be understood in terms of those dynamics. Hence, feminists rejected the maintenance of the privacy of the home that these conservative critics treasured. Ironically, consciousness-raising groups, which involved shared participation in the examination by women of their lives, explicitly rejected therapy as being a diversion from political action.[76]

Foucault and therapeutic discourses

Within academia, Michel Foucault's discursive methodology and conceptual framework has had an enormous influence. Nikolas Rose, whose concept of 'psy' culture has been a major influence on research into the history of psychology, began reading Foucault in translation in 1965.[77] Foucault had a complex and ambivalent, but essentially hostile, relationship to psychoanalysis and counselling.[78] In a 1982 interview, Foucault acknowledged that his conception of cultural epistemes involved constraints that were analogous to the repressions Rieff insisted were vital to society, but added that the crucial issue was 'whether the system of constraints in which a society functions leaves individuals the liberty to transform the system'.[79] The capacity to reject traditional authority and transform the system that the practice of therapy enabled was what Rieff had objected to in psychological man. As historians Lynn Hunt and Victoria Bonnell argued in 1999, however, within Foucault's methodology 'the self has been reduced to a constructed, and therefore empty and wholly plastic, nodal point in a discursive or cultural system . . . [This has] left little in the self to resist social or cultural determinations.'[80] Foucault's influence has contributed to the perception that belief in positive change is naïve, including change that might be produced through therapy or counselling, and has, arguably, reinforced within academia the cultural pessimism that is central to social conservatism.[81] From the 2000s, there have also been female-authored postmodern accounts in which this cultural pessimism is the starting point for analysis of therapeautic and emotional cultures.[82]

Critiquing therapy

There are important issues that need to be raised concerning therapy. Some scholars researching state provision of support, including personal counselling or therapy, have been extremely careful to delineate the benefits of such therapy for individuals, as well as the means by which therapy can become an element in the exercise of coercive state power. Karen Armstrong and Kristin Bullimer, who have undertaken research into sexual abuse and domestic violence respectively, identify with the women who are the recipients of therapy and their analysis is grounded in the circumstances in which actual abuse takes place or self-sacrifice and respect for duty is demanded of these women.[83] These scholars accept that there is often a necessity for 'intrusion' of officials into the family/intimate life/the home, but they are also aware of the vulnerability of the women and children to whom 'support' may be offered only on the basis of the redefinition of their problems by those officials. Legitimate, clearly specified criticisms of therapy emerge in these and similar contexts. There is a striking difference between this research and the generalisations about narcissism and the therapeutic society, and the often purely rhetorical links between different types of evidence, that Reiff, Lasch, Furedi – and even Foucault – use to construct their picture of society and the influence of therapy.

Conclusion

The complaints about medicalisation discussed in this chapter were directed toward society and not towards the medical establishment. The complainants were privileged, highly educated and successful men in secure academic positions who resented the decline in authority and status of those sectors of society with which they identified. They contrasted a nostalgic vision of relations between people in the past with their own times and attributed the changes they saw taking place to the medicalisation of the self and relations with others, which they claimed was produced by therapy. These earlier negative critiques and the values that inform them make up an unexamined sedimentary layer shaping analysis of changing emotional cultures in contemporary society. Lasch treated therapy as a self-indulgent search for a purely individual fulfilment and Furedi repeated the well-worn claim that people were better off with stoicism, the stiff upper lip and fortitude. Society has not responded to these largely masculine complaints; cheap, accessible counselling is increasingly widely available and sought out by people when they are distressed. The therapists and counsellors are part of a long tradition; previously advice had been sought from priests, lawyers and healers of all types. The major difference between therapists and these earlier figures, according to Rieff's conservative complaint, is that the practice of psychoanalysis encouraged autonomy and independence from traditional authority, while non-directive counselling, the most influential form of counselling, encouraged people to listen to themselves. How would we research therapy if we took Rieff's assessment seriously and accepted that the practice had the potential to contribute to social movements which undermined hierarchy and authority and contributed to the erosion of tacit norms of subordination and service?[84]

Notes

1 M. Foucault, *Madness and Civilisation: A History of Insanity in the Age of Reason* (London, 1965); M. Foucault, *Discipline and Punish: The Birth of the Prison* (Harmondsworth, 1979).

2 Examples include: J. Steadman Rice, *A Disease of One's Own: Psychotherapy, Addiction, and the Emergence of Co-Dependency* (New Jersey, 1996); A. Offer, *The Challenge of Affluence: Self-control and Well-being in the United States and Britain since 1950* (Oxford, 2006); Female historian E. Herman worked hard to reconcile this negative discourse with a positive appraisal of therapy in *The Romance of American Psychology: Political Culture in the Age of Experts* (Berkeley and Los Angeles, 1995). It is not until the 2000s, that a female authored account in this vein emerges: E. S. Moskowitz, *In Therapy We Trust: America's Obsessions with Self-Fulfillment* (Baltimore, MD, 2001).

3 E.g. Helena Deutsch, Anna Freud, Karen Horney, Melanie Klein, Sylvia Payne.

4 P. Halmos, *The Faith of the Counsellors* (London, 1965), p. 3. Note that Halmos was an internal critic who sought to improve counselling.

5 Note that this is a more limited category than Rose's definition of 'psy' experts. N. Rose, *The Psychological Complex: Psychology, Politics and Society in England, 1869–1939* (London, 1985).

6 Halmos, *Faith*, pp. 34–35.

7 M. Neve and T. Turner, 'What the Doctor Thought and Did: Sir James Crichton-Browne (1840–1938)', *Medical History*, 39 (1995), pp. 399–432; T. Turner, 'James Crichton-Browne and the Anti-Psychoanalysts', in H. Freeman and G. E. Berrios (eds), *150 Years of British Psychiatry*, volume II: *The Aftermath* (London, 1996), pp. 144–155.

8 E.g. B. Caine, 'The Stracheys and Psychoanalysis', *History Workshop Journal*, 45 (1998), pp. 144–169. See G. C. Bunn, A. D. Lovie and G. D. Richards (eds), *Historical Essays and Personal Reflections* (Leicester, 2001).

9 H. Cook, 'From Controlling Emotion to Expressing Feelings in Mid-twentieth-century England', *Journal of Social History*, 47 (2014), pp. 627–646.

10 N. Hale, 'From Berggasse XIX to Central Park West: The Americanization of Psychoanalysis, 1919–1940', *Journal of the History of Behavioral Sciences*, 14 (1978), pp. 299–315, pp. 303–304; N. Hale, *The Rise and Crisis of Psychoanalysis in the United States: Freud and the Americans, 1917–1985* (New York, 1995); E. Zaretsky, *Secrets of the Soul: A Social and Cultural History of Psychoanalysis* (New York, 2004).

11 M. Genter, *Late Modernism: Art, Culture, and Politics in Cold War America* (Philadelphia, 2010), p. 90.

12 Interview (1999) with the author in A. W. Zondervan, *Sociology and the Sacred: An Introduction to Philip Rieff's Theory of Culture* (Toronto, 2005), p. 14 and note 1, p. 168.

13 Zondervan, *Sociology*, p. 14.

14 P. Rieff, 'The Authority of the Past: Sickness and Society in Freud's Thought', *Social Research*, 21, 4 (1954), pp. 428–450, p. 450.

15 P. Robinson, *Freud and His Critics* (Berkeley, 1993), p. 3.

16 P. Rieff, *Freud: The Mind of the Moralist* (Chicago, 1959/1979), p. xi. See also Rieff, 'Authority', p. 445.

17 Rieff, *Freud*, pp. 31, 56–57. For an extended critique of Freud's biology, see F. J. Sulloway, *Freud, Biologist of the Mind: Beyond the Psychoanalytic Legend* (New York, 1979).

18 J. Z. Muller, 'Philip Rieff', in D. Murray (ed.), *American Cultural Critics* (Exeter, 1995), pp. 193–205, p. 197. See also Rieff's attack on Wilhelm Reich's beliefs in Reiff, *The Triumph of the Therapeutic: Uses of Faith After Freud* (Chicago, 1966/1973).

19 Muller, 'Philip Rieff', p. 198. Halmos, *Faith*, p. 5, p. 65.

20 Rieff, *Freud*, p. 277.

21 Rieff, *Triumph*, pp. 2–3.

22 C. Robin, *The Reactionary Mind: Conservatism from Edmund Burke to Sarah Palin* (New York, 2011), p. 4, pp. 21–22.

23 Rieff, *Triumph*, p. 3; Zondervan, *Sociology*, p. 14; For the great chain of meaning, see D. Rollison, *A Commonwealth of the People: Popular Politics and England's Long Social Revolution, 1066–1649* (Cambridge, 2010), pp. 181–183.

24 Zondervan, *Sociology*, p. 145.

25 P. Rieff, *Fellow Teachers* (Chicago, 1985), p. 94.

26 Robin, *Reactionary Mind*, pp. 42–43. E.g. Rieff, *Triumph*, p. 36.

27 Rieff, *Freud*, p. 33.

28 Ibid., pp. 32–33.

29 N. McLaughlin, 'Why do Schools of Thought Fail? Neo-Freudianism as a Case Study in the Sociology of Knowledge', *Journal of the History of Behavioral Sciences*, 34 (1998), p. 116.

30 Ibid.

31 C. R. Rogers, 'Introduction', in C. R. Rogers and R. F. Dymond (eds), *Psychotherapy and Personality Change: Co-ordinated Research Studies in the Client-Centered Approach* (Chicago, 1954), p. 4.

32 Rieff, *Freud*, p. 56.

33 K. Horney, 'The Paucity of Inner Experiences', *American Journal of Psychoanalysis*, 12, 1 (1952), pp. 3–9, p. 6.

34 F. Weinstein, *Freud, Psychoanalysis, Social Theory: The Unfulfilled Promise* (Albany, NY, 2001), pp. 34–40.

35 W. U. Snyder, 'A Short-term Nondirective Treatment of an Adult', *The Journal of Abnormal and Social Psychology*, 38 (1943), pp. 87–137, note 5, p. 90.

36 D. Murphy, M. Duggan and S. Joseph, 'Relationship-based Social Work and its Compatibility with the Person-centred Approach: Principled versus Instrumental Perspectives', *British Journal of Social Work*, 43 (2012), pp. 703–719, pp. 706–707.
37 O. Rank, *Will Therapy* (New York, 1936/1978, translated by J. Taft), p. 165.
38 R. C. Solomon, *What is an Emotion? Classic and Contemporary Readings* (Oxford, 2003), pp. 184–186.
39 H. Marcus, *Eros and Civilisation: A Philosophical Inquiry into Freud* (London, 1955/1987).
40 See Genter, *Late Modernism*, pp. 92–93; N. O. Brown, *Life Against Death: The Psychoanalytical Meaning of History* (London, 1959).
41 Rieff, *Triumph*, cited in Zondervan, *Sociology*, p. 3.
42 H. M. Ruitenbeek, *The New Group Therapies* (New York, 1970); J. Howard, *Please Touch* (New York, 1970).
43 R. D. Rosen, *Psychobabble: Fast Talk and Quick Cure in the Era of Feeling* (London, 1975), p. 4.
44 Ibid., p. 5.
45 Ibid., pp. 14–15.
46 C. Lasch, *The Culture of Narcissism: American Life in an Age of Diminishing Expectations* (New York, 1978), p. 7.
47 I. Tyler, 'From "The Me Decade" to "The Me Millennium": The Cultural History of Narcissism', *International Journal for Cultural Studies*, 10 (2007), pp. 343–363, p. 356.
48 Tyler, 'From "The Me Decade"', p. 356.
49 Muller, *Philip Rieff*, p. 193.
50 Lasch reviewed several of Foucault's works during the 1970s, e.g. *New York Times* (24 February 1974).
51 R. Kilminster, 'Narcissism or Informalization? Christopher Lasch, Norbert Elias and Social Diagnosis', *Theory Culture & Society*, 25 (2008), pp. 131–151, pp. 139–140.
52 Lasch, *Narcissism*, p. 82.
53 Ibid., p. 94. See also O. Kernberg, *Borderline Conditions and Pathological Narcissism* (New York, 1975); H. Kohut, *The Analysis of Self: A Systematic Approach to the Psychoanalytic Treatment of Narcissistic Personality Disorders* (New York, 1971).
54 Kilminster, 'Narcissism', p. 140.
55 Ibid., p. 140, citing Lasch, *Narcissism*, p. 82.
56 Lasch, *Narcissism*, p. 5.
57 Ibid., pp. xvii–xviii.
58 Ibid., p. 9.
59 C. Lasch, *Haven in a Heartless World: The Family Besieged* (New York, 1977).
60 D. Horowitz, *Consuming Pleasures: Intellectuals and Popular Culture in the Postwar World* (Philadelphia, 2012), pp. 314–316.
61 K. Piver, 'Philip Rieff: The Critic of Psychoanalysis as Cultural Theorist', in R. Porter and M. S. Micale (eds), *Discovering the History of Psychiatry* (New York, 1994), pp. 191–215, p. 201.
62 See J. B. Imber, 'Philip Rieff and Fellow Teachers', *Society*, 50 (2013), pp. 61–64, p. 64.
63 B. Fisher, 'Review: The Wise Old Men and the New Women: Christopher Lasch Besieged', *History of Education Quarterly*, 19 (1979), pp. 125–141, p. 133.
64 Ibid., p. 133.
65 Cited in Tyler, 'From "The Me Decade"', pp. 354–355.
66 Ibid., p. 357.

67 www.powerbase.info/index.php/Frank_F%C3%BCredi, accessed 20 December 2013.
68 J. Beer, 'Pieties of Silence', *American Conservative* (3 September 2006).
69 F. Furedi, 'The Silent Ascendancy of Therapeutic Culture in Britain', in J. B. Imber (ed.), *Therapeutic Culture: Triumph and Belief* (New Jersey, 2004), p. 24.
70 F. Furedi, *Therapy Culture: Cultivating Vulnerability in an Uncertain Age* (London, 2004), p. 101.
71 Furedi, 'Silent Ascendancy', 2004, p. 16.
72 Kilminister, 'Narcissism', p. 140.
73 Furedi, *Therapy Culture*, p. 70.
74 Ibid., p. 70.
75 Ibid., p. 149.
76 S. O'Sullivan, 'Passionate Beginnings: Ideological Politics 1966–72', *Feminist Review*, 11 (1982), pp. 70–71; D. Bouchier, *The Feminist Challenge: The Movement for Women's Liberation in Britain and the USA* (London, 1983), p. 44, p. 87.
77 Personal communication: N. Rose (11 December 2013); Rose, *The Psychological Complex*. Rose published the theory chapter of his thesis in 'The Psychological Complex: Mental Measurement and Social Administration', *Ideology and Consciousness*, 5 (1979), pp. 5–68. It is available at http://eprints.lse.ac.uk/622/.
78 J. Whitebook, 'Against Interiority: Foucault's Struggle with Psychoanalysis', in G. Gutting (ed.), *Cambridge Companion to Foucault* (Cambridge, 2012).
79 M. Foucault and J. O'Higgins, 'II. Sexual Choice, Sexual Act: An Interview with Michel Foucault', *Salmagundi* 58/59 (1982), pp. 10–24, pp. 16–17.
80 L. Hunt and V. E. Bonnell, 'Introduction', in V. E. Bonnell and L. Hunt (eds), *Beyond the Cultural Turn: New Directions in the Study of Society and Culture* (Berkeley, CA, 1999), p. 22.
81 D. Glenn, 'Prophet of the "Anti-Culture"', *Chronicle of Higher Education*, 52 (13 November 2005); R. Kimball, 'Christopher Lasch vs. the Elites', *New Criterion* (April1995).
82 E.g. E. Illouz, *Cold Intimacies: The Making of Emotional Capitalism* (London, 2007).
83 L. Armstrong, *Rocking the Cradle of Sexual Politics: What Happened When Women Said Incest* (Reading, MA, 1994); K. Bumiller, *In An Abusive State: How Neoliberalism Appropriated the Feminist Movement Against Sexual Violence* (Durham, 2008), pp. 69, 72–73.
84 For a therapeutic attempt to achieve these aims, see Cook, 'Controlling Emotion'.

3 A little learning *is* a dangerous thing

British overseas medical missions and the politics of professionalisation, *c.*1880–1910

Hilary Ingram

We won't ask about the diplomas or the degrees. With these or without them let us have the loving heart, the clear head, the cunning hand of consecrated Christian woman, to help us lift up this sinful, sunken race into fellowship with its Creator. It will be her best and dearest diploma to hear Him say at last – '*She hath done what she could.*'[1]

In the late nineteenth century, concerned medical professionals publicly denounced Protestant missionary organisations for deploying candidates as medical missionaries with little preparation or medical training. While physicians did not object to the idea of sending missionary labour, they did not support sending personnel as *medical* missionaries with only rudimentary training to draw on, arguing that such a dangerous practice could damage respect for the discipline. Such complaints promoted discussion within both medical and missionary circles and raised questions about the role of missionary medicine, what medical aid entailed on the mission field, and whether professional qualifications on par with British standards were required when working with non-European populations. In short, and as articulated by many of the chapters in this collection, complaints and the public debates that grew up around them – local, national and international – developed professionalisation and professionalism, and shaped general expectations of medicine and its practitioners.

Few historians have studied how the complaints of qualified medical professionals, both missionary and secular alike, influenced burgeoning professionalism in British medical missions.[2] The study of medical missions is an area often overlooked when examining the growth of the British medical community, yet it remains an important subfield of the history of medicine that encompasses key themes in the study of gender, race, missions and empire.[3] This chapter will examine the complaints registered against missionary organisations and situate them within a wider context of female professionalisation and the growth of British medical missions at the turn of the twentieth century.

A key development in the professionalisation of medicine in Britain can be traced to the passage of the 1858 Medical Act, which established the General Medical Council (GMC), the regulatory arm of the medical profession, and the British Medical Register. Prior to 1858, medicine in Britain remained largely unregulated, and community-based care was overseen by individuals claiming a variety of skills and expertise. This was not solely the domain of men, for women often filled important roles within their communities as midwives and healers. With the passage of the Medical Act, a legal definition for the term 'qualified practitioner' was established, supported by named entry on the Medical Register, and the processes by which new candidates could qualify were outlined. The Register enabled the public to clearly differentiate between trained doctors and 'quacks', a pejorative term to describe 'unqualified' medical aid. Midwives, alongside other practitioners of alternative methods of healing, were relegated to this 'unqualified' status.[4] To be entered on the Medical Register, candidates were required to pass an examination set by an approved examining body.[5] For nearly 30 years following, women were unable legally to practise medicine in Britain as no examination route was open to them.[6] Medical education was only gradually opening in the 1870s to permit women to take a complete medical training.[7] The passage of the 1876 Enabling Act finally allowed women to sit examination and be entered to the Medical Register.[8]

For medical women, challenges to practising medicine did not cease with their entry into the medical profession. Women faced considerable opposition from the medical establishment (whose members remained largely critical of their inclusion), and, at first, found suitable employment competitive and difficult to obtain. As they fought for acceptance at home in Britain, mission work provided the first generations of qualifying female doctors with invaluable opportunities for personal and professional development overseas.[9] Over a quarter of the female doctors that qualified in Britain were working in India by 1900, and of the 258 women on the Medical Register in the same year, 75 were listed as missionaries, with 45 stationed in India alone.[10] It was within this context of hard-won accreditation and growing professionalisation that physicians, women especially, sought to prevent missionary recruits from calling themselves 'medical missionaries' or holding leadership positions as medical authorities without the appropriate education and training. Only individuals entered on the Medical Register, they argued, should hold the title.

British Protestant missionary efforts grew exponentially during the late nineteenth century, coinciding with an expansion in imperial investment overseas.[11] Women had long contributed to furthering missionary interests, both through home support and by working alongside male missionary relatives as unpaid assistants, though few were independently recognised for this work. The female presence on the mission field did much to support the Christian domestic ideal of the family unit, and wives often worked extensively to aid educational and evangelistic initiatives targeted at local women and children.[12] As the nineteenth century progressed, however, there was continued debate about the efficacy of recruiting single women as missionary agents with discussions focusing, though not exclusively, on female intervention in India. The zenana – the separate quarters for women within some Indian households – was used to support this new idea of 'women's work for women'. Secluded local females were portrayed as the victims of archaic traditions and customs, hidden away from the world, and out of reach of the ministering efforts of male missionaries. Only Western women, supporters argued, could penetrate this protected domestic space to influence the hearts and minds of India's mothers and daughters. The resulting call for Western women to come to the aid of their Indian 'sisters' provided females with a missional foray all their own, one which complemented and did not threaten male leadership and agendas. From the 1860s missionary societies in Britain began gradually to open their doors to single, middle-class women as paid employees, providing one of the first opportunities to pursue a professional and respected career outside of the familial home.[13]

Just as women were beginning to define a role for themselves as independent missionaries overseas, support for medical missions was also gaining prominence. Prior to the mid-nineteenth century, missionary work was primarily considered a solely evangelistic endeavour.[14] 'Pillbox ministries', where missionaries relied on their acquired knowledge and the medications and home remedies at their disposal, existed, but generally full-time medical work was discouraged as it was considered secondary to evangelistic goals. In 1860, a missionary conference in Liverpool issued a statement in support of the medical mission, endorsing it as 'a valuable auxiliary to the direct work of the gospel in densely peopled countries, as China and India, where deep prejudices against its teachers may be removed by their means, and where medical aid is largely needed'.[15] By the late nineteenth century, the value and evangelistic potential of medical work was no longer contested and, instead, was increasingly considered an elite missionary service. This change was influenced, in part, by a shifting emphasis in mission theology on the importance of ministering to the practical as well as the spiritual needs of mission communities and the recognition that, by doing so, missionaries could build relationships with individuals otherwise hostile to their intervention.[16] The increasing professionalised status of medical practitioners at home in Britain also impacted upon the professional trajectory of the medical mission movement, with calls to move away from informal 'pillbox' ministries in favour of more systematic approaches led by qualified medical doctors and assistants.[17]

Still, change was gradual and medical aid on the mission field remained largely unregulated. Some missionaries continued to argue that sending only those fully qualified for medical service overseas was unreasonable, complaining that there were too few qualified candidates available to address the need overseas, and raised issue with the expense and time associated with funding a full medical education, as both prevented an immediate presence in the field. 'The course of instruction for gaining medical degrees is too long and too expensive to be within the reach of more than a few who wish to become missionaries', an unnamed female missionary pursuing unqualified medical work in Syria commented in 1888.[18] Given the practical nature of medical work, Christian critics of medical missions noted that medicine afforded only limited opportunities for direct evangelism. While caring for the poor and sick was considered intrinsic to Christian teaching, the concern remained that medical missionary work could become indistinguishable from secular charitable aid. Suspicion was levelled against those believed to be pursuing medicine for professional and/or personal gain instead of through a clear spiritual calling. Dr Gideon de Gorrequer Griffith, founder of the London-based Zenana Medical College, cast doubt on the spiritual preparedness of trained doctors, cautioning missionary societies to question if a candidate's 'spiritual growth in grace and in the knowledge of God's word have kept pace with their scientific and secular instruction and education'.[19] As late as the 1890s, missionary societies spoke of the danger of 'focusing too much on the professional and not the spiritual' when recruiting medical candidates.[20]

Missionary societies acknowledged the value of equipping outgoing candidates with some medical training, not only to facilitate access into communities largely resistant to Christian teaching, but also to support health and longevity in the field. By the late nineteenth century, most societies had established or partnered with missionary training homes and institutes where a basic medical training, varying in length and intensity, was often part of the required curriculum.[21]

All missionary training schemes raised concerns from the medical establishment, keen to preserve their privileges, though perhaps none more so than the Zenana and Medical Mission Home and Training School for Ladies. The independent school was later named the Zenana Medical College (ZMC), possibly in an effort to convey increased professional legitimacy. Established in London in 1880, the school's educational mandate was to 'train ladies as Medical Missionaries', with the intention that 'these ladies, while relieving the sickness of the body, would carry the good news of the Gospel to women and children'.[22] The ZMC advertised itself as 'distinctly unsectarian' and welcomed women from all Protestant denominations. While the school initially only admitted women intending to pursue medical work in India, this was soon extended to include those assigned to China, Ceylon, Syria and Africa.[23] Classes included studies in anatomy, dermatology, dental surgery, bandaging, pharmacology, midwifery, ophthalmic surgery, tropical diseases and physiology.[24] Students trained for two years, about half the time required to obtain a full medical qualification; the college promoted its programme as cheaper, more spiritually focused and less time-consuming than a full medical training, while still embracing the same rigorous standards. 'We do not profess to make Lady Doctors', it outlined in the prospectus, 'but we desire, by giving as efficient instruction as can be done in two years, to fit ladies to be

Medical Missionaries, and thus to fill those gaps which have hitherto never been occupied from lack of workers – the harvest being plentiful, but the labourers few'.[25] In 1889, the ZMC boasted through its promotional material that the 'institution [supplied] a long-felt need . . . shown by the number of applications for admission, which have been far more than the Committee have been able to entertain'.[26] It was these claims in particular that irked missionary and secular medical professionals alike.

Women doctors were particularly invested in the debate surrounding the partial training of medical missionaries. Unqualified female aid workers far outnumbered their male counterparts in the field, in large part due to the attention paid to zenana missions.[27] As the medical profession was only just beginning to open up during this period, many women had left for the mission field with whatever practical experience and training they could acquire in nursing, midwifery, and dispensary work. Medical training schemes sucn as the ZMC continued to provide those intending to become medical missionaries with the opportunity and justification to forgo the time and expense of a full qualification. In seeking to maintain their reputation and position as trained professionals, missionary doctors argued that affiliation with unqualified aid could lead to unnecessary scrutiny. American medical missionary Dr Anna Kugler was quick to point out the particular vulnerability women faced if implicated in medical scandal. 'Notwithstanding the wonderful strides that have within my own memory been made in the standing accorded medical women', Kugler commented at an Indian missionary conference in 1893, 'the fact remains that a large number of medical men judge more leniently of a professional mistake if committed by a man than if committed by a woman'.[28] Such stratified dynamics played out in the apportioning of blame within other hierarchical systems of medical care, as identified in Kim Price's chapter in this volume.

The debate surrounding the qualification of female medical practitioners was primarily centred on aid workers in India – perhaps unsurprisingly, given that the majority of women working in overseas missions were stationed in India during this time. By the early twentieth century there were more British female missionary physicians than men practising in the country.[29] The reasons for focusing on unqualified practice in India were varied. Medical women and their supporters had long regarded the country as a site of great opportunity. The powerful image of the Indian zenana captured the British imagination and not only fuelled the recruitment of single women within the missionary ranks but helped to legitimise, in the eyes of the British public at least, the entry of single women to the medical profession.[30] Public support for zenana intervention provided women doctors with an established need and exclusive patients. As medical aid expanded beyond the confines of the zenana, women again wrote of the advantages that pursuing medical work in India provided. 'There are few places where such a variety of practice, and especially surgical practice, can be obtained by a medical woman as in our Delhi Hospital', Dr Charlotte Hull of the Society for the Propagation of the Gospel confirmed in 1901 of her work at St Stephen's Hospital in Delhi.[31] Indeed, male critics of female medical participation in Britain did not always object to their qualified involvement overseas. Dr E. Downes, a Church Missionary Society (CMS) employee working in India, commented in 1883 that, 'Whatever view may be taken on the subject of Lady Doctors in England, I think it is clear that they are much needed in India'.[32] Employment prospects, the chance to gain valuable experience independent of metropolitan pressures, and the opportunity to build a reputation for female medical professionalism were supported as reasons why medical women should establish and maintain a professional foothold in India.[33] The continued use of unqualified medical missionary labour was regarded as a clear threat to the professional advances that medical women had only just begun to secure.

The archives of the London School of Medicine for Women (LSMW) reveal the extent of staff, student and alumni participation in the ongoing qualifications debate. Founded in 1874, the LSMW remained the only medical school open to women in Britain until 1886 when Sophia Jex-Blake, prominent feminist, medical education advocate and co-founder of the LSMW, launched a similar school in Edinburgh. Antoinette Burton has demonstrated that, in seeking to establish a reputation as legitimate medical professionals, the medical women's movement distanced themselves from the work of medical missions, eschewing the religious emphasis on philanthropic aid, and instead 'linked their cause to the progress of science, medicine and civilization itself'.[34] In registering complaints against established missionary practice, female medical reformers encouraged public attention for their cause and provided justification for their own professional advance into the imperial enterprise.[35]

While it is clear that secular criticism influenced the growing call for professional qualifications among medical missionary workers, missionary physicians did much to encourage change themselves. Some of the most vocal critics against the sending of unqualified labour were doctors with previous mission experience.[36] Scottish missionary Jane Waterston left her South African mission post in 1873, one of several women among the first graduating classes of the LSMW to return from the mission field to pursue a full medical qualification. Complaining in a letter to Dr James Stewart, a mentor and missionary doctor stationed in South Africa, Waterston wrote in frustration about the sending practices of the Church of Scotland:

> They train so-called medical missionaries at some expense and send out continually agents to India, who are just as continually getting married, and then another succession of *raw hands* go out. But when a woman works for some years on a pittance and then spends hundreds on a complete, instead of a sham, medical training and at the end is a woman with a considerable

> knowledge of life as well as of Mission work, instead of a raw girl with no experience of any kind, there are no funds to send her out. Rawness, greenness and cheapness are the things they want and very dear they have proved to be.[37]

Medical women appealed to a wide audience to encourage support for their cause. Baptist missionary Dr Ellen Farrer echoed Waterston's sentiments and challenged mission supporters to encourage societies to properly fund medical initiatives by demanding change through petition and financial sponsorship. Speaking at a Baptist women's conference in Manchester in 1891, Farrer elaborated:

> I again insist upon the necessity for a thorough [medical] training. . . . Is it not a shame and disgrace to our Christian churches, if, in order to avoid the extra expenditure of time and money incurred, they send out as medical missionaries those who would not be considered fit to practice as doctors here? Surely Christ deserves better than this.[38]

A common complaint raised in support of full qualifications was that the inexperience of unqualified medical workers could lead to scandal, betraying trust and complicating newly forged relationships among indigenous communities, and potentially threatening the reputation of Christian missions at large. Prevalent in these discussions was a presumption about the 'civilising' opportunities Western intervention afforded, and that any knowledge of Western medical practice would be a vast improvement over existing forms of treatment. Medical women cautioned that it was unwise to assume that mission patients were unaware and unconcerned when in receipt of unqualified care. In 1881, Dr Elizabeth Garrett Anderson, then Lecturer and later Dean of the LSMW, wrote in *The Times* that rumours circulated of Indian women questioning the extent of training held by 'medical missionaries' prior to seeking medical advice.[39] Dr Anna Kugler expressed similar concern in 1893, stating:

> The people of India are quick to detect a sham. They can soon determine whether or not persons are qualified for the position they are trying to fill, and if they think we are indifferent to the quality of the medical relief afforded, so long as the religion we teach is pure, their respect for our religion will not be increased.[40]

Western critics were not alone in raising these concerns as Indian medical doctors, backed by public support, also spoke out against unqualified medical intervention in India.[41] In registering these complaints, qualified doctors, both missionary and non-missionary alike, highlighted the damage that inexperienced aid could wreak on the confidence and future direction of medical mission support.

Throughout late 1893 and early 1894, an attack against the professional standards of the Zenana Medical College unfolded in the pages of popular British newspapers and medical journals, including the *British Medical Journal* (*BMJ*) and *The Lancet*, with physicians writing in to publicly express their complaints. While criticism of the ZMC served as the catalyst for the debate, an underlying argument present throughout was a deep concern about the missionary practice of sending partially-trained women for overseas medical work.

Labelling the ZMC a 'cruel farce', the unnamed author of one *BMJ* editorial stated that the college should remember that '"Professional aid" means something very different from mere amateur help'.[42] From the 1880s, ZMC students were able to study for a diploma in midwifery offered through the Obstetrical Society of London. As this award was not recognised by the General Medical Council, their work was still considered 'unqualified', and critics argued that the diploma could engender false confidence and encourage graduates to attempt cases they were unprepared for on the mission field. An anonymous contributor wrote:

> Not only is all this ethically wrong, but it is bad as mere policy; few things could more add to the difficulty of providing women doctors for Indian women than this plan of preoccupying the ground by a shoal of unqualified practitioners and of native pupils even more feebly qualified still.[43]

Feminist and physician Sophia Jex-Blake responded in a subsequent issue of the *BMJ* to express her agreement, stating 'No course can be better calculated to discredit alike the missionary cause and that of medical women'.[44] Taking issue with financial supporters of the ZMC, Jex-Blake continued:

> If only the kind people who have been deluded into giving their names and their money in support of these wretched two-year courses could realise the harm they are doing . . . they would surely no longer allow themselves to be made instrumental in injuring the cause they have at heart, but divert their assistance into channels for thoroughly educating qualified medical women, instead . . . of spoiling a noble work by 'flooding the country with cheap shams'.[45]

ZMC lecturer and medical missionary Dr C. H. F. Routh defended the work of the College following Jex-Blake's comments, 'It is urged that in two years our lady students cannot know much. Granted; but two years well employed will often do as much as three or four carelessly consumed'.[46] In his defence of the ZMC, Routh challenged the necessity for women to pursue a complete medical education. 'Few wealthy ladies follow missionary life', he wrote to the *BMJ*;

'If Miss Jex-Blake and her friends will provide the funds, doubtless more medical missionaries will be qualified'.[47] Jex-Blake once again countered Routh's complaint directly, stating that he had not 'touched on the real point'.[48] For Jex-Blake, the argument against the ZMC's legitimacy was not about the quality or extent of training women received, but that these women were working overseas as if they were fully-trained medical professionals, invalidating the work and position of female physicians in the field. Routh responded with contempt, writing:

> Dr. Jex-Blake seems to have forgotten that vituperation in the mouth of an educated lady is not argument. To charge medical men and clergymen of known integrity with aiding and abetting 'defective education and fraudulent pretence of efficiency' is really puerile. . . . Does Dr. Jex-Blake think that the ignorant Chinese and Indians would understand or refuse to be attended by any but qualified M.D.'s [*sic*] or surgeons?[49]

Routh's statement, while sexist in his dismissal of Jex-Blake, also reflects prevalent racist assumptions about the inferiority of non-Western peoples. Claims like these, couched in imperial rhetoric, operated as ideological justifications for Western supremacy and lent confidence to the belief that any form of medical intervention on the foreign mission field would be an improvement over existing practices.[50]

The ongoing controversy surrounding the work of the ZMC and, more specifically, the continued use of partially-trained workers for overseas service did influence missionary discussion. At an Anglican missionary conference in 1894, the Rev. Watson King Ormsby, Mission Secretary for the Guild of St Luke, reported that he was reading the public debate unfolding in the press and admonished societies for not taking immediate action. 'Medical knowledge and science have advanced with gigantic strides', Ormsby stated; 'The Church must demand from her medical missionaries that their status shall be proportionate to the progress of science. Professional scandal must not be sheltered beneath a religious garb.'[51]

The ZMC found itself the subject of a professional domestic scandal when, in 1896, its founder Dr Griffith was called to the home of a London couple to assist on an obstetrical case. Instead of going himself, Griffith sent the College's matron, a midwife without qualifications, to attend the birth. The child did not survive, though there is no indication in the reports that the child's death was due to improper medical practice. Griffith was accused of facilitating 'quack' care and the work of the ZMC was further called into question, particularly for its option to obtain a diploma upon graduation.[52] While sending women for work as partially-trained medical missionaries overseas was grudgingly tolerated, the use and supply of unqualified medical aid in Britain was considered far from acceptable.

As home support for the medical missions movement grew, and complaints from both within and outside missionary circles mounted over the sending of unqualified workers, leading organisations which had not done so upon entering the field of medical missions worked to establish guidelines defining what level of training was required to assume the title 'medical missionary'. In 1892, for example, the CMS passed a resolution stating that only qualified medical doctors should hold the title though, in the absence of trained physicians or surgeons, lay missionaries were permitted to continue to service minor medical concerns in the field.[53] The following year, delegates attending the Decennial Indian Missionary Conference in Bombay passed the recommendation that 'men and women sent to India should invariably possess legal qualifications and that none other should be placed in charge of medical work'.[54] While missionary societies lent their support to the definition of 'medical missionary' as one fully qualified, these resolutions proved difficult to enforce in the field.

Missionary training institutions also began to establish clear definitions regarding the scope of training they provided. Bermondsey Medical Mission, for example, was founded by the CMS in 1901 to provide their non-medical female candidates with practical medical training prior to deployment. The mission trained women for up to three months with the intention that the experience would enable them, not to become medical missionaries, but to better 'take care of their own health and of that of their fellow-workers'.[55] Two interdenominational medical training programmes that grew up in London around the turn of the century were Livingstone College and The London Missionary School of Medicine, established in 1893 and 1903 respectively. Both schools were careful to state explicitly that they were not producing medical missionaries, but were equipping outgoing non-medical missionaries with the basic medical knowledge and skill necessary for life overseas in foreign climates.[56] Students of Livingstone College, where initially classes were only open to men, were required to sign a statement declaring that they would not, once overseas, establish their position as that of a qualified doctor.[57] While their work was regarded as subordinate to that of trained missionary physicians, in the absence of qualified staff and when the needs of the mission station dictated, these graduates did adopt medical roles. Historian Ryan Johnson has argued that 'many former students did, in fact, become seen as medical missionaries'.[58] Herein lay the problem, for, by the late nineteenth century, while most missionary societies were content to support the definition that 'medical missionary' should only apply to those men and women who held a full medical qualification, in practice, missionaries with only partial training could quite easily assume the title and responsibility in lieu of available help.

Though the practical realities of field work limited opportunities for professional recommendations affirmed in the metropole to be immediately adopted overseas, through the 1890s missionary organisations steadily emphasised the importance of recognised qualifications for medical missionaries. Irene Barnes, when detailing the work of the Church of England Zenana Missionary Society (CEZMS) in 1897, defended the use of the term 'doctor' to describe all medical personnel affiliated with the society, writing that it 'must be understood as the respectful title given by patients to each and all of our "medical missionaries"'.[59] Four years later, Barnes was careful to define the position of a 'true medical missionary' only as one fully qualified. 'The Society individually and collectively recognizes', she wrote, 'that Medical Missionary work in its true form, viz., as carried on by fully equipped physicians, is becoming an absolutely necessary adjunct to, or rather integral part of, each Mission Station'.[60] Still, while societies acknowledged the professional position held by the medical missionary, some organisations defended their continued reliance on unqualified medical aid by complaining that the need overseas far outweighed the supply of available help. As late as 1905, CMS Secretary Eugene Stock praised the 'excellent and useful' work of partially-trained female medical missionaries who operated small hospitals and dispensaries in the absence of qualified support.[61] But as criticism was levelled against this practice, and influenced by the continuing professionalisation of medicine in Britain, organisations worked to better define the education and training required to hold assistant medical posts. For example, the professional status and responsibilities accorded to trained nurses were defined over this period. While nursing had often been regarded as the purview of the partially-trained, by the early twentieth century it was generally expected that qualified missionary nurses would hold over three years' training prior to deployment overseas.[62] Qualified nurses worked to protect their position and, much as missionary doctors had done over 20 years earlier, led calls to limit the title 'missionary nurse' only to women in possession of the approved qualifications.

Within a generation, partially-trained missionaries charged with overseeing hospitals and dispensaries were largely replaced by qualified medical professionals. But what happened to the women who pursued full-time medical work without recognised qualifications? Understandably, as their leadership was threatened and they faced the prospect of being replaced, some missionaries did not leave without voicing their own complaints. Elizabeth Beilby, a former LSMW student and missionary to India, had warned of impending conflict should missionary societies continue to send unqualified recruits in the 1880s. 'One thing I am quite certain of', she stated, 'is that however good the unqualified lady was, she would mind very much such a state of things'.[63] After her work was taken over by a qualified physician, Miss E. Owles, a CEZMS medical missionary, wrote of the decision, 'None gave a heartier welcome to her rightful post than the "quacks" who now gladly hide their diminished heads for ever and a day'.[64] While Owles' comment was praised as demonstrating 'true self-effacement', resignation can be also read into her response, reflected in the use of the term 'quack' to purposely diminish her efforts over the years. In choosing to remain in the field, partially-trained medical missionaries negotiated a fine line between leader and subordinate and were eventually, in essence, left behind given the increasingly professionalised status of medical missions work.

The career of Sarah Secunda Hewlett can be examined through this lens. Born in 1849, the daughter of an English clergyman, Hewlett possessed only a partial medical training when in 1880 she opened a dispensary in Amritsar, India, under the support of the CEZMS. In 1881, Hewlett founded St Catherine's Hospital and worked to service the local community, while also training up Indian converts as medical assistants, several of whom left the hospital following their training to establish mission dispensaries under their own leadership. [65] 'There is a sore and pressing need of help', Hewlett wrote in 1881, referencing the need for qualified medical missionaries in India, 'but we shall do all we can till the help comes'.[66] Alluding to the criticism that not all mission doctors were motivated by a defined spiritual calling, Hewlett concluded with the caution, 'May the mission-field be saved from all lady-doctors who are not also desirous to heal souls!'[67] Hewlett spoke regularly at missionary conferences and published several books about her experiences in India. At a missionary conference in 1883, Hewlett argued that,

> while we would not hinder our favoured sisters from pushing on to degrees, we earnestly beg that no lady may be hindered from pressing into the work the first moment she can; the cry for relief is exceeding great and bitter, and we of humbler standing will do all that we can towards giving that relief until more accomplished aid can be found.[68]

With Hewlett's tongue firmly in her cheek, the language of hierarchy and position is apparent in her words as deference is paid to qualified medical missionaries, a position with which Hewlett did not identify, though she remained careful to assert professional legitimacy for her own work. In 1886, with the assistance of Annie and Frances Sharp, Frances herself being a ZMC graduate, Hewlett founded one of the first specialised centres for the visually impaired in India at Amritsar. By the late 1890s, while St Catherine's Hospital was lauded as 'the most remarkable of our [CEZMS] agencies', and her work remained highly praised, caveats defending the inclusion of non-qualified personnel in discussions of medical work began to appear alongside descriptions of Hewlett's efforts within the mission press.[69] She retired from the CEZMS in 1908 and was replaced in hospital by Charlotte Vines, a qualified missionary doctor. Hewlett continued to work independently as a medical missionary in India for four more years, retiring to England in 1912.[70]

Qualified medical professionals recognised that all manner of medical assistance was required in the mission field. Still, they believed that the title 'medical missionary' and the responsibility of overseeing medical work should only be held by those who had completed a full medical training. Through public complaints and petitions, medical physicians, both missionary and secular, led the call to better define positional hierarchies within the burgeoning professional framework of medical missions. While the dominant historical narrative suggests that tensions between medical and missionary circles regarding recruitment practices for female medical missions had largely subsided by the late 1880s, this chapter has demonstrated that complaints continued to persist.[71] Criticism was not solely directed against women, as male missionaries were also accused of assuming medical roles in the field, but the impetus to highlight the issue in metropolitan debates was often the result of female intervention in the years following their gradual entry to the medical profession as qualified physicians. In 1910, missionary leaders from all over the world assembled in Edinburgh at the World Missionary Conference. During the course of these meetings a pan-Protestant statement was produced, confirming that the term 'medical missionary' should apply only if the candidate, be it man or woman, was a fully-qualified entrant on the Medical Register.[72] By this time, most missionary societies had established medical mission auxiliaries and crafted clear definitions regarding what medical duties should be performed by the doctor, the qualified missionary nurse, trained native assistant and so on, working towards increased professional regulation and transparency. While it continued into the twentieth century, the public debate to consider qualified medical doctors as the only legitimate medical missionaries illustrates that medical physicians, women in particular, were active participants in this mission controversy and fought to define and protect their status and identity as trained professionals.

Notes

1 *Report of the Second Decennial Missionary Conference, 1882–3 held at Calcutta* (Calcutta, 1883), p. 422.

2 A. Burton, 'Contesting the Zenana: The Mission to Make "Lady Doctors for India", 1874–1885', *Journal of British Studies*, 35, 3 (1996), pp. 368–397; R. Fitzgerald, '"Clinical Christianity": The Emergence of Medical Work as a Missionary Strategy in Colonial India, 1800–1914', in B. Pati and M. Harrison (eds), *Health, Medicine and Empire: Perspectives on Colonial India* (London, 2001), pp. 88–136, pp. 124–126.

3 For information on the growth of British medical missions, see R. Fitzgerald, '"Clinical Christianity"'; D. Hardiman (ed.), *Healing Bodies, Saving Souls: Medical Missions in Asia and Africa* (Amsterdam, 2006).

4 A. Witz, *Professions and Patriarchy* (London, 1992), pp. 74–75.

5 E. Crofton, *A Painful Inch to Gain: Personal Experiences of Early Women Medical Students in Britain*, P. Raemakers (ed.) (Peterborough, 2013), pp. 1–2.

6 Crofton, *A Painful Inch to Gain*, pp. 2–3. Two women, Elizabeth Blackwell and Elizabeth Garrett Anderson, did manage entry to the Medical Register during this period. Both women accomplished this on technicalities that were quickly closed to prevent more women from following suit.

7 For information on women's entry to the medical profession, see E. Moberly Bell, *Storming the Citadel: The Rise of the Woman Doctor* (London, 1953); C. Blake, *The Charge of the Parasols: Women's Entry to the Medical Profession* (London, 1990); Crofton, *A Painful Inch to Gain*.

8 Witz, *Professions and Patriarchy*, p. 98.
9 For work on British women's involvement in medical missions, see R. Fitzgerald, '"A Peculiar and Exceptional Measure": The Call for Women Medical Missionaries for India in the Later Nineteenth Century', in R. A. Bickers and R. Seton (eds), *Missionary Encounters: Sources and Issues* (Richmond, 1996), pp. 174–196; R. Fitzgerald, '"Rescue and Redemption": The Rise of Female Medical Missions in Colonial India during the Late Nineteenth and Early Twentieth Centuries', in A. M. Rafferty, J. Robinson and R. Elkon (eds), *Nursing History and the Politics of Welfare* (London, 1997), pp. 64–79.
10 D. Gaitskell, 'Women, Health and the Development of Medical Missions: Some South African Reflections', in K. Hallencreutz (ed.), *Gender, Poverty and Church Involvement: Missio 20* (Uppsala, 2005), pp. 57–78, p. 61.
11 For a general overview of the British missionary movement, see J. Cox, *The British Missionary Enterprise Since 1700* (New York, 2008).
12 C. Midgley, 'Can Women Be Missionaries? Envisioning Female Agency in the Early Nineteenth-century British Empire', *Journal of British Studies*, 45 (April 2006), pp. 335–358, p. 339; J. Murray, 'The Role of Women in the Church Missionary Society, 1799–1917', in K. Ward and B. Stanley (eds), *The Church Mission Society and World Christianity* (Grand Rapids, MI, 2000), pp. 72–86, p. 69.
13 Fitzgerald, '"Rescue and Redemption"', pp. 68–71.
14 C. P. Williams, 'Healing and Evangelism: The Place of Medicine in Late Victorian Protestant Missionary Thinking', in W. J. Sheils (ed.), *The Church and Healing: Studies in Church History* (Oxford, 1982), pp. 271–285, p. 271.
15 *Conference on Missions held in 1860 at Liverpool* (London, 1860), p. 57. Also quoted in Williams, 'Healing and Evangelism', p. 275.
16 Fitzgerald, '"Rescue and Redemption"', p. 65.
17 A. Porter, *Religion vs. Empire? British Protestant Missionaries and Overseas Expansion, 1700–1914* (Manchester, 2004), p. 311; A. F. Walls, 'The Heavy Artillery of the Missionary Army: The Domestic Importance of the Nineteenth Century Medical Missionary', in W. J. Shiels (ed.), *The Church and Healing: Studies in Church History* (Oxford, 1982), pp. 287–297, p. 287.
18 'Zenana Medical College', *The Morning Post* (12 September 1888), p. 2.
19 G. De Gorrequer Griffith, 'Correspondence (Unqualified Medical Missionaries)', *Medical Missions at Home and Abroad*, 10 (October 1880), p. 157.
20 G. Spottiswoode (ed.), *The Official Report of the Missionary Conference of the Anglican Communion on May 28, 29, 30, 31, and June 1, 1894* (London, 1894), pp. 419–420.
21 M. J. M. Causton, *For the Healing of the Nations: The Story of the British Baptist Medical Missions, 1792–1951* (London, 1951), pp. 42, 46; G. Gollock, *Candidates-in-Waiting: A Manual of Home Preparation for Foreign Missionary Work* (London, 1892), pp. 78–79; Fitzgerald, '"Clinical Christianity"', p. 104.
22 'Hospital Training for Zenana Missionaries', *Medical Missions at Home and Abroad*, 8 (April 1880), pp. 119–120.
23 *The Missionary Year-Book for 1889: Containing Historical and Statistical Accounts of the Principal Protestant Missionary Societies in Great Britain, the Continent of Europe, and America* (London, 1889), pp. 200–201.
24 'Unqualified Medical Missionaries', *British Medical Journal* [hereafter *BMJ*] 2, 1714 (4 November 1893), p. 1010.
25 'Hospital Training for Zenana Missionaries', p. 120.
26 *The Missionary Year-Book for 1889*, p. 201.

27 Fitzgerald, '"Clinical Christianity"', p. 124.
28 *Report of the Third Decennial Missionary Conference, 1892–3 held at Bombay*, vol. 1 (Bombay, 1893), p. 328.
29 Cox, *The British Missionary Enterprise*, p. 218; Fitzgerald, '"Rescue and Redemption"', pp. 70–71.
30 Burton, 'Contesting the Zenana', p. 369.
31 C. Hull, quoted in J. Cox, *Imperial Fault Lines: Christianity and Colonial Power in India, 1818–1940* (Stanford, 2002), p. 175.
32 *Report of the Second Decennial Missionary Conference, 1882–3*, p. 417.
33 K. Michaelsen, 'Becoming "Medical Women": British Female Physicians and the Politics of Professionalism, 1860–1933', unpublished PhD, University of California, Berkeley, 2003, p. 146.
34 Burton, 'Contesting the Zenana', pp. 395.
35 For information about secular imperialist initiatives targeted to Indian women, like the Countess of Dufferin's Fund, see Burton, 'Contesting the Zenana', pp. 368–397; S. Lang, 'Colonial Compassion and Political Calculation: The Countess of Dufferin and Her Fund', in P. Bala (ed.), *Contesting Colonial Authority: Medicine and Indigenous Responses in Nineteenth and Twentieth-Century India* (Langham, 2012), pp. 81–96.
36 For several testimonies from missionaries who discussed various problems they encountered when sent out to the mission field without adequate training, see J. Lowe, *Medical Missions: Their Place and Power* (New York, 1886), pp. 190–193.
37 J. E. Waterston, *The Letters of Jane Elizabeth Waterston, 1866–1905*, L. Bean and E. Van Heyningen (eds) (Cape Town, 1983), p. 128.
38 E. Farrer, 'Women's Work among the Sick Poor', in *The Training of Women for Christian Work: Papers read at the Baptist Union, held in Manchester on Thursday October 3, 1891* (London, 1891), p. 11.
39 Burton, 'Contesting the Zenana', p. 384.
40 *Report of the Third Decennial Missionary Conference, 1892–3*, p. 328.
41 Fitzgerald, '"Clinical Christianity"', p. 125.
42 'Unqualified Medical Missionaries', pp. 1010–1011.
43 Ibid.
44 S. Jex-Blake, 'Unqualified Medical Missionaries', *BMJ*, 2, 1716 (18 November 1893), p. 1129.
45 Jex-Blake, 'Unqualified Medical Missionaries', p. 1130.
46 C. H. F. Routh, 'Medical Missionaries', *BMJ*, 1, 1724 (13 January 1894), p. 103.
47 Routh, 'Medical Missionaries', pp. 103.
48 S. Jex-Blake, 'Medical Missionaries', *BMJ*, 1, 1725 (20 January 1894), p. 159. See also 'Medical Missionaries', *BMJ*, 1, 1724 (13 January 1894), pp. 96–97.
49 C. H. F. Routh, 'Medical Missionaries', *BMJ*, 1, 1726 (27 January 1894), p. 219.
50 D. Hardiman, 'Introduction', in D. Hardiman (ed.), *Healing Bodies, Saving Souls: Medical Missions in Asia and Africa* (Amsterdam, 2006), p. 14.
51 Spottiswoode, *Official Report*, p. 414.
52 'A Midwife Posing as a Medical Practitioner', *The Lancet*, 147, 3786 (21 March 1896), p. 790; R. R. Rentoul, 'The Granting of Questionable "Diplomas"', *BMJ*, 2, 1869 (24 October 1896), p. 1263.
53 Spottiswoode, *Official Report*, p. 417.
54 W. J. Wanless, *The Medical Mission: Its Place, Power and Appeal* (Philadelphia, 1911), pp. 71–72.
55 'C.M.S. Medical Mission in Bermondsey', *Mercy and Truth*, 5, 50 (1901), p. 36.

56 R. Johnson, 'Colonial Mission and Imperial Tropical Medicine: Livingstone College, London, 1893–1914', *Social History of Medicine*, 23, 3 (2010), pp. 555, 557. Livingstone College was initially only open to male missionary candidates. Later, women were admitted to study on short-term courses only.
57 Johnson, 'Colonial Mission', p. 553.
58 Ibid., p. 559.
59 I. H. Barnes, *Behind the Pardah: The Story of C.E.Z.M.S. Work in India* (London, 1897), p. 179.
60 I. H. Barnes, *Between Life and Death: The Story of the C.E.Z.M.S. Medical Missions in India, China and Ceylon* (London, 1901), p. 143.
61 E. Stock, *Notes on India for Missionary Students* (London, 1905), p. 83.
62 Fitzgerald, '"Rescue and Redemption"', p. 73.
63 E. Bielby, quoted in Lowe, *Medical Missions*, p. 193.
64 Barnes, *Between Life and Death*, p. 148.
65 Barnes, *Behind the Pardah*, p. 179.
66 'Conferences: The Calcutta Conference', *India's Women: The Magazine of the Church of England Zenana Missionary Society*, 3, 14 (1881), p. 115.
67 'Conferences', p. 115.
68 *Report of the Second Decennial Missionary Conference, 1882–3*, p. 187.
69 Barnes, *Between Life and Death*, pp. 144, 164.
70 Cadbury Research Library, University of Birmingham, Church of England Zenana Missionary Society (CEZMS), 'Roll of Missionaries of the CEZMS with Particulars of Service', vol. 1, CEZ/C/AM 1/1.
71 Burton, 'Contesting the Zenana', p. 393.
72 World Missionary Conference 1910, *The History and Records of the Conference together with Addresses Delivered at the Evening Meetings* (Edinburgh, 1910), pp. 113–120, p. 117; World Missionary Conference 1910, Report of Commission V, *The Preparation of Missionaries* (Edinburgh, 1910), pp. 134–135.

Part II

Politics

4 Paying the piper and calling the tune?

Complaints against doctors in workers' medical schemes in the South Wales Coalfield

Steven Thompson

In May 1921, a woman from the mining village of Bedlinog, south Wales, attended the surgery of Dr Thomas, the practitioner attached to the medical scheme established by the miners of the village to serve themselves and their families. She had hoped to obtain something from the doctor for her daughter. When presented with a few pills and a powdery substance, however, she complained to the doctor that this was a curious way for him to dispense medicines and was told to 'go to hell'. She lost her temper, threatened to throw the esteemed doctor through his surgery window and left the surgery in high dudgeon. She subsequently submitted a complaint to the workmen's committee that administered the scheme of which Dr Thomas was the surgeon, insisting that Thomas was drunk and unfit to see patients on the day in question. Following the procedure – agreed by the doctor when he was first contracted to provide medical attendance – the committee called both parties to their next meeting, heard both accounts of the incident and then deliberated in private on the course of action to take. A proposal that both parties apologise for their parts in the disagreement was defeated and, instead, the committee resolved that Thomas be asked to apologise to the complainant. The doctor consented and apologised for his behaviour.[1]

While the threat of violence against the doctor was unusual, other aspects of this case were all too typical of the numerous grievances heard by the committees of workmen's medical schemes in south Wales in the late nineteenth and early twentieth centuries. Patients, fiercely non-deferential in their attitudes to the medical profession and sensitive to their own dignity, were keen, and indeed had the means, to hold doctors to account for any perceived failing in the care they provided or any slight done to them – findings which underscore those presented in the Introduction and in King's chapter in this volume. Furthermore, the workmen's committees that administered the medical schemes, which proliferated in the region, exercised a considerable degree of control over the appointment and working conditions of doctors in much the same way as the administrators discussed in Price's chapter in this volume (albeit the antithetical Poor Law Guardians). They also acted as the bodies to receive complaints from members dissatisfied with any aspect of the schemes' activities, including the conduct of their doctors. Indeed, as this particular case demonstrates, the medical professionals appointed by these workmen's schemes were forced to recognise the authority of lay committees, accept their judgements in cases of dispute, and, very often, accept the punishments meted out to them. This particularly striking example, like those presented by Pilar León-Sanz in Chapter 5 of this volume, highlights so many of the factors that conditioned the character of grievances, the mechanisms for dealing with them, and their outcomes in a distinct social, political and industrial context.

South Wales was one of the cradles of the industrial revolution and, during the nineteenth century, became one of the powerhouses of the British economy and part of the foundation on which Britain's international and imperial pre-eminence rested. The development of iron production in an arc of towns along the northern rim of the South Wales Coalfield in the northern parts of Glamorgan and Monmouthshire during the second half of the eighteenth century, and the development of the copper industry in the region around the town of Swansea in the western part of Glamorgan in the same period, meant that the region dominated the British and, indeed, global production of these two important industrial commodities by the early nineteenth century.[2] These metal-making industries had spurred the emergence of a small coal industry during the decades either side of the turn of the century, but it was the far more rapid increase in coal mining in the second half of the nineteenth century, largely for an export market, that made south Wales one of the centres of British industry and population in the modern period. Improvements in the techniques of deep-mining and chemical analyses of the coal, which showed the superiority of the various grades of coal found in the region, helped to bring about break-neck development in the coal industry in the decades after 1870.

The populations of the two counties of Glamorgan and Monmouthshire increased from 71,525 and 45,582 respectively in 1801 to 405,798 and 219,798 in 1871, and grew even more rapidly in the following years to number 1,120,910 for Glamorgan and 395,719 for Monmouthshire by 1911.[3] By 1913, the peak year in the production of south Wales coal, the industry employed over a quarter of a million men and boys, making it the largest coalfield in Britain.[4] It was also one of the most militant, particularly following the formation of the South Wales Miners' Federation in 1898, as socialism, syndicalism and communism became important elements within the labour movement during the early decades of the twentieth century, and as significant levels of solidarity and unity were forged between workers.[5] It was in this environment that distinctive workers' medical schemes were formed which possessed large numbers of members, offered a broader range of medical services than workers' schemes elsewhere, and were characterised by a significant degree of lay control.[6]

Workers' medical schemes in south Wales were as old as industrialisation itself, with the appointment of surgeons by ironmasters, coal owners and copper industrialists in the late eighteenth and early nineteenth centuries to treat their workers. The industrialists retained the power to dismiss such surgeons at will, despite their being funded from compulsory deductions from workers' wages. The compulsory nature of these schemes and the inability of members to choose the doctor or manage the funds that accumulated from wage deductions was a source of dissatisfaction and tension throughout the 1800s and came to be challenged by workers and their representatives, especially in the last few decades of the century and the early part of the twentieth. In many schemes, workmen's committees, elected directly by the workmen whose subscriptions paid the physicians' salaries, gained the right to obtain the 'doctor's money' from the colliery office and then appoint the medical men. In other schemes, workmen's committees were able to go a step further and employ the doctors on set salaries, using the surplus to provide other medical benefits.[7]

Many of these committees were to evolve into comprehensive, sophisticated and robust medical aid societies that covered large populations and provided a range of medical and para-medical services in addition to hospital care, convalescent facilities, travel assistance, maternity services and the provision of an array of medical and surgical equipment. By the time of the 1911 National Insurance Act, it was estimated that 189,000 miners in south Wales were covered for medical attendance through these organisations; if their dependent wives and children are added to this total, it is clear that the schemes were highly significant in the provision of primary care in the region.[8] Furthermore, many of the largest schemes, particularly in northern Monmouthshire, were expanded beyond the workers employed in pits or foundries and came to include 'town' subscribers from among commercial, professional and other occupations; in some places, this meant that almost the entire population of a town or district were enrolled in the medical schemes established by workers.[9]

Many progressives and reformers in the 1930s and 1940s saw in organisations such as the Tredegar Workmen's Medical Aid Society models for a national health service that they wished to see introduced at that time.[10] For its part, the medical establishment viewed such schemes as the worst examples of the lay control of medical expertise that they were so opposed to, and south Wales was considered a problem area by the British Medical Association (BMA), the professional association that represented the interests of British doctors, throughout the early decades of the 1900s.[11] It is within this political economy of medical provision that the complaints from patients about their doctors need to be understood.

Very few of the numerous medical schemes that existed in south Wales during the second half of the nineteenth century or the early decades of the twentieth have left much in the way of source material, and fewer still have left minute books in which complaints, and the hearings that deliberated such grievances, are recorded. Three schemes that have done so are the Ebbw Vale Workmen's Medical Aid Society, the Maesteg Medical Fund and the Bedlinog Medical Committee; the records of all three schemes document complaints and so can be used as a good indication of the culture of complaining in this particular context.[12] These organisations, all of them intended to secure medical attendance for workers and their families, have some similarities but also certain important differences. Bedlinog was a classic south Walian colliery village, in a small tributary of the Taff Valley, just to the south-east of Merthyr Tydfil, with terraced housing clustered around a single colliery that employed over a thousand men just before it closed in 1924. Its medical scheme consisted of a single doctor who provided attendance to the workmen and their families. Maesteg, in contrast, is a small town in the Llynfi Valley in the central part of the coalfield around which was clustered a number of collieries in which roughly three-quarters of the district's working population was engaged.[13] Its medical scheme was correspondingly larger than that at Bedlinog, with 6,500 members by 1912; medical attendance was provided by four doctors and institutional care granted as a result of the scheme's subscriptions to the local hospital and the Cardiff Royal Infirmary.[14] The town of Ebbw Vale, situated in north-east Monmouthshire, was larger again, with a population of 35,000 in 1921, and was so dominated by a single steel and coal firm, in which over 50 per cent of employed men worked, that it might be described as a 'company town'.[15] Its medical scheme was one of the largest in south Wales, with 24,000 individuals covered by 1920, when it employed 10 practitioners, offered a nursing service and a masseuse, subscribed to numerous hospitals in Wales and England, and offered artificial limbs and other surgical appliances to injured members.[16] The nature of these three communities and their respective medical schemes created distinctive dynamics in doctor–patient relations in the three locations, though their nature as industrial communities also led to certain similarities as far as complaints are concerned.

In common with most other medical schemes in the region, a clause commonly appeared in the agreements between doctors and workmen's committees in these three cases that placed the responsibility for investigating grievances on the committees. It is evident from the minute books of the schemes that there were a large number of complaints. Indeed, apart from the usual administrative work of collecting money and paying bills, the investigation of grievances turned out to be one of the major tasks of committees. In each of the three schemes, complaints had to be submitted in writing to the committee which would then, in most cases, call the complainants, the doctors and any witnesses to a meeting. All parties were questioned by committee members, and required to leave the room while the case was discussed. Judgement was then communicated by the secretary or individual committee members. Occasionally, the secretary of the scheme or another committee member would be instructed to investigate a complaint, but this was relatively rare. A further refinement of these mechanisms was brought about in larger schemes in south Wales, such as those at Ebbw Vale and Tredegar, whereby a chief surgeon assumed supervisory functions over the other medical staff and investigated grievances under the direction of the committee. In such cases, the chief surgeon would report his findings to the committee who decided what, if any, action to take against a doctor, though, in practice, cases investigated by the chief surgeon tended to be limited to those where doctors were absent from their surgeries or else unfit to carry out their duties; any complaints made about the chief surgeon were investigated by the committee itself, as were most grievances of a more serious nature about the other doctors.[17]

Nevertheless, despite the presence of complaints mechanisms in the rules of these schemes, there continued to be a struggle over the professional autonomy of doctors and the lay authority of workmen's committees. A case in point is a dispute that arose between the workmen's committee and physicians at Ebbw Vale in 1913, occasioned by a complaint against one of the practitioners. Councillor George Davies, a member of the committee, opined that 'he for one would not sit on a committee which was simply there as a collecting centre for the doctors', and instead intended to extend the provision of services as broadly as possible and bring the physicians under the authority of the workmen's committee.[18] In this way, the authority of committees to receive and consider complaints was resented and occasionally challenged, though it is also clear that workmen's committees were able to withstand such pressures and continued to receive large numbers of grievances.[19]

The complaints received by workmen's committees varied in content and, following social scientist Rudolph Klein's useful categorisation of complaints about the quality of professional medical care, can be grouped into three main areas: the technical, the organisational and the stylistic. Technical aspects refer to the particular skills of the individual doctor and the extent to which s/he could apply a body of professional knowledge to patients, while the organisational characteristics refer to a physician's availability to patients and his or her 'ability to apply his skill in the right place at the right time'.[20] Stylistic aspects of the quality of professional attention relate to the doctor's manner with patients and the relationship that was formed with patients. Dissatisfaction at the organisation of medical attendance was the most common cause of grievance in workmen's medical schemes in industrial south Wales and, within this category, the basic failure to provide medical attendance was the cause of most disgruntlement. This came about in a variety of ways. In many cases, a practitioner was requested to attend by the patient, a member of the patient's family, a friend, or a member of the committee, but did not attend promptly or, in some cases, at all. In other instances, doctors were absent from the surgery when patients called or when messengers were sent to request their attendance. In both scenarios, efforts were often made to obtain the attendance of another physician, where it was possible, and the minutes of complaint hearings can give a vivid impression of the panicked and frustrating attempts to obtain assistance in dire circumstances. One member of the Ebbw Vale scheme was sent by a midwife attending his wife to fetch a doctor in November 1915 when problems arose during the birth. The doctor, Sullivan, was not home. As a result, he went to the surgery of another medical man employed by the scheme, Cowie, and was told that he would attend in place of Sullivan but for the fact that he was not available. The husband went back to Sullivan's surgery, obtained no response there, returned to Cowie's, but he too was still out. The husband then resorted to approaching a committee member who arranged for a third physician, Hood, to attend. Fortunately, Hood was at home but, unfortunately, he refused to attend since it was by then 6 p.m. and the patient's doctor, Sullivan, would now be at his surgery for his evening consultations. Hood was censured for his refusal to attend.[21]

More problematic still were the many instances in which doctors refused requests to attend cases. This derived, in part, from the commercial nature of medical practice in Britain before 1948, in which each individual patient was a direct source of income to a physician, and from the professional obligation that medical practitioners did not poach each other's patients. On a number of occasions in the Ebbw Vale practice, for example, doctors refused calls to attend cases, claiming that the patient was registered on a colleague's list.[22] It needs to be noted that this was not always a mere administrative or bureaucratic nicety on the part of the practitioners in relatively minor cases, and that it could involve a refusal to offer care and assistance in quite desperate situations. In November 1913, an accident at the Victoria Foundry in Ebbw Vale left two men seriously injured, but a messenger to Dr McCaig was met by a refusal to attend the badly injured men because the two workers concerned were patients of another physician on the scheme. One of the men had an arm and a leg amputated, such was the severity of his injuries, and died the following day. McCaig was subsequently forced to realise the gravity of his mistake in not attending the injured, partly as a result of representations made to him by his fellow medical men on the scheme and the criticisms of the coroner in the case, and only very narrowly escaped losing his position.[23] In yet other incidents, complaints arose when doctors failed to attend a sick child or a woman in labour and, while some cases were very serious in character and resulted in the death of an individual, it is possible to speculate that the anxieties of a parent or a husband in such difficult situations were the cause of the grievance in other cases, as much as any failing in the professional behaviour of the physician.[24] Indeed, it is fair to assume that the committee thought as much, at least some of the time.[25]

One of the reasons for the failure of doctors to attend to members of the schemes, and frequently a cause for complaint in and of itself, was insobriety on the part of the practitioner; using Klein's categorisation of the quality of professional case, this was both an organisational and a stylistic failing. Drinking was a considerable problem for many workers' schemes in south Wales and crops up repeatedly in the minutes of the three organisations. Some schemes attempted to prevent the problem and questioned doctors very carefully about their drinking habits before making appointments; the applicants for a position with the Dowlais Workers' Medical Fund in 1913 were obliged to appear before a packed public meeting of over 400 people and state whether they were teetotallers or mere abstainers. Other schemes inserted a specific clause in contracts that insobriety constituted gross misconduct and was an offence that gave grounds for dismissal.[26]

Despite such efforts to prevent the problem arising, committees were forced to deal with complaints over doctors' drunkenness. There were even cases in which physicians appeared before committees to defend themselves against complaints of insobriety while in an inebriated state, and in one instance an applicant for a position with the Ebbw Vale scheme was intoxicated at his interview, which was not successful.[27] Patients, understandably, had little faith in the ability of intoxicated practitioners to treat them effectively. In Ebbw Vale in 1908, for example, the continual drunkenness of one assistant doctor, Cowan, was brought to the attention of the committee by another of the scheme's practitioners and he stated that not only had 50–60 patients refused to have the physician attend them, but one sick child had been prescribed a dose of medicine that would have killed him had he taken it; Cowan was dismissed.[28]

This problem of insobriety derived in part from the nature of practice in this industrial district. Doctors in the region faced large, and often unmanageable, workloads, went without the facilities and services available to their counterparts in better-provisioned areas, and complained of the social isolation they felt in overwhelmingly proletarian communities. Considerable strains were experienced by these physicians in the course of their work. James Mullin, an Irish doctor worked as an assistant in a number of industrial districts in south Wales before establishing his own practice in Cardiff, discussed this in his autobiography: 'Good people who have never undergone the temptation begotten of fatigue and insomnia find it very easy to blame the victim', he commented, 'but those who, like myself, have undergone it must substitute pity for blame'.[29] In addition, the particular character of general practice in this industrial region meant that south Wales was not a particularly attractive option and could not compete with the many attractions of practice in more salubrious and better-paying districts, with the effect that it tended to be considered as a last resort by doctors seeking positions. This is borne out to some extent by the experience of the Ebbw Vale scheme as it struggled to attract a sufficient number of assistants to staff the scheme in the early twentieth century, which itself placed greater strains on the existing staff and thereby increased the likelihood of complaints.[30]

The result of these various structural factors was that south Wales attracted what one doctor described as the 'flotsam and jetsam of the profession', or what A. J. Cronin, a general practitioner and later successful novelist, referred to as the 'rag-tag and bobtail of a glorious, a truly noble profession'.[31] Again, this was most evident in Ebbw Vale, where constant attrition with the BMA, and indeed calls by the association at various times before the First World War for members to boycott the scheme and not apply for vacancies that arose, led to a high turnover of doctors.[32] In such circumstances, it is possible to speculate that the workmen's committee was faced with a diminishing and inferior pool of applicants and that it perhaps tended to be doctors who lost positions in other localities as a result of insobriety that defied the BMA and sought positions with the society.[33]

The case at Bedlinog which opened this chapter, in which the woman threatened the doctor with violence, was a rare occurrence, but it nevertheless points to a more general situation in which complaints arose from the robust or even fractious nature of doctor–patient relations in south Wales. Quite a large number of complaints arose from the perceived rudeness of physicians. In certain cases, it is possible to discern the effects of tiredness, illness and overwork behind such incivility and, when in better mood, many practitioners were in fact willing to apologise for their behaviour.[34] In other instances, incivility was perhaps a character failing: Dr Taylor, the head surgeon of the Ebbw Vale scheme, for example, apologised for his abrupt manner with patients after a complaint in 1913 and characterised it as a 'manner acquired by habit and army training and not of temperament'.[35] Indeed, in the early 1900s, many members of the labour movement in south Wales who wished to bring medical schemes under lay control and exercise a greater level of authority over medical personnel pointed to the manner of doctors in their dealings with working-class patients as another reason why lay control should be asserted. One correspondent to a Rhondda Valley newspaper in 1902 claimed that, 'Now and again I have seen big slices of Hooliganism chucked at women and children, and respectable workmen treated as veritable Shonies in the surgery.'[36] Accusations of rudeness were the cause, or an exacerbating factor, in a number of complaints. In the case of a complaint brought against Dr Aviss of the Ebbw Vale Society, J. Evans alleged that the physician had behaved in a rough manner towards his dying sister, that

> he had insisted that the patient should walk across her room, although in a very weak state, he commanded her to look in glass and examine her own tongue, in fact that his whole conduct was brutal, and that they had called in another Doctor.

In the event, Aviss was dismissed by the committee for his conduct.[37]

For their part, the members of these medical schemes could be quite as rude and inconsiderate as their doctors. Such was the abuse directed at him by one woman in 1905 that Dr Donovan wrote to the Ebbw Vale committee to complain and ask that it take action against her; he also refused to attend her again, giving rise to a counter complaint from her husband.[38] This treatment meted out to doctors by club members was utilised by the medical establishment in their attempts to demonstrate the undesirable nature of lay control. In his autobiography, published in 1921, James Mullin belittled the medical complaints and expectations of the miners he treated:

> If only the little finger of a collier ached, or a thimbleful of recalcitrant wind lost its way in the corridors of his colon, it was 'Off for the doctor immediately; why shouldn't he come and cure me at once? Are we not his master, do we not keep the roof over him, the clothes on his back, feed his family and provide him with a horse when he ought to tramp around like the rest of us?'[39]

As far as members were concerned, such comments perhaps reveal a desire to bring physicians under lay-patient control, but they were clearly intended by practitioners as evidence of the harmful effects of lay control. Francis Maylett Smith, a doctor who practiced near Aberdare in the years before the First World War, later left south Wales to work in the Staffordshire coalfields and found that the colliers and their families there were not as demanding as those in south Wales: 'They did not ask for much', he commented, 'and were grateful for little'.[40] The medical secretary of the BMA, Alfred Cox, a vehement critic of workers' schemes in south Wales, similarly differentiated miners there from their counterparts in other British coalfields and opined in 1920 that 'The South Wales miner is notorious as being the most dissatisfied and restless workman in the kingdom'.[41] This lack of deference on the part of patients in south Wales was the cause of friction between members of the schemes and their doctors, but was also perhaps one of the underlying reasons for so many other grievances that committees heard through these years. Members of the schemes were very demanding of their physicians, were prepared to claim what they saw as their rights, and were sensitive to any slights they perceived in the doctors' behaviour.

In some ways, the most significant grounds for complaint were the quality of care provided to the patient by his or her physician and the questioning of medical judgement. This type of grievance lies in Klein's technical category and, while the number of such complaints was small relative to other types of complaints, they are significant in political terms. This was an area loaded with tension and significance in south Wales because it formed a central plank in the BMA's struggles with lay control in the region. The Association insisted that medical expertise should be respected and take precedence over lay opinion, and that the result of the extension of lay control would be the setting aside of professional expertise and its replacement with lay ignorance.[42] Such claims were, of course, rhetorical strategies on the part of the medical establishment to garner support and generate opposition to lay authority; on the other hand, the evidence relating to complaints perhaps bears out the accuracy of such accusations, albeit to a very limited extent. Doctors, it is clear, were protective of the 'dignity' and 'honour' of their profession, and did not like the fact that committees of workmen sat in judgement of their professional expertise when complaints arose.[43] If Rudolph Klein is to be believed, the introduction of a complaints mechanism in the National Health Insurance scheme of 1911 was not an attempt to protect patients' interests, but rather was a means by which the medical establishment was able to take complaints out of the influence of such workmen's committees and capture control of the process for themselves.[44]

Many grievances relating to medical judgement arose where the drunken state of the doctor was an exacerbating factor and, in such cases, it was easy for lay committees to point out the errors of judgment made by the doctor, often with support from other members of the medical staff; upon investigation, the physicians in these cases were forced to admit their errors.[45] Far fewer instances of dissatisfaction about medical judgement alone are evident in the minutes, but they do exist. In February 1911, Dr Irwin of the Ebbw Vale scheme was the cause of two complaints from members dissatisfied with the treatment offered their two respective children. In the first case, Irwin had misdiagnosed the patient and had therefore treated the child incorrectly until a second diagnosis of 'Croupus Pneumonia'. Another physician had been called in, but the child had died. In the second case, the complaint revolved around the failure to prescribe the correct medicines. In the event, the doctor was dismissed from the scheme, though it should be noted that the committee judged him no longer physically capable of carrying on his practice and so his failure of judgement might have been attributable to illness or old age.[46] Irwin had a reprieve, but provoked further complaint in June of that year and was dismissed for failing to treat a broken arm properly.[47] In another example, in the same year, Irwin's colleague, Dr Rains, similarly received notice to terminate his contract for underestimating the seriousness of a case and failing to attend the child sufficiently, the child dying as a result.[48]

While the lay knowledge of patients could be used to bring complaints against doctors, and the lay understandings of committee members were the basis of any decisions taken, it also needs to be noted that professional expertise was drawn upon on occasion in the submission or deliberation of complaints relating to professional competence. An instructive case comes from the records of the Ebbw Vale Society in 1900. John Griffiths of Beaufort, Ebbw Vale, brought a complaint of negligence against Dr D. R. Bowen following the death of his wife from puerperal fever, a virulent bacterial infection contracted by women in childbirth. Griffiths alleged that Bowen had failed to attend promptly or sufficiently regularly after being called and had diagnosed 'milk fever', when a subsequent diagnosis had in fact confirmed puerperal fever. Crucially, Griffiths had called in another physician, Dr Smith from nearby Sirhowy, as a result of his dissatisfaction with Bowen. Smith had insisted that the death of his wife was due to the negligence of the practitioner who had treated her before he was consulted; he even went so far as to claim that Griffiths' wife would not have died had she been treated properly and that Bowen deserved to be horse-whipped for his negligence. The workmen's committee interviewed Smith as part of their investigation and subsequently decided to dismiss Bowen from their service.[49]

As this case suggests, there were clearly situations in which patients within workers' medical schemes were willing to question professional decisions and raise charges against the competence of their doctors. As importantly, such grievances were often upheld and the doctors concerned punished by lay committees of workmen. Alcohol abuse, as previously noted, was occasionally an exacerbating factor but not in all cases, and the sober, considered judgments of physicians were also questioned and gave rise to complaints. At times, the opinions of other doctors were drawn upon to inform or support lay complaints, though these were few in number and it is possible that professional courtesy, and even solidarity, prevented this from happening on a larger scale. At the same time, cases in which professional judgement was questioned and was the cause of disgruntlement were not numerous, and certainly not as common as the failure to attend or the manner of the practitioner in his dealings with his patients, but were seized upon by members of the medical establishment, locally and nationally, as a means to raise fears over lay control. Whatever the impact of such rhetorical strategies and professional aggression elsewhere in the public sphere, the result in industrial south Wales was to sensitise the labour movement more generally and its individual members specifically, as patients, to the dignity of labour and the rights due to workers from their medical servants. Medical attendance was a burning issue in south Wales through the last decades of the nineteenth century and the early decades of the twentieth, and local newspapers of the time are full of articles and correspondence treating the 'doctors' question', as the struggle over control was usually termed in such periodicals. In such an environment, sensitivities were heightened and complaints more numerous.

The outcomes of these various complaints about practitioners varied from dismissal of the doctor to censure, as well as to the exoneration of the physician. Perhaps inevitably, given its size and the number of practitioners it employed, not to mention its particularly strained relations with the medical establishment, Ebbw Vale was the scheme that dismissed most doctors; it experienced a particularly high turnover in medical staff in the decade or so before the outbreak of the First World War.[50] Interestingly, no doctors were dismissed from the scheme during the war years, though this, of course, was a time when the scheme was short-staffed as a result of the enlistment of medical men in the armed forces, and physicians found guilty of misdemeanours in these years were merely censured for behaviour that would previously have resulted in their dismissal.[51]

An interesting feature of cases in which dismissal was decided, and one that demonstrates the very subjective nature of evaluations of a doctor's worth, was that in a few instances, decisions to terminate a physician's position were criticised or appealed by sections of the doctor's patients and committees were requested to rescind their decisions. The sociologist Charles F. Hanna, in his study of the 'complaint form of association', noted the integrative and disintegrative consequences of complaint and, while the integrative consequences are immediately obvious in the numerous collective actions taken by the members of medical schemes against their doctors, it is also possible to discern instances in which complaint caused the disintegration of consensus among associations of working people.[52] This happened at Bedlinog in 1921 when the committee's decision to ask for Dr Evans' resignation or, if that was not forthcoming, to dismiss him, was appealed by some members. After a great many public meetings of the membership and a series of ballots, the decision was overturned; the committee resigned *en masse* and was replaced by a new committee of Evans' supporters,[53] which demonstrates (as does Newsom Kerr in this volume) the impact a collective may have on complaints and decisions. A few months later, the new committee was also forced to hear grievances against Evans, but the doctor died before action could be taken against him and the committee was again replaced.[54]

In the case of Dr Irwin at Ebbw Vale in 1911, mentioned above, a public meeting was held at Victoria, the district in which his practice was situated, after the decision to dismiss him and a majority voted in favour of a resolution calling on the committee to rescind its ruling. Significantly, the committee meeting at which this result was discussed also received a deputation from the minority at that public meeting, who had voted against the appeal that the decision be rescinded, and each member of the deputation had a grievance against Irwin.[55] Similarly, in the case of Dr D. R. Bowen, also at Ebbw Vale and also discussed previously, a public meeting called by the committee to discuss the appointment of a successor to Bowen and a proposed reorganisation of the scheme in Beaufort resolved by a large majority that the committee be asked to withdraw its resolution to dismiss Bowen; it was found that members who voted for this resolution 'admitted his [Bowen's] faults but were prepared to overlook them'. The Beaufort residents formed their own board and presented a petition with 645 signatures to the committee that demanded that Bowen be reinstated. They declared that they would not accept any doctor in place of Bowen and threatened to leave the scheme if the jury upheld its resolution. In the event, the jury refused to rescind their decision and Bowen was subsequently dismissed.[56]

Such cases emphasise the very personal nature of doctor–patient relations and the extent to which approval or disapproval of a physician was based on the individual, particular and subjective face-to-face meetings between patients and practitioners. It also serves as a reminder that despite the strained doctor–patient relations in south Wales and the considerable amount of struggle and disagreement between doctors and workmen's committees, many practitioners were held in high esteem by innumerable patients who remained loyal to them notwithstanding the criticisms or complaints levelled at them by other individuals.

A good standard of care, or a kindness done to a patient by a doctor, could inspire tremendous loyalty in the face of disastrous or negligent conduct suffered by other patients.

Conclusion

The distinctive workers' medical schemes in industrial south Wales gave rise to a situation in which large numbers of complaints were brought by patients against their doctors. This was a product, perhaps an inevitable outcome, of the organisational characteristics of the schemes. These were, in many cases, sizable practices with large numbers of working-class patients, many of whom worked in dangerous occupations in which minor impairments were a daily occurrence and major injuries very common. As Klein notes, illness was an everyday matter to a doctor, to be dealt with in a routine manner; for the patient, on the other hand, and as León-Sanz contends, it was a 'unique event, charged with emotion'.[57] This difference in perspective was exacerbated by the dominant, labourist perspective that health and working capacity were crucially important to the well-being of the worker's family and therefore even more charged with significance. Furthermore, larger medical schemes possessed greater numbers of (often overworked) doctors who were subject to considerable strain and prone to alcohol abuse. In this particularly febrile environment, the large volume of daily doctor–patient interactions perhaps inevitably led to a large number of complaints.

It is also the case, however, that the schemes were characterised by a distinctive political economy of healthcare in which members, or patients, exercised a significant degree of control through their representative committees. Furthermore, these councils were prepared to utilise what Aneurin Bevan – a trade unionist and later MP from south Wales who became Minister of Health and architect of the National Health Service – described as that 'bump of irreverence' that was determined to subordinate professional expertise to lay control and authority.[58] Due to the bitter struggles waged between members and doctors for control of these medical schemes in the late nineteenth century and the early twentieth, workers were very sensitive to their position within these organisations and were determined that if they paid the piper, they should call the tune. This stands in stark contrast to the relative powerlessness of patients' groups in the second half of the twentieth century, identified by Alex Mold in this volume, and it might be argued that the complaints of workers, at least in such schemes, had greater force than those of patients, citizens or consumers in the later period. Complaint was one of the means by which workers and their representatives exercised authority over professional expertise and status.

Notes

1 South Wales Coalfield Collection, Swansea University, Bedlinog Medical Committee, Minutes [hereafter BMCM], 1, 3 June 1921.
2 D. J. V. Jones, *The Last Rising: The Newport Chartist Insurrection of 1839* (Cardiff, 1999), pp. 7–8; J. Davies, *A History of Wales* (London, 1993), pp. 351–352; S. Hughes, *Copperopolis: Landscapes of the Early Industrial Period in Swansea* (Aberystwyth, 2000).
3 *Comparative Account of Population of Great Britain, 1801, 1811, 1821 and 1831*, 348 (1831), xviii, pp. 407–408; Census of England and Wales, 1871, Population tables, Vol. II: Registration counties, p. 527; Census of England and Wales, 1911, Vol. 1: Administrative areas, pp. 5, 7.
4 E. W. Evans, *The Miners of South Wales* (Cardiff, 1961), pp. 237, 241; J. Benson, *British Coalminers in the Nineteenth Century: A Social History* (London, 1980), pp. 216–217.
5 K. O. Morgan, *Rebirth of a Nation: Wales 1880–1980* (Oxford, 1980); H. Francis and D. Smith, *The Fed: A History of the South Wales Miners in the Twentieth Century* (London, 1980); C. Williams, *Capitalism, Community and Conflict: The South Wales Coalfield 1898–1947* (Cardiff, 1998).
6 On workers' medical schemes in south Wales, see R. Earwicker, 'Miners' Medical Services before the First World War: The South Wales Coalfield', *Llafur*, 3, 2 (1981), pp. 39–52; S. Thompson, 'A Proletarian Public Sphere: Working-class Self-provision of Medical Services and Care in South Wales, *c.*1900–1948', in A. Borsay (ed.), *Medicine in Wales, c.1800–2000: Public Service or Private Commodity?* (Cardiff, 2003), pp. 86–107; D. G. Green, *Working-Class Patients and the Medical Establishment* (Aldershot, 1985).
7 Earwicker, 'Miners' Medical Services'; Thompson, 'A Proletarian Public Sphere'; Green, *Working-Class Patients*.
8 *Report for 1912–13 on the Administration of the National Insurance Act, Part 1 (Health Insurance)* [Cd.6907], 1913, xxxvi, p. 480.
9 At Tredegar, for example, it was estimated that roughly 22,800 of the urban district's 25,110 people were members of the scheme by the 1920s; M. Foot, *Aneurin Bevan, A Biography*, Vol. 1 (London, 1963), p. 63; H. Finch, *Memoirs of a Bedwellty MP* (Newport, 1972), pp. 33–35; Green, *Working-Class Patients*, p. 174.
10 See Political and Economic Planning, *Report on the British Health Services* (London, 1937), pp. 151–152.
11 For contemporary accounts, see *British Medical Journal* [hereafter *BMJ*] (22 July 1905), Supplement; *BMJ* (11 September 1920), Supplement, pp. 73–76. On BMA efforts to organise to meet the challenges posed by 'contract' or 'club practice', see P. Bartrip, *Themselves Writ Large: The British Medical Association 1832–1966* (London, 1996), pp. 133–150.
12 The minutes are excellent sources on the particular character of individual complaints but cannot be used to count the numbers of complaints. Too often, the minutes mention that 'numerous complaints' had been received about a particular doctor or else that the secretary or another committee member was investigating complaints without exact details being entered into the minutes.
13 The population of the Maesteg Urban District was 28,917 by 1921 and, of the 10,838 occupied males, 7,213 were engaged in coal-mining; Census of England and Wales, 1921: County of Glamorgan, pp. 1, 35.
14 *Report for 1912–13 on the Administration of the National Insurance Act*, p. 658.

15 Census of England and Wales, 1921: County of Monmouth, pp. 1, 21, 23.
16 A. Gray-Jones, *A History of Ebbw Vale* (Risca, 1970), p. 245.
17 For examples, see Gwent Archives, Ebbw Vale Workmen's Medical Aid Society Minutes [hereafter EVWMASM], 3 September 1910; *Rules of the Tredegar Workmen's Medical Aid Society* (Tredegar, 1913), p. 7.
18 *Merthyr Express* (22 November 1913).
19 For cases of doctors resigning in protest during the investigation of a complaint or refusing to appear when summoned by a workmen's committee, see EVWMASM, 22 April 1905, 1 May 1905, 26 April 1919.
20 R. Klein, *Complaints Against Doctors: A Study in Professional Accountability* (London, 1973), pp. 43–44.
21 EVWMASM, 27 November 1915.
22 EVWMASM, 27 April, 18 September 1918.
23 Ibid., 8, 11, 13, 15, 19, 24 November 1913; *Merthyr Express* (22 November 1913).
24 See the case of Edgar Jones, who complained that Dr Irwin had suggested that his wife rise from her bed, but was then told by Dr O'Sullivan that she should remain there; his case was dismissed without investigation; EVWMASM, 7 May 1910.
25 As an example, a complaint against Dr McDermott at Ebbw Vale in 1909 was dismissed chiefly as a result of the complainant having taken his son out of hospital against the recommendation of McDermott; EVWMASM, 15 September 1909.
26 *Merthyr Pioneer* (18 October 1913); BMCM, 24 June 1922; Copy of agreement between committee and Dr W. David Jenkins, 1 July 1922; EVWMASM, 2 December 1913.
27 EVWMASM, 2 August 1907.
28 EVWMASM, 4 February 1908.
29 J. Mullin, *The Story of a Toiler's Life* (London, 1921), p. 151.
30 It was stated by one of the scheme's doctors in 1900 that a recent General Medical Council requirement that assistant doctors in such schemes be fully qualified had made it more difficult to appoint sufficient numbers of assistants and that large salaries needed to be paid to attract them as a result; he also claimed that the scheme paid less to assistants than other schemes in the region; EVWMASM, 26 May 1900.
31 F. Maylett Smith, *The Surgery at Aberffrwd: Some Encounters of a Colliery Doctor some Seventy Years Ago* (Hythe, Kent, 1981), p. 88; A. J. Cronin, *The Citadel* (London, 1937/1949), p. 12.
32 For examples, see Glamorgan Archives, BMA, South Wales and Monmouthshire Branch, minute book (hereafter SWMBMB), 2 May 1899, and Monmouthshire Division of the BMA, minute book (hereafter MDBMAMB), 17 April 1905; EVWMASM, 16 April 1905. A regular series of 'Warning Notices' was published in the *BMJ* to discourage prospective applicants from applying for positions in schemes that did not meet the BMA's approval, while 'black lists' of doctors willing to go against the BMA and accept positions on such schemes were drawn up by the regional branches. Some such doctors, described as 'black legs', were eventually expelled from the BMA, as happened to Dr R. A. Neilson, one of the Ebbw Vale scheme's doctors in 1906; BMA, SWMBMB, 13 December 1906.
33 Indeed, A. J. Cronin claimed in his autobiography that practices in south Wales attracted 'a draggled succession of "dead beats", doctors who had failed elsewhere, fallen into disrepute, or even been struck off the register for professional misconduct'; A. J. Cronin, *Adventures in Two Worlds* (London, 1952), p. 125.
34 BMCM, see 3 June 1921; EVWMASM, 21 May 1910.

35 EVWMASM, 22 November 1913.
36 *Rhondda Leader* (11 January 1902), p. 6 ('Shoni' was a colloquial Welsh term for a less than respectable individual); for a similar accusation of rudeness, especially to women and children, see *Merthyr Express* (11 January 1902), p. 3.
37 EVWMASM, 2 December 1912.
38 EVWMASM, 21 January 1905.
39 Mullin, *The Story of a Toiler's Life*, p. 152.
40 F. Maylett Smith, *A G.P.'s Progress to the Black Country* (Hythe, Kent, 1984), p. 127.
41 A. Cox, 'The Future of Colliery Practice in South Wales and Monmouthshire – Servitude or Independence', *BMJ* (11 September 1920), Supplement, p. 74.
42 For examples of such rhetoric, see *BMJ* (22 July 1905), Supplement, p. 5, which lists a number of difficulties caused by 'government by non-medical committees', including 'The ignorance of non-medical committees concerning the conditions which are central to efficiency of a medical service'; also, *The Lancet* (7 October 1905), p. 1065; *The Lancet* (25 November 1905), pp. 1573–1574; MDBMAMB, 1 September 1905.
43 For an example, see the disdain of Dr Cluich, who resigned from service in the Ebbw Vale scheme rather than continue to defend himself to a committee of workmen that was not prepared to accept him at his word; EVWMASM, 22 April 1905.
44 *BMJ* (22 July 1905), Supplement, p. 89; Klein, *Complaints Against Doctors*, p. 60.
45 BMCM, see 1, 3 June 1921; EVWMASM, 13 July 1907.
46 EVWMASM, 4 February 1911.
47 EVWMASM, 17 June 1911.
48 EVWMASM, 17, 26 August 1911.
49 EVWMASM, 17 November 1900, 1 December 1900. For another example, see 22 August 1896.
50 From 1900 to 1909, nine doctors were dismissed by the Ebbw Vale Workmen's Medical Aid Society, a rate of one doctor per year; in 1910, two doctors were dismissed and this increased to three in 1911; EVWMASM, 1900–11, *passim*.
51 EVWMASM, 1914–18, *passim*.
52 C. F. Hanna, 'Complaint as a Form of Association', *Qualitative Sociology*, 4, 4 (1981), p. 303.
53 BMCM, 5 October, 4, 10, 14, 17 November, 2, 16 December 1921.
54 BMCM, 9 March, 22 May 1922.
55 EVWMASM, 25 February 1911.
56 EVWMASM, 14, 23 February, 11, 23, 26 March 1901.
57 Klein, *Complaints Against Doctors*, p. 47.
58 *Tribune* (13 May 1938).

5 From claims to rights

Patient complaints and the evolution of a Spanish mutual aid society (Sociedad Protectora de Obreros La Conciliación, Pamplona, 1902–36)

*Pilar León-Sanz**

Compulsory health insurance was not formalised in Spain until the 1940s. Before that, approximately two-thirds of Spanish workers and their families entrusted their healthcare to diverse mutual assistance societies, mutual insurance associations and other private institutions.[1] An analysis of the assistance offered by these organisations illuminates the social climate that led to requiring citizens to procure obligatory insurance coverage. This chapter focuses on worker members' complaints about the medical service given by the Spanish mutual insurance association Sociedad Protectora de Obreros La Conciliación in Pamplona between its establishment in 1902 and 1936, in order to elucidate key issues in medical service at the time; indeed, in comparing these issues to those discussed in Steven Thompson's chapter about a similar scheme in south Wales, further insights may be drawn into the particularity of place and the nature of complaint.

Mutual benefit societies and mutual insurance associations such as La Conciliación were a collective means of voluntary provision that developed separately from the state. Some of these societies had their roots in the old trade guilds, but the majority were new, promoted by the 1887 Spanish Law on Associations. In general, the mutual societies were classified according to their sponsors' ideologies and their social composition.[2] La Conciliación (1902–84) was founded in Pamplona as an exclusively male Catholic society (women were first admitted in 1936). It was composed of workers, employers and protector members,[3] with labour, healthcare and economic objectives, and was under a governing 'Mixed Board' (see Figure 5.1) with representatives from the three cohorts. The worker members were grouped into guilds, including carpenters, cobblers, tailors, shop assistants, bakers, typographers, and chocolate makers.

Pamplona is the capital city of Navarra, a region of northern Spain. The population of Pamplona remained unchanged during the first two decades of the twentieth century. This stagnation was due, among other reasons, to the difficulties caused by the fact that it was a walled town, and, particularly, to the slow process of industrialisation, which was held back by the Carlist Wars. Moreover, between

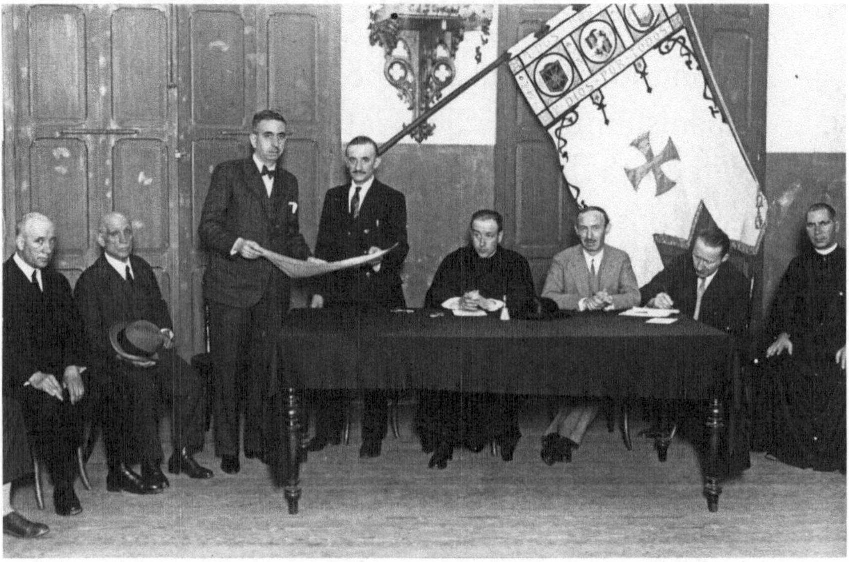

Figure 5.1 The board of La Conciliación, the body that dealt with complaints, on the feast day of La Conciliación, 14 June 1931. The five figures at the table are, from left to right: D. Luis Ortega Angulo (former president) receiving a diploma from Mr Justo Garrán y Mosso (president) in recognition of his work for La Conciliación; Mr Pablo Goñi (chaplain); Mr Jesús Ruíz River (provincial government representative); and Mr Pedro José Arraiza (secretary) (photograph by José Gallego Galle, 1931; courtesy of the Archivo Municipal de Pamplona).

1900 and 1920, a large number of Navarrese migrated.[4] Pamplona also suffered high unemployment.[5] The early twentieth century saw Spain in general, and Pamplona in particular, marked by social crisis and political and labour unrest, which resulted, *inter alia*, in problems of food distribution.

The 'foral' regime and the Diputación (provincial government) were of particular importance to the political landscape of the area, as Navarra was unusual in having administrative autonomy from the central government. The Diputación Foral de Navarra was therefore directly responsible for matters such as the social welfare of the region. In the early part of the twentieth century, conservative parties held power in both the local and regional government.[6] Although not all of these supported La Conciliación,[7] the Society had government backing and institutional aid because, La Conciliación argued, 'the Association saved these corporations a great deal of money in beneficence and other expenses'.[8] For example, the Society co-operative helped ensure that the price of milk, coal and other basic supplies were reduced, an initiative promoted by the Town Council. Of particular importance in this area were the personal contacts of the Society's protector-members (who might be termed subscribers in the context of British charities); they produced synergies with government bodies, which helped La Conciliación to participate in the political life and the physical and social construction of the city.[9]

Pamplona had the same medical healthcare systems as in the rest of Spain. Mutual benefit societies and mutual insurance associations provided medical assistance to over one-third of the city's population, which at the time was 30,000. As we will see, assistance in an urban area was made up of a patchwork of different systems and organisations, together with the less formal initiatives and activities promoted by individuals and families. Several studies have analysed the situation of medical and social associations in Navarra in the period under consideration.[10] Catholic inspiration lay behind many of the workmen's institutions.[11] There is unanimity that, in Pamplona, socialism did not become a social force until 1923, which explains why the number of members in La Conciliación at the time was far higher than those of the socialist Federación.[12] On issues of medical care for its members, La Conciliación habitually co-operated with the mutual aid societies and guilds in Pamplona, including the Craftsmen's Guild (the oldest in the city, founded in the latter half of the nineteenth century), the Workers' Union and the Sodality of the Passion. Even so, La Conciliación was fiercely independent in its criteria and actions.

Between 1902 and 1936, political structures ultimately transformed La Conciliación from a mixed mutual aid society into a workers' association and, finally, into a mutual insurance association. Changes in the association happened gradually, reflecting the growing role of the worker members. The transformations shed light on the relationship between the organisation and current labour conditions, as well as changes in social and labour legislation.[13] La Conciliación existed until 1984, although it underwent major shifts in the number of members and structure during the Spanish Civil War (1936–39). For this reason, the present study centres on the years before the Civil War in order to examine the progress of the original project, the members' sense of the association's identity, and the role that complaining played in the shaping of local medical services.[14]

In general, an analysis of the complaints about physicians shows us the complexity of social relations between the Society's management and the doctors employed by them on the one hand, and on the other hand those entitled to social and medical assistance: the worker members and their families.[15] By 1936, the Society had over 1,000 members. The sources reveal the lifestyles and medical experiences of the Society's members, contributing to our understanding of workers', employers' and protector-members' attitudes as articulated in the nature of the issues they raised.

The stories behind these complaints also reveal the emotional lives of those involved in La Conciliación. To paraphrase historian Barbara Rosenwein, emotions appear when what happens affects our wellbeing; they arise from our values and assessments. In the stories on complaints about medical attention, social groupings were characterised by common interests and objectives and exemplify Rosenwein's notion of 'emotional communities', which

> are precisely the same as social communities – families, neighbourhoods, parliaments, guilds, monasteries, parish church membership – but the researcher looking at them seeks above all to uncover systems of feeling: what these communities (and the individuals within them) define and assess as valuable or harmful to them; the evaluations that they make about others' emotions; the nature of the affective bonds between people that they recognize; and the modes of emotional expression that they expect, encourage, tolerate, and deplore.[16]

The worker members of La Conciliación, a group with common interests and goals, demonstrated similar appreciations of emotions and manners of expression in the complaints found in the Society's records. This chapter will briefly consider particular epistemological aspects discerned from the perspective of studies of emotions because 'the history of emotions likewise rewrites the narrative of class formation and class relations', making 'emotional style ... an important marker of class identity'.[17]

Although important professional issues are noted in the sources, this study focuses on when and how early-twentieth-century labourers complained about medical assistance; their most common complaints and how these were dealt with; and the influence and leverage of patients' emotions in the issues they raised and in their demands. The Society's archives contain its regulations, accounts, correspondence, invoices and minutes, including those of the Mixed Board's weekly meetings, which reported on its medical team and medical assistance. From these documents the manner in which complaints were formulated is explored, taking note of the expressions of the feelings and intentions of the worker members and the measures taken by the board to resolve grievances. Following the ideas of the historian Peter Stearns, an emotional culture may be identified among the workers which, far from being irrational, sought improvements for the healthcare beneficiaries.[18]

The complaints procedure at the mutual assistance association La Conciliación

La Conciliación initially offered its members labour mediation, economic subsidies and medical assistance, expanding to pharmaceutical services (from 1910), a Chronic Fund and midwifery service (from 1914), and post-mortem aid (from 1918). It also founded a savings bank and a co-operative (1912 and 1922, respectively). In addition, it organised educational and recreational activities for its members.[19] The Society covered only ambulatory medical assistance for the workers and their families' common illnesses, unless this was covered by another organisation such as a beneficence institution. Association physicians received members in their consulting rooms and made house calls.[20]

Between 1902 and 1936, La Conciliación employed the services of four physicians at any one time. The first group was composed of Agustín Lazcano, Joaquín Gortari, Teodoro Lizasoain and Santiago Abadía. In February 1905, Joaquín Gortari was replaced by Saturnino Martínez. From February 1907, Pedro Subelza took the place of Santiago Abadía, to assist the member families who lived up to 10 kilometres outside the city.[21] From 1914 and in the 1920s, the four physicians were Pedro Subelza, Sergio Lazcano, Saturnino Lizarraga and Ramón Sanz, who was replaced by José Alfaro in 1926.[22] Studies have shown that La Conciliación was an established part of Pamplona's medical healthcare network.[23]

The physicians employed by La Conciliación were paid 6.25 pesetas per family for those within the city and 9 pesetas for the families outside.[24] Pamplona was divided into four areas: in the two districts with the greatest number of families, the doctor's annual pay was approximately 3,000 pesetas (£155 annually), and in the smaller districts (such as the one attended by Dr Sanz) only 700 pesetas (£36).[25] This system and the salaries were similar to those of other mutual benefit societies in Spain at the time.[26]

From the beginning, periodically, the Mixed Board decided 'to advise these people [the worker members] that those who have complaints about the doctors should make their complaints to the Board in writing, so that, if fitting, the appropriate measures can be taken'.[27] Expressions of dissatisfaction by La Conciliación's members tended to be associated with complaints, which illustrates Klein's idea that complaints are only the visible tip of the iceberg of discontent.[28]

While patients' complaints generally focused on medical or pharmaceutical assistance, this chapter will examine only the claims made against medical care. A comparative reading of the complaints reveals patterns in the sites and sources of complaint and therefore suggests the characteristics of medical care and consequent patient behaviour. As a rule, when a complaint was filed, the person against whom it was made was given the opportunity to provide their version of the event. When the complaint was of particular importance, such as serious suspicions of malpractice, a commission was set up or an individual entrusted with the investigation. On other occasions, the parties involved were summoned to testify to the Board. If the situation could not be resolved in this manner, other physicians were called upon to give their opinion.[29] A protector-member of the Mixed Board always took part in the examination of medical-pharmaceutical issues. Finally, the result of the investigation was made known to the complainant. Similar procedures were followed in other European healthcare organisations.[30] A 1909 example may be considered a typical case:

> The President reported in a letter that Don Ángel Guerrero, a member of the Farmers' Guild, made a complaint about the conduct of the Society physician Don Ramón Sanz. The Board agreed to contact R. Sanz and ask him to explain to them what he considered appropriate in his defence on the subject of the accusations made in said letter.[31]

The minutes of the following meeting read:

> The official note presented by the physician Don Ramón Sanz was read out. It presented reasonable statements on the accusations presented by the member Ángel Guerrero. The Board agreed and sent a copy of the official note to the member.[32]

The majority of the members' complaints were focused on what they perceived as physicians' lack of attention, lack of punctuality or failure to resolve health problems. These complaints forced the Board to remind doctors of their obligation to 'fulfil the exact conditions of all parts of the regulations', which established the duties and responsibilities of the physicians.[33] At the same time, the Board reminded the members that they 'should ensure the suitability in time and form' of the complaints they made.[34] Apart from these complaints, the Board enforced an inspection demand system: 'the Inspector [would] observe if the La Conciliación patients [received] proper medical care and [would] inform the Board of the result of his inquiries'.[35]

Complaints about medical assistance: the case of Dr Ramón Sanz

Records show that complaints were made about all the physicians. But there was one general practitioner, Ramón Sanz, whose irresponsibility and carelessness became so notorious that some Society members threatened to cancel their membership if he was permitted to continue as their doctor. Members repeatedly tried to alter his contract through verbal and written complaints, and finally managed to terminate his appointment. The process of complaints and replies shows us how the Society operated, again illustrating the social climate of the time. What the case and discussions in the following section also illustrate – as do Wall, Thompson, Mold and Newsom Kerr in this volume – is the impact of a collective on the outcome of the complaint; the case similarly reveals how effective (or not) an internal inquiry may be and serves as a useful counterpoint to both McHale's independent inquiries and many of those complaints made under the glare of the media.

Sanz began working as a substitute physician for La Conciliación in 1908. From December of that year until December 1914, he attended to the patients who lived outside Pamplona. Later, he worked in the city, taking charge of the smallest group of members, thus making him the Society doctor with the lowest wages. In October 1913, a La Conciliación member, Pío Pérez, complained about what he considered 'insufficient attention paid to a member of his family by the physician Don Ramón Sanz'. When he was informed of this complaint, Sanz replied that 'he mislaid the call note and forgot about this patient among the many he had to visit, but that he had returned to attend the person in question before receiving the President's summons'. At the time, the Board accepted his explanation and closed the inquiry.[36] Other complaints against Sanz noted that he did not respond to summons, and that he delayed giving patients their sick notes. Aid depended on being given a sick note that stated the diagnosis, which had to be signed by one of La Conciliación's doctors. If a sick note was not presented on time, there was an investigation to see if this was due to the physician or the member.[37]

In 1917, a verbal complaint against Sanz was made by the delegate of the Bakers' Guild. When the President of the Board took him to task about these complaints, Sanz justified his neglect of these patients by declaring that he had 'simultaneously been called by another patient and had later called another physician'. In the case of the baker, he 'had not received the message, which might have been mislaid by his serving woman'. The President considered that, given the diversity of opinions, the differences could only be settled in a face-to-face meeting, but despite the meeting the problem was not resolved.[38]

Other complaints were more serious and appear to refer to harmful decisions by Sanz. Specifically, for example, two complaints were read at a meeting in 1916: One described how the physician had been urgently summoned in the afternoon of 9 March to attend to the son of a member, but did not appear until about 10.30 p.m. because he had been at the handball court. By the time Sanz arrived at the house, the boy was dead.[39] The other complaint was lodged by a locksmith who asked for his medical service to be cancelled because, despite Sanz having seen his son 10 times about a nasal problem, the doctor refused to operate on the boy. The locksmith then went to another physician who immediately 'operated and four days later the boy was cured'. The affair cost the plaintiff 25 pesetas, but he preferred to pay the new doctor rather than have to deal with Sanz again. Both demands, and the Board's displeasure, were communicated to Sanz. Indeed, the Board stated that 'he did not possess the qualities required of a physician for La Conciliación'.[40] Sanz responded with a lengthy letter which insisted that:

> First, the letters of cancellation are groundless, they are non-specific complaints; second, his presence at the Euskal-Jay handball court is not at all incompatible with his visits to patients, he goes when he is called; third, he should be excused for the delay in writing the sick notes for three patients and the discharge of another.

The Board settled the matter with a laconic 'Seen', indicating that the issues had been discussed, but that nothing had been resolved.[41]

Together with the written grievances, there was a trail of individual and collective verbal complaints. At a meeting of the Mixed Board in January 1916, Mr M. Aramendía stated that he would cancel his membership if Dr Sanz were not dismissed.[42] A few months later, the minutes again refer to two locksmiths who wanted to cancel their memberships if Ramón Sanz continued to work there; they would remain in La Conciliación only if they were allowed to choose another physician.[43] The recurrence of the complaints divided the Board: the worker members wanted to dismiss Dr Sanz; others, although in agreement, said this could not be done without a formal accusation, as he had been warned twice and had defended his behaviour. The Board feared appearing foolish a third time.[44] And again, after finding Sanz guilty of delaying the submission of a sick note,[45] the Board sent him a 'brisk Official Note' reminding him of their regulations and expressing their displeasure with his work, stating that it 'will not permit' this behaviour.[46] Sanz's reply is surprising, as he insisted that 'All the members and their families are satisfied with his services and that he always writes the sick notes within the time set down by the Regulations'. The Board filed the manuscript, with a 'No comment'.[47]

Matters did not improve in 1918. In February, the records tell the case of a bricklayer member who complained about Dr Sanz's improper medical care of his son. Apparently, 'he said it was nothing' and, as the boy did not improve, they took him to see Dr Joaquín Gortari, who explained that he needed urgent treatment. As a result of Sanz's neglect, the patient 'died six days afterwards'. The family insisted that 'they would never call him [Sanz] again'. The gravity of the situation forced the Board to set up a commission to examine the case. Sanz admitted to his 'error of diagnosis' and offered to apologise to the bereaved family. He was also given a formal admonition and told that the Board did not wish to receive any more complaints and that, if there was another, 'it would be fatal for him'.[48] But in June, facing the delay in the presentation of a sick note, the Board further warned Sanz not to break the regulations.[49] In December 1918, the President had to speak to him again because he did not attend to a member in an urgent situation; the man died without receiving medical attention. The President stressed the innumerable complaints about his work and urged him to mend his ways, 'threatening' him with expulsion from the Society. Sanz replied that he was aware of dissatisfaction with his work. He insisted that he was fond of the member who had died but that he was not informed of the urgency of the case, so he had visited an hour after receiving the call and on the way had been told of the death.[50] Indeed, Sanz's notoriety led some workers to try to make the most of the situation. In 1919, the Board issued a warning to the member Epitamio Vidaurre because he had not paid his membership fee while waiting for a solution to his complaint about Dr Sanz. In this case, the Board reminded the member that the open case could not serve as 'an excuse for not fulfilling his [the member's] obligations'.[51]

The situation was partially resolved in 1921, when the Society decided that its members could choose freely from among its physicians. Four months after the new regulations came into effect, in May 1921,

> a letter from the physician Don Ramón Sanz was read out, in which he expressed his surprise at the considerable drop in his reimbursement for the month of May, and stated that he should have been given a list of all the members he had to visit with their names and addresses well in advance.[52]

The Board then delivered to Dr Sanz the substantially shorter list of the members who had chosen him as their doctor, together with their agreement that he should act in accordance with 'the new list which was in his hands exclusively for the present'.[53]

The Mixed Board of La Conciliación unanimously agreed to dismiss Dr Sanz in October 1926. However, this decision was challenged, leading to the resignation of several protector members. This explains why the Board had not made the decision earlier, in spite of over a decade of complaints against Sanz, who was supported by powerful members of Pamplona society at the time (none of whom were his patients). The Board stated, in his defence, that 'The secretary of the Guild of Clerks was responsible for the campaign against Dr Sanz, and the reason for this ill-will was that one of the Secretary's daughters had died' while under his care. The Mixed Board of La Conciliación was forced to give an explanation to the College of Physicians of Navarra and send an official note to the Provincial Governor. But the decision was made, and on 23 November 1926, Dr Ramón Sanz was replaced by Dr José Alfaro.[54]

Analysing the medical complaints

The complaints found in the 1902–1936 records reveal marked similarities in patient dissatisfaction. As the case of Dr Sanz suggests, although some of the complaints discovered in the archives of La Conciliación refer to unspecified 'poor care', most can be divided into three groups: improper medical attention (delays in the doctor's arrival, failure to make home visits or the medical problem not being resolved); delays in writing or delivering sick leave certificates or discharge notes; and issues regarding the payment of medical fees in extraordinary circumstances or when the patients were attended to by physicians from outside the Society.[55]

The most frequent complaint made by the doctors was associated with members seeking medical attention from external sources. The regulations passed in December 1902 state that 'members who are attended by other societies will lose their rights to medical attention by La Conciliación, although all members will receive the same monetary aid'.[56] This issue led to discontent and unease between members and physicians, as the latter claimed they were frequently summoned by members who did not have the right to assistance. Dr J. Gortari, for example, abandoned La Conciliación's medical team following a complaint by a member who, according to the physician, had no right to healthcare from the Society.[57]

On other occasions, complaints were made when physicians refused to make house calls, as they thought patients could travel to their clinics. This led to the dismissal of Dr S. Abadía who, in spite of 'having been called twice', refused to visit the home of the member Juan Cilveti to attend to his wife and daughter. In his defence, Abadía argued that patients with skin rashes could come to his clinic. When Dr A. Lazcano, who had been sent instead, was asked if the women could have gone to the clinic, he replied that 'the girl with the rash could indeed have gone, but the patient also had bronchitis, and Dr S. Abadía had not been informed about this point by the family'.[58]

As was the case for Dr Sanz, when it came to paying a La Conciliación physician or any other doctor in the city, there was always a demand from a labourer eager to recover his money. In 1907, the Farm Workers' Guild reported that Agustín Lazcano had wanted to charge a fee of 23 pesetas for his assistance to a member, Juan Cilveti, who argued that his dues were paid. Lazcano claimed that this was an additional consultation, as he was not the family doctor and had attended to Cilveti only because the President of the Mixed Board had specifically asked him to.[59] In 1915, the Secretary of the Bakers' Guild complained about Agustín Lazcano because he had charged 25 pesetas for assisting his wife in childbirth. Apparently, Sergio Lazcano had sent his father, Agustín, by then retired, to assist this woman, and then charged the family a fee.[60] The following year, another member, José Martínez, wrote an irate complaint regarding Pedro Subelza. He accused the practitioner of not attending to his daughter properly, making it necessary for Martínez to call another doctor, who subsequently charged him 52 pesetas. To prove his discontent, the labourer abandoned the Society; this action was counterproductive because, although the Board interviewed Subelza to study the issue, as Martínez was no longer a member the Board did not bother to reimburse him the monies demanded.[61] Similar objections are recorded in the 1930s. For example, in 1934 a member of the 'Artes blancas' (Bakers') Guild protested to the Mixed Board about its physician, Mr Repáraz, because 'He refused to attend his wife who had an injured hand'. This meant that the member had to pay 50 pesetas to the Casa de Socorro (the First Aid Station).[62] In this case, the doctor's response to the Board was satisfactory and the incident was filed away.[63]

From their responses to the complaints presented, it appears that the Board was prudent in making judgements, particularly with regard to individual physicians. On the one hand, many of the Society's doctors were also prominent actors in civil life, which made any sanctions taken against them potentially scandalous. Also, members of the Mixed Board were often socially and politically connected with the practitioners, which may have led them to look upon their friends with leniency or to fear the repercussions of strong actions, even when the evidence was overwhelming, as in the case of Dr Sanz.

The language and tone of complaints: the paradigms of emotional communities

Many of the patient complaints archived in the Society's files contain specific references to emotions. Patients expressed 'grief' at not receiving assistance after having 'asked for it twice'.[64] In other cases, like that of Pío Pérez, the attention received by a member of his family from the La Conciliación physician was considered 'deficient', leading to family distress.[65] Another member stated that the doctor 'did not assist his wife properly'.[66] When complaints worsened, members angrily threatened to 'abandon the service', or declared that 'they [would] never call ... [the doctor] again'.[67] The words the members used when complaining include pain, sorrow, insecurity or sadness. Generally, they emphasise their feelings of helplessness or vulnerability because of the doctors' indifference to their summons; distress and anger at what they perceived as superficial attention; and resentment, anguish and grief at what they considered the preventable death of family members, many of them children.

The language deployed by the worker members in their letters of complaint reveals the workings of emotional practices, and conveys a sense of emotions as 'social facts'. Emotions are constitutive of human nature and by inference constitutive of social life. At the same time, social facts combine emotional valence, cultural meanings and institutional arrangements. Both facts and actions can be explained and justified by narratives.[68] Traditionally, historians of emotions believe that emotional practices are habits, or rituals that aid people in achieving certain emotional states. They are part of what is often referred to as 'emotional management', and emotions are, perhaps most obviously, practices involved in communication. In this case, the worker members of La Conciliación used them as a means of exchange in a specific social context.[69] Arguably, emphasis on emotions in medical complaints was an effective tool for the kind of recompense or solutions that the members sought.[70]

The similarities in the objectives pursued and the language utilised in these narratives allow us to classify the claimants as an emotional group: they expressed the concerns of a collection of people and the general perspective reflected the interests of each of the individual complainants. In her work on medical narratives, Rita Charon has explained how these texts support the singularity, temporality and intersubjectivity of each medical encounter.[71] So we need to read the workers' complaints on both a personal and a collective level to comprehend the nature and possibilities of a community of emotions.

The language used in the complaints reveals the petitioners' worries for themselves, other members, and the Society itself. These cases often condemned the Society's perceived incompetent management, not only on the complainants' own behalf, but also for the whole organisation. Though complaints were most often personal, records show instances of collective action, notably in June 1917 when, apart from specific individual complaints, the Master of the Bakers' Guild demanded a solution for the faulty pharmaceutical service that affected many members.[72] Here, collective action served to support the workers' autonomy and agency, as they wielded their complaints as a weapon to defend themselves against specific practices such as physicians' control of sick-leave permits. These social interactions and group relations became a source of rules, norms and mechanisms of control, which led to a heightened capacity to make decisions and to act.

Between 1902 and 1936, the number and tone of the complaints changed. In the 1920s, the members' views of the Board's indecision or delays in response led to an escalation in the tone and nature of the threats aimed at forcing the Board to act on their behalf.[73] Many members threatened to leave the Society if their grievances were not addressed; others noted the scandal caused by inaction. At the end of the period studied, not only was the consideration of the Board requested, but a solution for the repeated lack of adequate response was required. This view highlights the key connections between emotions and economy. In numerous cases studied, issues related to fees for medical attention provoked the complaints, stressing the connection between the choices made by the members and their views regarding the assistance they received. Workers who filed complaints were exercising their right to choose. It has been said that in the late nineteenth century and the early twentieth, institutions such as La Conciliación blended emotional and rational perspectives on society.[74]

Changing attitudes in La Conciliación

The Mixed Board of La Conciliación was well aware of the members' complaints. Their responses might be understood as a way to retain member confidence in the institution. Trust is a judgment made about actions, so the Board's efforts to respond rapidly to queries and complaints illustrate its desire to transmit confidence. In this sense, trust is not so much an emotional response as a perception, which is acquired through the actions of individuals or institutions. In effect, a dossier was opened for each complaint and the responses were negotiated. This attitude may have been conditioned by the need to justify the organisation's performance. Replying to the complaints, the Board regularly expressed 'its desire that the members should have as much professional assistance as is their due', an expression that confirms the association's paternalistic nature. Importantly, the Society's economic viability depended on donations, so they needed to ensure the workers' satisfaction.[75] But sometimes the Mixed Board questioned the complaints made by workers by carrying out their own examination and critique of the circumstances surrounding the cases presented.[76]

The archives reveal the Mixed Board's pragmatism. It did not oppose members' demands if the complaint did not imply additional expenses for the Society; it authorised visits to other physicians or folk healers in the town, although it did not cover the treatment of the latter. Due to a complaint made in 1907 about Dr Gortari's inattention, the Mixed Board granted the President of the Society the power to take any necessary measure to resolve problems arising from conflicts between practitioners and worker members. Consequently, the President could entrust any physician belonging to La Conciliación or from Pamplona to attend a member or his family if no other doctor was already attending to them.[77]

Moreover, it is clear that complaints both changed and shaped practice. When, in 1914, a doctor defended himself against a charge of negligence in childbirth by claiming that this service was not included in the regulations, the Society created a position for a midwife.[78] Thereafter, the midwife was responsible for all deliveries, only calling for a physician if the delivery was complicated.[79] The case of the Diverse Services Guild member Florencio Jiménez's complaint confirms the procedure. After Jiménez argued that Dr Pedro Subelza did not attend to his wife properly after the delivery of their child, Subelza explained

> that he had not seen the patient again because the La Conciliación physicians are under no obligation to attend the woman in labour unless they had already been called by the midwife. They see the patient again only if the midwife so demands and this is habitual practice in private cases.[80]

Other changes were provoked by members' claims regarding the procedures for the distribution of sick notes. A lawsuit by the Master of the Bricklayers' Guild was registered because member Felipe Ciaurriz was ill and off work for four days, but was not visited by the physician again. These cases are useful not only to understand the complexities of everyday life but also because they illustrate ordinary people's agency.[81]

From 1916 onwards, the Board began admitting discharges given by doctors who did not belong to La Conciliación.[82] So, towards the end of 1916, when a member complained that the treatment prescribed by Agustín Lazcano had not made him any better and asked for permission to see another practitioner and still receive aid, the Board did not hesitate to approve this demand, but reminded the complainant that 'the La Conciliación physicians must watch over everyone'.[83]

Conclusion: new rights and benefits

The analysis of the medical complaints of worker members of La Conciliación promotes an understanding of how, during the first third of the twentieth century, medical assistance was structured and perceived by physicians and workers. The dissatisfaction of La Conciliación members with the medical services does not appear to be unique. Similar situations of discontent are described in other places and in the context of professional sources at that time.[84]

Clearly, members' individual and collective complaints led to changes in the form and quality of assistance the Society provided. Examples of these include the employment of a midwife, greater flexibility in the control of sick leave, and the freedom to choose one's physician. The prerogatives which resulted from the worker-members' complaints were soon incorporated as rights within La Conciliación's healthcare services. The sources support the idea that, at this time, the worker members of a Spanish mutual aid society took an active role in decisions about their own or their family's healthcare. Though the term 'patient empowerment' did not exist at the time, we have observed that workers members' agency regarding doctors was generalised.[85]

Protests conditioned the professionals' attitudes in a period of debate on the characteristics and development of professional structures. They also provoked significant changes in La Conciliación's medical staff. Indeed, the attitude of the Mixed Board changed over the years. At the outset, the Society was firm with its doctors: members' complaints led to the resignation of two of its physicians (Dr Gortari in January 1905, and Dr Martínez in December 1914).[86] Another (Santiago Abadía) was summarily dismissed by the Mixed Board in 1907, because of a formal complaint about his inattention.[87] Later, the Board became more compliant and ineffective, subject to social and political influences, as noted in its dealings with Dr Sanz. This shift in attitude may have contributed to the increase in complaints in the second decade of the Society's existence.

Examining these case histories allows us to hear the voices of the patients and physicians and to recover subjective experiences. We can understand the everyday ways in which people coped with dissatisfaction and the decisions that followed the claims and grievances. These narratives chart the social experience of illness because, as historian of medicine Roy Porter noted, each patient's story is nuanced by his/her age, gender, social class or economic standing, and many other significant variables.[88] Further, as Rosenwein suggests, since the 1960s, historians have become skilled at writing history from 'the bottom up', uncovering the lives and ways of ordinary people. But

> with the growth of the history of emotions, more and more scholars are trying to write the history of these men and women's subjectivity, to

reconstruct their internal states, for they are committed to writing history not just from the bottom up but from the inside out.[89]

In contrast to tendencies in other areas of social history that focus on large-scale social strata or classes, the analysis of these narratives offers insight into the complexities of social relations within guilds, or between the patients and their families and the professionals involved. This analysis concedes greater importance to people than to places, to quality of life rather than to topographical peculiarities. The patients' stories contribute, at the same time, to our knowledge of the social dimension of the time. Engaging the micro level of doctors' responses to these and other complaints and how they coped with them has implications for a wider debate on socio-political welfare systems. It is here, then, and through the examination of complaints, that the study of patients' stories – read individually and collectively – enhances an understanding of physicians, patients and society, and the relationships forged among them.[90]

Notes

* This study is part of the research project 'Emotional Culture and Identity' (Institute for Culture and Society at the University of Navarra). I am grateful to colleagues in the area of History of Medicine at the University of Navarra for their advice.

1 For the introduction of obligatory insurance in Spain, see M. Vilar-Rodríguez and J. Pons-Pons, 'The Introduction of Sickness Insurance in Spain in the First Decades of the Franco Dictatorship (1939–1962)', *Social History of Medicine*, 26, 2 (2013), pp. 267–287; J. Cuesta, 'El proceso de expansión de los seguros sociales obligatorios. Las dificultades, 1919–1931', *Historia de la acción social publica en España: Beneficencia y previsión* (Madrid, 1990); S. Castillo (ed.), *Solidaridad desde abajo: Trabajadores y socorros mutuos en la España contemporánea* (Madrid, 1994).

2 P. León-Sanz, 'Professional Responsibility and the Welfare System in Spain at the Turn of the 19th Century', *Hygiea Internationalis* 5, 1 (2006), pp. 75–90.

3 Patrons or protector members were those who donated to the institution and were part of the society's Board of Directors.

4 A. García Barbancho, *Las migraciones interiores españolas* (Madrid, 1967); S. Anaut Bravo, *Cambio demográfico y mortalidad en Pamplona (1880–1935)* (Pamplona, 1998).

5 Ángel García-Sanz Marcotegui, 'El Ayuntamiento de Pamplona ante la 'crisis obrera', *Gerónimo de Uztariz: Boletín*, 3 (1989), pp. 26–39.

6 J. Andrés-Gallego, *Navarra cien años de historia* (Pamplona, 2003).

7 J. Andrés-Gallego, *Historia contemporánea de Navarra* (Pamplona, 1982); I. Olabarri Gortazar, 'Notas en torno al problema de la conciencia de identidad colectiva de los navarros en el siglo XIX', in *Congreso de Historia de Euskal Herria* (San Sebastián, 1988), pp. 339–356.

8 Archive of the University of Navarra, *La Conciliación*: *Minute books (1902–1936). Pro manuscript* [hereafter LCBM], 1915, vol. 5, p. 152.

9 P. León-Sanz, 'The Strategies of Interrelations between Assistance Associations and Other Agencies in Pamplona, 1902–1936', in P. León-Sanz (ed.), *Health Institutions at the Origin of the Welfare Systems in Europe* (Pamplona, 2010), pp. 167–192.

10 M. Ferrer Muñoz, 'Panorama asociativo de Navarra entre 1887 y 1936', in *Congreso de Historia de Euskal Herria* (Vitoria, 1988), pp. 49–65.
11 J. Andrés-Gallego, *Pensamiento y acción social de la Iglesia en España* (Madrid, 1984).
12 J. Andrés-Gállego, 'Sobre el inicio de la política obrera contemporánea en Navarra, 1855–1916', *Príncipe de Viana*, 39, 150 (1978), pp. 335–375; J. M. Pejenaute Goñi, 'La Federación Católico Social de Navarra y los partidos políticos del momento (1910–1916)', *Príncipe de Viana*, 5 (1986), pp. 37–51; M. Tuñón de Lara, 'Navarra en los movimientos sociales de la historia contemporánea de España', *Príncipe de Viana*, 5 (1986), pp. 9–22.
13 Such as the Corporative Organisation of Labour (1926) and Professional Associations (1932).
14 For La Conciliación and the influence of the Civil War and the political changes, see P. León-Sanz, 'Medical Assistance Provided by *La Conciliación*, a Pamplona Mutual Assistance Association (1902–84)', in B. Harris (ed.), *Welfare and Old Age in Europe and North America: The Development of Social Insurance* (London, 2012), pp. 137–166.
15 The importance of these sources for studying medical care is analysed by A. Borsay and P. Shapely (eds), *Medicine, Charity and Mutual Aid: The Consumption of Health and Welfare in Britain, c.1550–1950* (Aldershot, 2007); R. Klein, *Complaints against Doctors: A Study in Professional Accountability* (London, 1973); L. Mulcahy and J. Q. Tritter, 'Pathways, Pyramids and Icebergs? Mapping the Links between Dissatisfaction and Complaints', *Sociology of Health and Illness*, 20, 6 (1998), pp. 823–845, p. 826; D. G. Green, *Working-class Patients and the Medical Establishment: Self-help in Britain from the Mid-nineteenth Century to 1948* (New York, 1985); see also A. Lüdtke (ed.), *Histoire du quotidien* (Paris, 1994, translated from the German by O. Mannoni), p. 9; J. C. Häberlen, 'Reflections on Comparative Everyday History: Practices in the Working-Class Movement in Leipzig and Lyon during the Early 1930s', *The International History Review*, 3, 4 (2011), pp. 687–704.
16 B. Rosenwein, 'Worrying about Emotions in History', *American Historical Review*, 107 (2002), pp. 821–845, p. 842.
17 S. J. Matt, 'Current Emotion Research in History: Or, Doing History from the Inside Out', *Emotion Review*, 3, 1 (2011), pp. 117–124, p. 121.
18 J. Plamper, 'The History of Emotions: An Interview with William Reddy, Barbara Rosenwein and Peter Stearns', *History and Theory*, 49 (2010), pp. 237–265, p. 263.
19 P. León-Sanz, 'Creando identidad: Educación y recreación en *La Conciliación* (1902–1984)', in S. Castillo (ed.), *Mundo del trabajo y asociacionismo en España. Congreso VII Congreso de Historia Social 24–26 Octubre 2013* (Madrid, 2013).
20 The medical care offered by La Conciliación was similar to that available in other European institutions. See J. Lane, *A Social History of Medicine: Health, Healing and Disease in England, 1750–1950* (Routledge, 2001), pp. 68–81; B. Harris and P. Bridgen (eds), *Charity and Mutual Aid in Europe and North America since 1800* (New York and London, 2007).
21 Arts. 10 and 22, respectively, of the published regulations of La Conciliación (Pamplona, 1902).
22 For the relationship between the physicians and La Conciliación, see P. León-Sanz, 'La concertación de la asistencia en la enfermedad en La Sociedad de Obreros *La Conciliación* (1902–1919)', *Navarra: Memoria e Imagen*, Volume II (Pamplona, 2006), pp. 97–108. For the professional profile and the hygienic–social ideas of these physicians, see P. León-Sanz, 'Private Initiatives against Social Inequalities and Health

Vulnerabilities', in P. Bourdelais and J. Chircop (eds), *Vulnerabilities, Social Inequalities and Health* (Évora, 2010), pp. 93–108.
23 León-Sanz, 'The Strategies of Interrelations'.
24 LCBM, 1903, vol. 1, pp. 17–18.
25 J. María Serrano, M. Dolores Gadea and M. Sabaté, 'Tipo de cambio y protección: La peseta al margen del Patrón Oro, 1883–1931', *Revista de Historia Industrial*, 13 (1998), pp. 83–102.
26 E. Rodríguez Ocaña, 'La asistencia médica colectiva en España, hasta 1936', in *Historia de la acción social pública en España: Beneficencia y previsión* (Madrid, 1990), pp. 321–361.
27 LCBM, 1904, vol. 1, pp. 197–200. For a description of the notion of medical mishap, dissatisfaction, voiced grievances and complaints or claiming, see L. Mulcahy, *Disputing Doctors: The Socio-legal Dynamics of Complaints about Medical Care* (Maidenhead, Berkshire, 2003).
28 Klein, *Complaints against Doctors*, p. 105. However, Mulcahy and Tritter explain that voiced dissatisfaction and formal complaints are different expressions which are not necessarily linked; Mulcahy and Tritter, 'Pathways, Pyramids and Icebergs?'.
29 As Klein explains, there was often no professional consensus about what should be done; Klein, *Complaints against Doctors*, p. 56.
30 Complaint literature shows that similar processes became common in the complaints procedure: M. Gorsky, J. Mohan and T. Willis, *Mutualism and Health Care: British Hospital Contributory Schemes in the Twentieth Century* (Manchester, 2006), pp. 130–139; W. B. Howie, 'Complaints and Complaint Procedures in the Eighteenth- and Early Nineteenth-century Provincial Hospitals in England', *Medical History*, 25 (1981), pp. 345–362; E. Kalff, 'Les plaintes pour insalubrité du logement à Paris (1850–1955) miroir de l'hygénisation de la vie quotidienne', in P. Bourdelais (ed.), *Les hygiénistes: Enjeux, modèles et pratiques* (Paris, 2001), pp. 118–144; Klein, *Complaints against Doctors*; Green, *Working-class Patients and the Medical Establishment;* C. Brock, 'Risk, Responsibility and Surgery in the 1890s and Early 1900s', *Medical History*, 57, 3 (2013), pp. 317–337.
31 LCBM, 1909, vol. 3, p. 46v.
32 LCBM, 1909, vol. 3, pp. 46v–47v.
33 LCBM, 1913, vol. 4, p. 78v.
34 LCBM, 1913, vol. 4, p. 111.
35 LCBM, 1912, vol. 4, p. 44.
36 LCBM, 1913, vol. 4, p. 111.
37 LCBM, 1917, vol. 7, p. 44.
38 LCBM, 1917, vol. 6, p. 355. Our sources affirm that conflict between lay and technical judgements happens most frequently when complaints include the doctor's refusal to visit the patient or when there is a delay in medical assistance. Klein, *Complaints against Doctors*, p. 53.
39 LCBM, 1916, vol. 6, p. 223.
40 LCBM, 1916, vol. 6, p. 223.
41 LCBM, 1916, vol. 6, pp. 225–226.
42 LCBM, 1916, vol. 6, p. 15.
43 LCBM, 1916, vol. 6, p. 174.
44 LCBM, 1916, vol. 6, p. 210. There are more complaints against Sanz in the records: LCBM, 1916, vol. 5, p. 193; 1917, vol. 6, p. 284; 1917, vol. 6, pp. 343–47; 1918, vol. 7, p. 346.

45 LCBM, 1917, vol. 7, p. 75.
46 LCBM, 1917, vol. 7, p. 79.
47 LCBM, 1917, vol. 7, p. 86.
48 LCBM, 1918, vol. 7, p. 166.
49 LCBM, 1918, vol. 7, p. 229.
50 LCBM, 1918, vol. 7, p. 359. The quotations confirm the idea that doctors attributed any failure on their part to external circumstances, rather than admit malpractice; see J. Allsop and L. Mulcahy, 'Maintaining Professional Identity: Doctors' Responses to Complaints', *Sociology of Health and Illness*, 20, 6 (1998), pp. 802–824, pp. 811 and 815.
51 LCBM, 1919, vol. 8, p. 213. Later, Klein also describes reciprocal complaints among patients and doctors (*Complaints against Doctors*, p. 69).
52 LCBM, 1921, vol. 9, pp. 23–24.
53 LCBM, 1921, vol. 9, p. 25.
54 LCBM, 1926, vol. 11; copies of the letters exchanged regarding the dismissal of Dr R. Sanz are in the University of Navarra Archive, La Conciliación, Folder 'Médicos'. At that time, it was quite common in several European countries for professional associations (such as the British Medical Association in the UK or the Colegios de Médicos in Spain) to participate in negotiations between friendly societies, medical insurers and physicians. A. Albarracín Teulón, *Historia del Colegio de Médicos de Madrid* (Madrid, 2000); León-Sanz, 'Professional Responsibility and the Welfare System'; Klein, *Complaints against Doctors*, pp. 64–66 and 87–93.
55 Similar categories are identified by J. Allsop, 'Two Sides to Every Story: Complainants' and Doctors' Perspectives in Disputes about Medical Care in a General Practice Setting', *Law and Policy*, 16, 2 (1994), pp. 149–183; Klein, *Complaints against Doctors*, pp. 52, 115 and 136; C. Hawkins, *Mishap or Malpractice?* (Oxford, 1985), p. 273.
56 LCBM, 1903, vol. 1, p. 14.
57 LCBM, 1904, vol. 1, pp. 267–268. Several studies show the discontentment among doctors hired by friendly societies or medical aid societies. See Klein, *Complaints against Doctors*, p. 62; Green, *Working-class Patients and the Medical Establishment*; J. José Llovet, 'Problemática e ideologías de la responsabilidad médica en España (1850–1949)', *Asclepio*, 44 (1992), pp. 71–94; P. León-Sanz, 'El poder de los médicos: Un análisis de el ejercicio profesional de la medicina en nuestros días (Madrid, 1906)', *Estudos do Século XX*, 5 (2005), pp. 223–241.
58 LCBM, 1907, vol. 3, p. 47v. It was afterwards noted that better communication with the patient helps avoid malpractice processes. Klein indicates that 'trivial or tragic all [complaints] are important', because complaints 'raise some complex issues about the nature of general practice and the doctor–patient relationship' (Klein, *Complaints against Doctors*, p. 52).
59 LCBM, 1907, vol. 3, p. 47v.
60 LCBM, 1915, vol. 5, p. 156.
61 LCBM, 1916, vol. 6, p. 195.
62 LCBM, 1934, vol. 14, p. 7v.
63 LCBM, 1934, vol. 14, p. 11.
64 LCBM, 1907, vol. 3, p. 47v.
65 LCBM, 1913, vol. 4, p. 111.
66 LCBM, 1922, vol. 9, p. 146.
67 LCBM, 1918, vol. 7, p. 166.
68 S. Fineman, *Understanding Emotion at Work* (London, 2003).

69 M. Scheer, 'Are Emotions a Kind of Practice (and is That what Makes Them Have a History)? A Bourdieuan Approach to Understanding Emotion', *History and Theory* 51, 2 (2012), pp. 193–220, p. 209.
70 Expressions of dissatisfaction and the transformation of discontent into complaints have been studied by Mulcahy and Tritter, 'Pathways, Pyramids and Icebergs?'.
71 R. Charon, *Narrative Medicine: Honoring the Stories of Illness* (Oxford, 2006).
72 LCBM, 1917, vol. 7, p. 25.
73 The appropriate response to complaints is an important factor for achieving satisfaction on the part of complainants. Cf. S. Lloyd-Bostock and L. Mulcahy, 'Social Psychology of Making and Responding to Hospital Complaints: An Account Model of Complaint Processes', *Law and Policy*, 16, 2 (1994), pp. 123–148.
74 M. Berezin, 'Exploring Emotions and the Economy: New Contributions from Sociological Theory', *Theory and Society*, 38 (2009), pp. 335–346.
75 León-Sanz, 'Private Initiatives'.
76 N. Crossley, *Reflexive Embodiment in Contemporary Society* (Maidenhead, Berkshire, 2006).
77 LCBM, 1909, vol. 3, p. 46v.
78 LCBM, 1914, vol. 5, p. 27v.
79 LCBM, 1915, vol. 5, p. 67v.
80 LCBM, 1922, vol. 9, pp. 146, 150–151.
81 LCBM, 1916, vol. 6, p. 115. See S. Castillo, 'En torno al mutualismo español contemporáneo: Solidaridad desde abajo revisited', in E. Maza (co-ordinator), *Asociacionismo en la España Contemporánea: Vertientes y análisis interdisciplinar* (Valladolid, 2003), pp. 61–88, p. 66.
82 LCBM, 1916, vol. 6, p. 71. This change was motivated also by the increase of morbidity; see P. León-Sanz, 'The Mutual Benefit Societies' Responses to the 1918–19 Influenza Pandemic in Pamplona', in M. Isabel Porras and R. A. Davis (eds), *Emerging Infection, Emergent Meanings: The 'Spanish' Influenza Pandemic of 1918–1919* (Rochester, NY, forthcoming). This question is framed within the interesting debate at the time regarding patients' free choice of physicians. See Supplement to the *British Medical Journal*, 10 (June 1911); Green, *Working-class Patients and the Medical Establishment*; Klein, *Complaints against Doctors*, p. 76.
83 LCBM, 1916, vol. 6, p. 114v. Green (*Working-class Patients and the Medical Establishment*) and Klein (*Complaints against Doctors*, pp. 64–66) insist on the financial problem that led to the free choice of physicians by patients without supervision by friendly societies.
84 Green, *Working-class Patients and the Medical Establishment*; Cuesta, 'El proceso de expansión de los seguros sociales obligatorios'; Kalff, 'Les plaintes pour insalubrité'.
85 S. Wilde, 'Truth, Trust, and Confidence in Surgery, 1890–1910: Patient Autonomy, Communication, and Consent', *Bulletin of the History of Medicine*, 83, 2 (2009), pp. 302–330. For the evolution of the patient's role, see A. Mold, 'Repositioning the Patient: Patient Organizations, Consumerism, and Autonomy in Britain during the 1960s and 1970s', *Bulletin of the History of Medicine*, 87 (2013), pp. 225–249. Mulcahy and Tritter conclude for a latter period that 'The voicing of dissatisfaction in complaints is an example of consumer activism which has generally been overlooked by medical sociologists and those interested in the interface between sociology, law and medicine' ('Pathways, Pyramids and Icebergs?', p. 826).
86 LCBM, 1904, vol. 5, pp. 18v, 267–268.
87 LCBM, 1907, vol. 3, p. 80.

88 R. Porter (ed.), *Rewriting the Self: Histories from the Renaissance to the Present* (London, 1997). For the importance of narrative voices for these studies, see J. Klein, 'Open Moments and Surprise Endings: Historical Agency and the Workings of Narrative in The Social Transformation of American Medicine', *Journal of Health, Politics, Policy and Law*, 29, 4–5 (2004), pp. 621–642.

89 Plamper, 'The History of Emotions'.

90 A. Wear, 'Interfaces: Perceptions of Health and Illness in Early Modern England', in R. Porter and A. Wear (eds), *Problems and Methods in the History of Medicine* (London, 1987), pp. 230–255.

6 The shape of the iceberg

Doctors and neglect under the New Poor Law, *c.*1871–1900

Kim Price[1]

Overview

England has a long history of inspecting and reporting standards of care under state medicine, which is affirmed by this vibrant collection of essays.[2] One of the country's most recent administrative incarnations has been the national Care Quality Commission (CQC). According to the CQC, there were 1.25 million National Health Service (NHS) 'incidents' reported in the year of 2010–11, which had continued a 'year-on-year' increase.[3] In turn, a leading British newspaper, *the Guardian*, reported that negligence claims were 'soaring and payouts to patients or their families [had] hit unprecedented levels' – even the chairman of the world's oldest medical defence organisation, the British Medical Defence Union (MDU), has commented that the 20 per cent rise in legal action between 2009 and 2010 was 'unmatched in the company's 126-year history'.[4] Such alarmist observations are omnipresent throughout the social history of modern medical practice.[5] A thin red line of medical defence lawyers keeping a tide of litigating patients at bay has been a pervasive image in modern British medicine.

Historians, though, have been slow to counter the disingenuous, but persistent, claim of historically unprecedented levels of litigation and complaining in the NHS. For example, the MDU was itself inaugurated in the 1880s due to a perception of increasing charges of negligence and libel,[6] but – then, as now – the court records reflect discouragement, not encouragement, for aggrieved patients. It has long been recognised that, relatively speaking, very few cases of medical negligence reach the courts. Moreover, the need for accountability in litigation tends to mask the relationships between systemic faults and the (blameworthy) 'active' neglect of individual medical practitioners.[7] As Jean McHale reminds us in her chapter in this volume, public inquiries, policy responses to high-profile negligence and litigation statistics have often obscured the latent faults of healthcare environments. This chapter will therefore question the 'active' neglect by pre-NHS poor law doctors, in order to reveal some historic contrasts and commonalities in dealing with negligence under British state healthcare.

The first part of this chapter will argue that over the 126-year period of rising litigation, ascribed above, the practice of medicine has altered significantly. Though numbers of claims for recompense have clearly risen since the nineteenth century, this belies the changing nature of medical negligence throughout that time and across very different healthcare loci. Concomitantly, the ways that negligence is understood, conceived, defined and applied (in law, medicine and society) have continually changed and evolved. However, the history behind the deceptively simplistic etymologies of 'negligence' and 'complaining' remains unwritten.[8] As June Jones and Andy Shanks emphasise in this volume, the extremes of patient neglect tend to be highlighted, which obscures analyses. Likewise, socio-legal studies have focused on the law of medical negligence since the mid-twentieth century, but there has been almost no comparable research into the centuries of mixed healthcare systems in Britain before the NHS was introduced in 1948.[9] Because of this, it is difficult to quantitatively measure progress and accurately trace the meaning of any rises over time. In part, this difficulty has stemmed from a fixation on litigation, which has meant that administrative structures for dealing with patient dissatisfaction are overlooked.[10]

The second part of this chapter will thus use negligence under the Victorian poor law as a case study in pre-NHS complaint handling. Poor law neglect should have been a non-event; it was confined to a setting in which pauperised patients had few rights and no income to bring a charge against a doctor. Yet paupers could, and did, make complaints, which were sometimes investigated in official inquiries.[11] Historians have begun to detail the agency of pauper narratives, but there remains no framework for understanding the administrative process for investigating and dealing with complaints. As this chapter will demonstrate, the volume of official inquiries, the irregular judicial process and the consequent outcomes together make poor law negligence a unique episode in legal, medical and social history. Charges of neglect against medical officers from the 1830s to 1900 provide an ideal example of the transitory factors involved in defining what constitutes negligence; as this chapter will argue, under the New Poor Law it was as much defined by contemporary policy and funding as it was caused by an individual doctor's negligent practice.

The submerged 'shape' of medical negligence

Recent legal studies demonstrate that the 'vast majority' of medical dissatisfaction and grievances remain unvoiced.[12] Historians therefore face a problem in choosing what to measure. As Rudolf Klein, a leading sociologist, has said, 'the total number of complaints tells us nothing about their content'.[13] Then there is the difference between complaining about medicine and making a claim for medical negligence. People complain about medicine on differing levels; from grumblings in the community (leaving few extant documents) to making an official complaint about negligence and pursuing litigation (and leaving an 'official' source for analysis). This led Klein to describe an 'iceberg' of unmeasured patient dissatisfaction.[14] He estimated that for each patient that stepped forward to make a formal written complaint, there were 400 more cases of 'friction', not to mention approximately 100 'grumbles'.[15] Writing in the 1970s, but looking back over the development of a complaints mechanism in the NHS, Klein observed:

> The statistics of complaints that appear in the annual reports of the Department of Health and Social Security tell us very little about what is happening in general practice and the attitudes of the patients towards it. Because the system for dealing with complaints is designed to police the contract between the practitioner and the NHS, rather than to deal with the dissatisfaction of the patient, it does not deal with the major causes of stress and friction. . . . To the extent that the complaints machinery filters out the 'trivial' grievance, so it gives a misleading picture of the general situation.[16]

Perhaps it is impossible to accurately measure dissatisfaction with medicine over time. People in the past may have been dissatisfied with the medical care that they received, but chose to say nothing. Others may have complained verbally or started rumours (as Steven King argues in Chapter 7 of this volume). Neither group sued for recompense or framed their treatment legally as negligence. Moreover, some patients may not have had access to legal representation, or may have been denied 'rights' due to social or cultural norms which excluded, for example, their class or gender. In the absence of accurate records or a measurable paper-trail of complaining, a pre-NHS history of patients' rights – meaning the unfettered ability to express and resolve dissatisfaction – is like staring into the abyss.[17]

In view of this, charges of medical negligence against doctors can present a tangible litmus paper for measuring substandard medical practice in history. Yet as a quantitative measure, negligence may only indicate the extremes of substandard care or temporal patterns of cultural and legal preference. For example, the highest numbers of today's negligence cases in the UK stem from inaccurate (or non-) disclosure of information to patients or from a failure to use modern technology correctly – a statistic that shrouds the human story that each year around 400 people die or suffer a serious injury from an adverse event involving the use of equipment or medical devices.[18] This is a modern trend, founded on developments in medicine *and* society. First, social and legal changes (such as advances in education, legal aid and the system of medical jurisprudence) have come together under a loose agenda of patients' rights and patient-borne knowledge – a movement that Alex Mold deals with in Chapter 8 of this volume. Second, the medical world has become a sophisticated wonderland of bio-medicine, scientific engineering and medical technology. In contrast, before the NHS, technical medical machinery was uncommon in state medicine and 'disclosure' was almost non-existent as a motivation for complaint or as a cause for litigation.[19]

Given the differences in judicial guidance before and after Bolam (which McHale discusses in Chapter 12) – and the contrasts between pre- and post-NHS healthcare – historians of law and medicine have argued that charges against doctors in the UK were relatively rare until the twentieth century.[20] This may be true for litigation, but it does nothing to appraise the extent and shape of a possible 'iceberg' of dissatisfaction, complaining and negligent practice at this time. For a start, historically, doctors did not have the financial and professional security that they gained in the twentieth century. Before then, doctors had to arrange for their defence themselves. It was a costly procedure and most doctors would dismiss libellous action or public slurs because they could not afford the defence fees (a further confounding factor in charting the 'rise' of complaining before and after the formation of medical defence insurance). Normally, it was only through public appeals – in newspapers and journals – that a charge could be properly defended. According to the legal historian Clifford Hawkins, 'If a victim of slander or libel, [a doctor] had to sue his prosecutor himself or suffer in silence – and lack of expert advice might prejudice his case'.[21]

However, the same financial inability of doctors to defend themselves applied equally – indeed, more so – to the vast general populace of England and Wales. Legal historians have argued that as a result of this, 'in the late-nineteenth and early-twentieth centuries it was very unusual for patients to sue their doctors. Conventionally considered an almost presumptuous thing to do, it was in any event beyond the means of all but a tiny minority.'[22] Thus, it tended to be in extreme cases, such as manslaughter, that the Victorian public brought charges of medical negligence to English courtrooms. In spite of public misgivings – and a consistent mistrust of doctors throughout the nineteenth century – there was only a slight rise in court actions against doctors per se towards the end of the century.[23] What, then, do we make of the apparently anomalous English poor law, where doctors were being charged with neglect in surprising numbers throughout the latter Victorian period?

A doctor of the poor *law*

Since Elizabethan times, the poor law had existed in England to alleviate extreme want from destitution or sickness, but debates had continuously raged over the manner and extent of relief. In 1834, the New Poor Law ushered in a more systematic 'workhouse' deterrent system than had hitherto existed. At its heart were local 'unions', each with a board of guardians who oversaw the administration of indoor relief – workhouse, asylum and infirmary – and outdoor relief, paid to the poor in their own homes. Likewise, from the 1840s, the state (through the locally administered system) employed doctors as medical officers *en masse* to treat paupers.

Neither doctors nor the authorities, however, were prepared to lay aside private practice and have the medical officers become full-time 'State doctors'.[24] This, it cannot be overstated, was the greatest impediment to welfare reform (under any guise) in the nineteenth century and a key component in poor law medical negligence. Doctors consistently failed to balance their time between their private practice and poor law duties.[25] The former had the potential to be lucrative; the latter provided a reliable income, kept out competition and advertised the doctor's skill. The crowded field of nineteenth-century medicine ensured a constant supply of eager and qualified medical professionals, which, in turn, suppressed wages throughout the whole of the nineteenth century. Medical historians have noted this irony of Victorian capitalism and condemned the New Poor Law 'for insisting on gross understaffing with medical officers and consequent neglect of the sick poor', at the same time that there was an overabundance of general practitioners.[26] Yet the lack of unity or foresight among medical practitioners lay behind much of the atrophied poor law medical reform.

Contemporary politicians, medical professionals and poor law administrators alike understood the problem, but the majority were against uniform, workable salaries.[27] This state of affairs was acceptable to Victorians within the context of 'free trade'. For example, Sir John Trollope was president of the Poor Law Board (PLB) – the central national authority – in 1852, and he reasoned that 'perhaps the medical gentlemen themselves are somewhat to blame for this state of things. Under the operation of excessive competition they have been induced to take contracts at a lower scale than they can afford to do'[28] – as is clearly reflected in Figure 6.1. As the *British Medical Journal* observed in 1864, 'It seems to us hoping beyond hope to expect that a free trade House of Commons will ever force ratepayers to pay more for the services of an official than the official himself demands for his services'.[29]

Despite the clear suppression of salary levels, as shown in Figure 6.1, belief in the 'free market' and competition governed employment procedure.[30] By far the greatest number of medical officers received a salary of under £50 per annum – not infrequently placing them on a salary less than that of the workhouse master (or matron) and similar to that of less skilled workhouse staff such as nurses, porters or instructors. Expenses and the supply of medicaments also came from their salary, which was supposed to be supplemented by their income from private practice. The difference between life and death for some of Britain's poorest sick therefore hung in the balance sheets of a local private practice. Throughout the nineteenth century, though, doctors took poor law appointments on salaries that were far too low for them to practise without detriment within the bounds of their professional obligations.

William Golden Lumley, an influential civil servant, replied to 'comments' that the PLB had supported guardians in suppressing doctors' salaries:

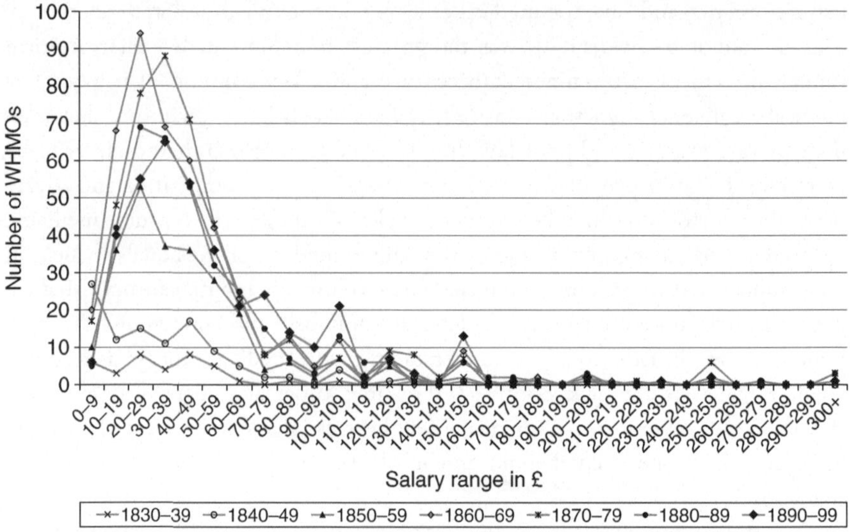

Figure 6.1 Distribution of the starting salaries of workhouse medical officers (WHMOs), 1830–99 (source: TNA MH9 Series, in K. Price, *Medical Negligence in Victorian Britain: The Crisis of Care under the English Poor Law, c.1834–1900*, London, 2014).

> the medical profession have the remedy in their own hands, let them decline to offer for the office at the remuneration proposed. The guardians must elect duly qualified practitioners, and, if their offers be really insufficient, must acquiesce and raise their terms.[31]

While it may be true that the PLB were ensuring value for money, they were also using political obfuscation to shift around the problem – they admitted that medical officers were unable to fulfil obligations, but shirked responsibility for a system that would inevitably lead to neglect. Legally, this was defensible. The theoretical basis of medical practice and law reflected the strong market values at this time.

The ethical considerations of doctors were centred on corporate self-interest, not the doctor–patient narrative centred around patients' rights that we are now familiar with.[32] Medical professionals in the nineteenth century were more concerned with the establishment of trust than with philosophical precedents in ethics. Without trust, there was no patient and therefore no business income.[33] For example, ethics was described by *The Medical Practitioners' Legal Guide* (1870) as 'a code of etiquette, upon the due observance of which the profession most properly relies for the cultivation of a high tone of character among its members'.[34] Ethics – both within and outside of the poor law – was about formulating a framework for the division of labour and a code of 'etiquette' between working practitioners.[35] Doctors were warned to avoid 'officious intercourse in a case under the charge of another' and 'impeaching the professional skill or knowledge exhibited in the primary treatment of [a] case, though such treatment may have been unsuccessful'.[36] They were advised to keep disputes in-house, away from public scrutiny and arbitrated by 'higher' members of the profession: 'The adjudication should not be made public, but submissively acquiesced in and accepted *con amore*.'[37]

Notwithstanding a robust and widespread loyalty to the profession, there were regular public disputes and wrangles between medical practitioners over fees and practice jurisdictions in the nineteenth century.[38] This was a feature of medical practice that continued into the twentieth century, as Steven Thompson and Pilar León-Sanz's chapters in this volume demonstrate. The in-fighting was missed neither by the public nor by the PLB. Indeed, the PLB demanded a much more egalitarian practice of medicine than was the norm for the times or was expected between the lowly medical officer and his higher-ranking poor law employers. From 1849, special rules were created for the employment and regulation of medical officers. The 'professional etiquette' of doctors, it was said, must not interfere with a medical officer's duties. Guardians were to be the ultimate arbiter of any dispute, and physicians were to have no special place. Medical officers were not 'bound to supply any medicines which might be prescribed by the physician'.[39]

Though understandably set to minimise outside interference, this approach was tantamount to setting medical professionals against one another. It also undermined the authority of physicians. Despite physicians being ostensibly less qualified than the lowly general practitioner, their gentlemanly background, cultural elitism and classical education held sway and they lorded it over the rest of the profession.[40] The PLB thus cared little for the medical profession's limited and self-interested 'ethics'. In over-ruling the medical profession's guidance, such as it was, the permanent officials of the poor law had also gained the upper hand. They, not the medical profession, were the ultimate authority in decisions over medical treatment and allocation of resources. In turn, guardians, relieving officers and overseers were able to confront, question and undermine medical officers' actions.

Negative attitudes to medicine at this time were largely – and somewhat justifiably – born from its 'trade' characteristics, questionable treatments and long history of charlatans, fakers and quacks[41] – a matter that directed professionalisation into the twentieth century, as Hilary Ingram's chapter in this volume suggests. Though doctors sought individually to claim the moral and ethical high ground in the 1800s, they struggled to escape the strictures and image of a trade – especially with the sorts of public complaints discussed elsewhere in this collection by Steven King. Moreover, a lack of convincing medical science underpinned a limited curative ability; these factors helped to sustain an ongoing ambivalence towards the medical profession, a circumstance arguably influenced by the 'culture of complaint' in its psychiatric branch (described in Andrew Scull's contribution to this volume). This contemporary backdrop informed and hardened the attitudes of many high-ranking poor law officials in both governmental and local administration.[42]

Likewise, the law in this period reflected public ambivalence, providing no special rights for doctors who were judged by comparison to what an 'ordinary man' would do under the circumstances (as McHale describes in this volume, this was later surmounted by Bolam).[43] Doctors had few exceptional rights under the law. Thus UK court precedents tended to overrule medical claims to exclusive knowledge: 'It [was] for the judge to direct the jury what standard to apply and for the jury to say whether that standard [had] been reached . . . the law requires a fair and reasonable standard of care and competence.'[44] Courts were directed to assess whether a defendant had exercised due care and diligence, but there was little uniformity.[45] The power to decide on courtroom medical matters, and what an acceptable 'standard of care' was, remained in the hands of laymen throughout the nineteenth century. As the Introduction to this collection suggests, politicians, court officials, local dignitaries and parish overseers – even poor law guardians and workhouse masters – were all therefore backed by the law to confront and question medicine.[46] The tension between lay authority and a rising medical profession is the key to understanding why the neglect of patients – and their complaints – readily led to high numbers of charged medical officers.

Lumley, for example, was clearly set against medical officers achieving a 'higher' social position. This 'destiny may await them', he said, but in the meantime 'they must be considered as they are'.[47] This attitude was visible in the rules of employment for doctors under the poor law, which expanded slowly from the late 1840s but underwent an overhaul in 1871, the year that the Local Government Board (LGB) was inaugurated.[48] The LGB absorbed its predecessors, the PLB and medical officers of the Privy Council, which brought new political powers to the permanent officials of the poor law. Joseph Rogers (a famous medical officer and reformer and the leader of the Poor Law Medical Officers' Association from 1869) said that, from that time, they had 'usurped' the poor law with 'powers they were not entitled to' and pushed forward their own agenda.[49] It signalled a restrictive time for poor law medicine, when the rules of medical officers' employment were used by the LGB inspectorate to control their union and hold back their push for systemic reforms.[50]

A catch-22

While 1871 may have been a prime moment for doctors to come under the wing of a major aspect of national health policy and (ostensibly) to ensure improved medical welfare, the LGB does not seem to have taken this course. As the *Lancet* had lamented in 1869, the 'perversity' of 'appointing barristers rather than medical men shows the deep hatred to the profession which has existed at the Poor Law Board'.[51] The rules of 1871, written by none other than William Lumley, the Board's assistant secretary and legal expert, are the most explicit examples of the LGB's intention, from that time, to stamp down on the medical officers' association. It had been gaining momentum from the mid-nineteenth century and agitating for reforms in medical provision, conditions of employment and remuneration.[52] According to Lumley, the medical profession was backed by 'considerable political influence' and there was an 'energetic [and] intelligent association of medical officers earnestly engaged in furthering the interests of their order'.[53] He pointed out that their association was supported by the press and that 'much success [had] attended these various efforts'.[54] Lumley pulled few punches in the preface to the 1871 rules of employment, where he issued a stark warning:

> Men do not seek for that which they do not consider it to be for their advantage to possess. No one is compelled to be a medical officer. The salary and duties are clearly disclosed to every candidate before he obtains the office, and he ought to consider calmly and cautiously whether the remuneration is compensatory for the services; and if he accept the office he ought not complain if he finds he is mistaken. He should in that case take the earliest opportunity of retiring from his position.[55]

Lumley's opening salvo is representative of the times. Expanding medical power, knowledge and – albeit slowly – curative ability were motivating the profession to have more influence in public life, including poor law administration.

The rising status of the wider medical profession was in direct contrast, though, to their lowly position in the poor law, reflected in their appallingly low remuneration. Lumley issued a further warning: '[medical officers] are liable to be dismissed for incompetency or unfitness, or for disobedience of the orders of the commissioners, and must submit to the various consequences which attend upon dismissal.'[56] In other words, 'bite the bullet or else'. This effectively set up the medical officers as the nation's scapegoat wherever and whenever poor law medical scandals and neglect occurred. At this time, Lumley also expanded the rules governing official inquiries into medical negligence:

> The decision of the [Board] is conclusive, and cannot be opened by any court of law. . . . The questions which are inquired into are such as relate to mala praxis, negligence in regard to the paupers whom he [the medical officer] may be ordered to attend, either by not visiting promptly, or omitting to visit with regularity, want of sobriety, absence from his district or the workhouse without adequate provision of a substitute, improper conduct towards

> pauper patients under his charge, insubordination in regard to the board of guardians, or wilful disobedience of their orders or those of the [Board].[57]

The list of charges was vague. Creative guardians – wishing to rid themselves of a troublesome doctor – could invent virtually groundless charges and distort the duties and rules of a medical officer's engagement. Moreover, the LGB held all the cards and a judicial ace up their sleeve: their decisions could not be opened by any court of law, and inspectors superseded and could overrule the decisions of guardians.[58]

The LGB had the legal jurisdiction to indict their employees, but, essentially, inspectors were also the judge and jury of an official inquiry. Moreover, it was the law of contracts, not tort (as it is in most Western countries today), which was used by the LGB to legally bind their decisions. Inspectors were keen to ensure that a contract was binding because it formed the basis of their legal powers. Their inquiries gave the air of a thorough investigation, but the cynical way that the LGB used contract doctrine implies that doctors' fees, attendance and obedience were their predominant concerns. Despite regular orders, circulars and (occasional) legislation throughout the nineteenth century, the contractual basis of official inquiry judgments continued and doctors bore the brunt of failings in poor law medical practice. This was at no time more apparent than during the first three decades of the LGB, when they drove forward a crusade against outdoor relief.

The rules of 1871 were a shrewd move by a department making dangerous cutbacks in welfare expenditure. From then, charges of negligence against medical officers became symptomatic of tensions in administering and funding the poor law's medical services. After the successful agitation which led to the Metropolitan Poor Act of 1867, the poor law inspectorate was keen to avoid further costly alterations to the system of medical relief at a time of recession, growing distress and destitution.[59] Under the Longley Strategy (pursued between the 1870s and 1890s), the LGB instigated a policy to cut back welfare expenditure and diminish reliance on poor law outdoor relief – a period characterised by historians as a crusade.[60] By removing essential funds for nutrition, housing and medical care, the crusade against outdoor relief lowered the health of many families and increased the number of individuals who could no longer be supported at home.[61] Elizabeth Hurren has led research into this policy, and she argues that the 'crusade . . . drove those in deepest poverty to enter a system in which they were shuffled about to save costs', and that it 'deterred those most in need'.[62] It unintentionally drove up the numbers of institutional dependents and increased the workload of workhouse medical officers.[63] The crusade also encouraged guardians and relieving officers (who assessed a claimant's means) to cut back on expensive medical procedures and fees, as discussed below. In short, it dovetailed with prevailing systemic problems of medical officer employment and increased medical officers' exposure to complaints about negligent practice.

The consequent rise in charges against doctors under the poor law affected the fortunes of medical officers as a professional group. It also undermined the threat posed by Rogers' leadership in the 1870s and 1880s. In 1882, he described the dire situation:

> within the last two years, in consequence of certain occurrences, he had made up his mind to abandon, so far as he was individually concerned, the idea of appealing to the Local Government Board, and had determined to endeavour to mould the Association into a Mutual Defence Association.[64]

Despite a copious poor law literature, no historian has yet singled out charges of negligence against medical officers and the association's shift in focus to 'defending' medical officers.

The rising tide of charges of negligence against medical officers in the 1870s (demonstrated in Figure 6.2) implies that Rogers was right to do so: there was something unusual occurring within poor law medicine. Rogers used the rapidly increasing numbers of charges of negligence against medical officers as a means to expose and reform the system. In essence, this became *the* chosen reform method of Rogers and the association during the 1870s and 1880s.[65] The timing of this has much to do with the attitude and policies of the LGB in this period.

During the cutbacks of the crusade, the authorisation of medical extras and emergency treatment were particularly affected at a localised level. A widely

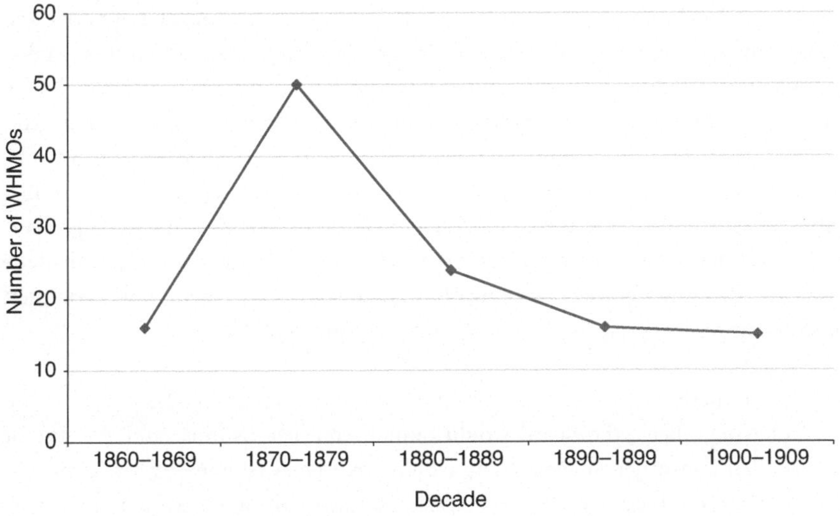

Figure 6.2 Peak in (known) forced resignations and dismissals of workhouse medical officers (WHMOs) in the 1870s (source: TNA MH9 Series, in Price, *Medical Negligence in Victorian Britain*).

reported case of neglect in the Isle of Wight workhouse in 1877 led various publications to question the relationship between 'crusading' and, as the *Lancet* described it, 'systematic mismanagement and neglect': 'when an accident occurs inspectors hold an inquiry, censure what they previously sanctioned, supersede certain of their approved agents, and, in this pleasant way, appease the clamour of public opinion'.[66] During the crusade, cases of starvation and neglect (often due to withholding relief) were reported with shock but were not uncommon.[67] Most importantly for negligence and complaints, orders for emergency attendance were increasingly withheld. In turn, guardians could, and frequently did, veto payments for medical officers who had attended an urgent case, or treated paupers without an order. The problem was compounded by the fact that a parish overseer could give an order for a medical officer to attend an emergency, but that guardians could legally refuse to pay for this type of attendance. Medical officers, who also worked in private practice, were thus faced with a costly choice: whether or not to attend emergency cases. The double bind of medical officers meant that they daily walked a tightrope in decision-making. Their rules of employment perpetuated the problem:

> a medical officer may render his aid promptly without an order, relying upon the due acknowledgement of his services; but he must remember that he has no absolute legal claim upon [guardians], as they are to make compensation in any such case only if they think proper to do so.[68]

In the Stratford-on-Avon Union in the English Midlands, for example, the workhouse medical officer wrote to the Board in 1870, complaining about the non-payment of his emergency fees in a case where rapid intervention was needed to mend the dislocated bone of a pauper child. In the words of the LGB, the doctor had 'reduced the dislocation without having previously received any order' and was not, therefore, due the nominal fee. Although they accepted there were subsequent orders for his attendance, those were 'merely applied so as to require [his] subsequent attendance on the child'.[69] The LGB recommended that the guardians pay a 'reasonable remuneration' for the medical officer's attendance, but made it clear that this was a gratuity. The neatly-framed role of overseers in this complex legal construct was clear in the LGB's closing words to the doctor:

> you remark as to the difficulty experienced in obtaining the order of the relieving officer, the Board would remind you that, as [this case] was one of sudden and urgent necessity, it would have been competent for a churchwarden or overseer of the Parish to have given an Order for your attendance.[70]

However, guardians could refuse to pay that type of order.

Despite the obvious financial risk of attending gratuitous orders for attendance, the official guidance in 1866 was to 'attend first and raise the question afterwards'; otherwise a medical officer might find himself 'in a situation from which he would find it difficult to extricate himself, however unknowingly his neglect had arisen'.[71] In turn, the LGB advised that if guardians refused to pay, medical officers should try to recover their fees from the overseer in the courts.[72] As described above, this was expensive and time-consuming. General practitioners were unable to afford legal costs or unwilling to lose time spent chasing claims in court. This aspect of the medical welfare system left little room for manoeuvre. The rules legally covered the LGB and guardians from all directions: officers and overseers, even paupers, could request the medical officer without paperwork. In practice, this meant that medical officers commonly ignored 'requests' for their attendance, hoping that the outcome bias would be in their favour. If they did not attend to an overseer's order and the outcome was unfavourable – resulting in death or serious injury – then the absentee could be charged with negligence.

The 1866 guidance warned: 'In case of the Medical Officer refusing or neglecting to afford such attendance, it will be incumbent upon him to prove that he was justified in the course he may have adopted.'[73] Alfred Sheen's experience of this, at Cardiff Union, led him to publish a guide for workhouse medical officers in 1890. It forewarned doctors about over-zealous orders for regular (free) attendance and obstruction over emergency cases, which involved a fee.[74] In effect, the doctors were caught up in a contractual 'catch-22' that echoes the black humour of Joseph Heller's military conundrum. Too many orders had created a situation where medical officers ignored calls for aid, or came when it suited them – delays that could result in a fatality, and a charge of negligence against a medical officer. The view of most medical officers in the 1870s was clearly described in a letter of 1873 to the *British Medical Journal*:

> The poor must be given to understand that in all sudden cases they must go at once to the medical officer, without an order. If the latter attend to the case, and then claim the regulation fee, he is politely asked for the order, and having none, is told by the board to go about his business. If, on the other hand, he decline to go to a case before the order is obtained, he is held to do so at his own risk; and should such a case terminate fatally, down comes the coroner upon the medical officer like a hatchet.[75]

The expenses of 'sudden cases' – or rather, the doctor's fees they incurred – led to widespread interference from guardians and to cutbacks in emergency treatment. One medical officer wrote to the *British Medical Journal* after fighting his employers for payment: 'From a humane point of view, it is impossible for a medical man to refuse to attend an urgent case until an order is first procured, although this conduct of the guardians would almost drive one to it.'[76] In fact, 'good' doctors, such as Sheen and Rogers, did ignore some orders, as a means of protest against excessive requests for their attendance.[77] As a result of his actions – and, arguably, his public involvement with reformers – Rogers was forced to resign from his post as workhouse medical officer to the Strand Union.[78] Nonetheless, the central authority was legally entitled to charge individuals with negligence (whatever their motives), even if this avoided correcting the systemic faults that led to the neglect of patients.

Conclusion

Charges of negligence against medical officers were hinged on accountability, but this often meant misconduct or disobedience under the New Poor Law. It therefore had little in common with the UK's modern tort-based system of medical jurisprudence. It was an employment tribunal, thinly disguised by legal prowess, elements of judicial procedure and the use of contract law. Medical officers recognised that there was a serious problem and that they were caught in a catch-22, but as a professional group they were unable to prevent the cascade of charges of neglect against them in this period. Moreover, those charges played a devastating role in breaking up their reform movement, forcing thousands of doctors, such as Rogers, into a defensive position. In this way, the poor law may have been instrumental in hardening doctors' attitudes at the turn of the twentieth century and, in turn, forcing a power shift in the lay–medical symbiosis. This circumstance may even be an overlooked but important aspect of the transition from poor law to welfare state, and a formative element in the shaping of complaints structures under the early NHS.

It is difficult not to adopt a cynical view and criticise the LGB for their lack of humanistic endeavour. Lumley's 'guidance' occasionally reads like a declaration of war on the medical profession. Certainly, they sought lower rates and value for money, using the free market to their advantage to obtain cheap doctoring. This was unexceptional and typically corporate Victorian financial management. Nevertheless, it was a direct conduit to negligence when coupled with the 'crusading' policy. The inspectorate's roles as both a lynchpin of the crusade and the legal overlords of official inquiries are in need of more attention from historians. Ultimately, the poor law provides an important case study in pre-NHS and pre-Bolam medical law. Above all, it demonstrates that *a priori* reasoning should be avoided at all costs when discussing the statistics of complaining and medical negligence.

Notes

1 I would like to thank the Wellcome Trust for funding the research that underpins this chapter and express my gratitude to Bloomsbury Academic for their permission to adapt parts of my forthcoming book for this edited volume: K. Price, *Medical Negligence in Victorian Britain: The Crisis of Care under the English Poor Law, c.1834–1900* (London, forthcoming 2014).
2 For example, see T. Crook, 'Sanitary Inspection and the Public Sphere in Late Victorian and Edwardian Britain: A Case Study in Liberal Governance', *Social History* 32, 4 (2007), p. 369.
3 Care Quality Commission, *The State of Health Care and Adult Social Care in England:. An Overview of Key Themes in Care in 2010/11 – Summary* (September 2011), p. 7.
4 S. Bosely and D. Campbell, 'Negligence Claims against GPs Rising', *Guardian* (29 July 2011), www.guardian.co.uk/society/2011/jul/29/negligence-claims-gps-rising, accessed 5 May 2014; C. Evans, *The Medical Defence Union Limited Report and Accounts 2011: Including Cautionary Tales*, p. 2, www.themdu.com/~/media/Files/MDU/Publications/Annual%20reports/2011%20annual%20report%20and%20accounts.pdf., accessed 1 May 2014.
5 For further discussion, see T. Reader and A. Gillespie, 'Patient Neglect in Healthcare Institutions: A Systematic Review and Conceptual Model', *BMC Health Services Research* 13, 156 (2013), www.biomedcentral.com/1472–6963/13/156, accessed 1 May 2014; M. L. Millenson, 'Pushing the Profession: How the News Media Turned Patient Safety into a Priority', *Quality and Safety in Health Care*, 11 (2002), pp. 57–63.
6 C. Hawkins, *Mishap or Malpractice?* (Oxford, 1985), pp. 2–17.
7 J. Reason, *Human Error* (Cambridge, 1990), p. 211; J. Reason, *Managing the Risks of Organizational Accidents* (Aldershot, 1997), pp. 9–15.
8 L. Mulcahy, *Disputing Doctors: The Socio-Legal Dynamics of Complaints about Medical Care* (Maidenhead, 2003), pp. 4, 58; K. Price, 'Towards a History of Medical Negligence', *Lancet*, 375, 9710 (16 January 2010), pp. 192–193.
9 For introductory articles by two of the foremost historians of the NHS, see F. Honigsbaum, 'The Evolution of the NHS', *British Medical Journal*, 301 (3 October 1990), pp. 694–699; C. Webster, 'Conflict and Consensus: Explaining the British Health Service', *Twentieth Century British History*, 1, 2 (1990), p. 151.
10 Mulcahy, *Disputing Doctors*, p. 34.
11 National Archives, MH10/92: Circular of 27 September 1866, complaints of inmates, offering suggestions for guidance of guardians.
12 Mulcahy, *Disputing Doctors*, p. 4.
13 R. Klein, *Complaints against Doctors: A Study in Professional Accountability* (London, 1973), p. 104.
14 Klein, *Complaints against Doctors*, pp. 60–120.
15 Klein observed that potential complaints were 'choked off'; for every complaint there were 100 'grumbles' and for each patient who publicly grumbled 'there were four who changed their doctor' ('friction'). Klein, *Complaints against Doctors*, pp. 105–106.
16 Klein, *Complaints against Doctors*, p. 119.
17 The key work on 'iatrogenic' harm remains I. Illich, *Limits to Medicine – Medical Nemesis: The Expropriation of Health* (London, 1976/2002), *passim*. Historians have been slow to counter the medicalised view with that of the patient. See R. Porter, 'The Patient's View: Doing Medical History from Below', *Theory and Society*, 14, 2 (1985), pp. 175–198; F. Condrau, 'The Patient's View Meets the Clinical Gaze', *Social History of Medicine*, 20, 3 (2007), pp. 525–540.

18 J. Herring, *Medical Law and Ethics* (Oxford, 2006), p. 38.
19 Klein, *Complaints against Doctors*, pp. 70–71.
20 R. G. Hodgkinson, *The Origins of the National Health Service: The Medical Services of the New Poor Law, 1834–1871* (London, 1967), pp. 415–427; M. A. Crowther, 'Paupers or Patients? Obstacles to Professionalization in the Poor Law Medical Service before 1914', *Journal of the History of Medicine and Allied Sciences*, 39, 1 (1984), p. 40; Hawkins, *Mishap or Malpractice?*, p. 15.
21 Hawkins, *Mishap or Malpractice?*, p. 15.
22 H. Teff, *Reasonable Care: Legal Perspectives on the Doctor–Patient Relationship* (Oxford, 1994), p. 17.
23 For public animosity towards doctors, see C. Hamlin, 'Edwin Chadwick, "mutton medicine" and the fever question', *Bulletin of the History of Medicine*, 70, 2 (1996), pp. 233–265.
24 S. Webb and B. Webb, *The State and the Doctor* (London, 1910), pp. v–ix.
25 For an introduction to their 'divided loyalties', see M. A. Crowther, *The Workhouse System 1834–1929: The History of an English Social Institution* (London, 1981), p. 156.
26 I. Loudon, *Medical Care and the General Practitioner, 1750–1850* (Oxford, 1986), p. 248.
27 For contemporary views on this, see R. Griffin, 'The Grievances of the Poor Law Medical Officers' (1859), p. 29; 'Poor-law Medical Reform', *British Medical Journal*, 20 (1861), p. 530.
28 Quoted in R. Griffin, 'The Grievances of the Poor Law Medical Officers Elucidated in a Letter to the Members of the Legislative and a Commentary on the Proposed Act of Parliament for Redress' (London, 1858), p. 12.
29 'Poor-law Medical Relief', *British Medical Journal*, 184 (1864), p. 38.
30 R. Griffin, 'The Grievances of the Poor Law Medical Officers Further Elucidated in the Report of the Proceedings of the Deputation to the Poor Law Board' (Weymouth, 1859), p. 31.
31 W. G. Lumley, *Manuals of the Duties of Poor Law Officers: The Medical Officer*, third edition (London, 1871), p. xxxiv.
32 A. Jonsen, *The Birth of Bioethics* (New York, 1998), pp. 368–371; R. Charon, 'The Ethicality of Narrative Medicine', in B. Hurwitz, T. Greenhalgh and V. Skultans (eds), *Narrative Research in Health and Illness* (Oxford, 2004), pp. 23–36; R. Richardson, 'Narratives of Compound Loss: Parents' Stories from the Organ Retention Scandal', in Hurwitz *et al.*, *Narrative Research*, pp. 239–256; C. Vincent and L. Page, 'Aftermath of Error for Patients and Health Care Staff', in B. Hurwitz and A. Sheikh (eds), *Health Care Errors and Patient Safety* (Oxford, 2009), pp. 179–192.
33 For discussions of 'trust' and 'sympathy' as tools of the medical trade, see L. B. McCullough, *John Gregory's Writings on Medical Ethics and Philosophy of Medicine* (London, 1998), p. 170.
34 H. Weightman, *The Medical Practitioners' Legal Guide; or, the Laws Relating to the Medical Profession* (London, 1870), p. 147.
35 M. Fissell, 'The Medical Market Place, the Patient, and the Absence of Medical Ethics in Early Modern Europe and North America', in R. B. Baker and L. B. McCullough (eds), *The Cambridge World History of Medical Ethics* (New York, 2009), p. 533; I. Waddington, *The Medical Profession in the Industrial Revolution* (Dublin, 1984), pp. 153–175.
36 Weightman, *Medical Practitioners' Legal Guide*, p. 149.
37 Ibid., p. 151.
38 Waddington, *Medical Profession*, pp. 153–175; P. Vaughan, *Doctor's Commons: A Short History of the British Medical Association* (London, 1959), p. 35.

39 W. G. Lumley, *Manuals of the Duties of Poor Law Officers: The Medical Officer* (London, 1849), p. 31. See also W. G. Lumley, *Manuals of the Duties of Poor Law Officers: The Medical Officer*, second edition (London, 1857), p. 40.

40 The life of Thomas Wakley serves as a paragon for intra-professional struggle: J. Hostettler, *Thomas Wakley: An Improbable Radical* (Chichester, 1993), pp. 50–51.

41 For trade in the dead, see E. Hurren, 'A Pauper Dead-house: The Expansion of the Cambridge Anatomical Teaching School under the Late-Victorian Poor Law, 1870–1914', *Medical History*, 48, 1 (2004), pp. 69–86; R. Richardson, *Death, Dissection and the Destitute* (London, 1987). For 'orthodox' versus 'quack' medicine, see I. Loudon, 'The Vile Race of Quacks with which this Country is Infested', in W. F. Bynum and R. Porter (eds), *Medical Fringe and Medical Orthodoxy, 1750–1850* (London, 1987), pp. 106–128; R. Porter, *Quacks: Fakers and Charlatans in English Medicine* (Stroud, 2001).

42 For example, see Hamlin, 'Edwin Chadwick, "mutton medicine"', pp. 233–265.

43 J. L. Montrose, 'Is Negligence an Ethical or a Sociological Concept?', *The Modern Law Review*, 21, 3 (1958), p. 261.

44 The summing-up of an early twentieth-century judge, from Teff, *Reasonable Care*, p. 180.

45 Montrose, 'Is Negligence an Ethical or a Sociological Concept?', p. 261.

46 C. H. [Charles Holmes – a surgeon who was a poor law medical officer for a time before becoming established], *Sick Paupers and their Medical Attendants: An Exposé of the Fraud Inflicted on the Sick Poor and the Ratepayer, in the Employment by Poor-Law Medical Officers of Unqualified Assistants* (London, 1878), pp. 1–24.

47 Lumley, *Manuals*, third edition (1871), pp. xxviii–xxix.

48 Lumley, *Manuals* (1871).

49 J. Rogers, *Reminiscences of a Workhouse Medical Officer*, Foreword by T. Rogers (London, 1889), p. 91.

50 A cursory comparison of Lumley's manuals demonstrates the 1871 expansion: Lumley, *Manuals* (1849); Lumley, *Manuals* (1857); Lumley, *Manuals* (1871).

51 Nunquam Dormio [pseudonym], 'Poor Law Medical Inspectors', *Lancet*, 2366 (1869), p. 27.

52 K. Price, 'A Regional, Quantitative and Qualitative Study of the Employment, Disciplining and Discharging of Workhouse Medical Officers of the New Poor Law throughout Nineteenth-century England and Wales' (PhD thesis, Oxford Brookes University, 2008), pp. 31–103.

53 Lumley, *Manuals* (1871), p. xxxv.

54 Ibid., p. xxxv.

55 Ibid., p. xxxii.

56 Ibid., p. xxxi.

57 Ibid., p. 37.

58 Ibid., p. 37.

59 Price, *Medical Negligence in Victorian Britain.*

60 E. Hurren, *Protesting about Pauperism: Poverty, Politics and Poor Relief in Late-Victorian England, 1870–1900* (Woodbridge, 2007), *passim.*

61 K. Waddington, 'Paying for the Sick Poor: Financing Medicine under the Victorian Poor Law – the Case of the Whitechapel Union, 1850–1900', in M. Gorsky and S. Sheard (eds), *Financing Medicine: The British Experience Since 1750* (London, 2006), pp. 102–105; Hurren, *Protesting about Pauperism*, p. 253; E. Hurren, 'Poor Law versus Public Health: Diphtheria, Sanitary Reform, and the 'Crusade' against Outdoor Relief

1870–1900', *Social History of Medicine*, 18 (2005), pp. 399–418; K. Williams, *From Pauperism to Poverty* (London, 1981), pp. 91–144; M. MacKinnon, 'English Poor Law Policy and the Crusade against Out-relief', *The Journal of Economic History*, 47 (1987), pp. 603–625; C. Smith, 'Family, Community and the Victorian Asylum: A Case Study of the Northampton General Lunatic Asylum and its Pauper Lunatics', *Family and Community History*, 9 (2006), p. 116; K. Price, '"Where is the fault?": The Starvation of Edward Cooper at the Isle of Wight Workhouse in 1877', *Social History of Medicine*, 26, 1 (2013), pp. 21–37.

62 Hurren, *Protesting about Pauperism*, p. 56.

63 A. Borsay, *Disability and Social Policy in Britain since 1750: A History of Exclusion* (London, 2005), pp. 31–36.

64 'Poor Law Medical Officers' Association', *British Medical Journal*, 1130 (1882), p. 380.

65 For example, see National Archives, MH 12/13388 1877–79 Coventry Union Correspondence: 1879, official inquiry into the charges against Mr Thomas Millerchip, district medical officer (who received the association's full support).

66 'The "Starvation Case", Isle of Wight', *Lancet* (16 June 1877). For further context, see Price, '"Where is the fault?"', pp. 21–37.

67 For example, see 'Letters to the Editor: Who is in Fault?', *The English Labourers' Chronicle* (12 May 1877), p. 5; 'The Starvation Case at Sunderland', *British Medical Journal* (17 March 1877), p. 340; 'Out-door Relief', *Reynold's Newspaper* (5 August 1877).

68 Lumley, *Manuals* (1871), p. 19.

69 National Archives: MH 12/13514 Stratford-on-Avon Union, 1870.

70 Ibid..

71 N. C. Walsh, *The Medical Officer's Vade-Mecum or Poor Law Surgeon's Guide* (London, 1866), p. 7.

72 Lumley, *Manuals* (1871), p. 19.

73 Walsh, *The Medical Officer's Vade-Mecum*, p. 30.

74 A. Sheen, *The Workhouse and its Medical Officer*, second edition (Bristol, 1890), p. 7.

75 Letter from Dr Campbell, 'Fees in Cases of Urgency', *British Medical Journal*, 658 (1873), p. 176.

76 Letter from W. Blenkarne, 'Medical Relief in the Bridgnorth Union', *British Medical Journal*, 1275 (1885), p. 1179.

77 Rogers, *Reminiscences*, p. 19.

78 For further context, see Price, *Medical Negligence in Victorian Britain*.

Part III

Patients

7 The role of complaint in establishing the rights of the patient and the duties of the doctor, 1800–70s

Steven King

Introduction

The nature of the relationship between a doctor and his middle-class and aristocratic patients in the nineteenth century is now well established for the British case. In a medical market where cure was often elusive, the role and aspiration of the doctor was as much socio-cultural as medical. Moneyed patients with plenty of choice – and the knowledge and desire to execute it – demanded prompt personal and written attention, easy financial terms, and (notwithstanding a wider sense of the disappearance of the patient narrative) an active role in what modern medical professionals would label a 'care package'.[1] Local medical societies helped to create a collective and increasingly national identity among doctors and a wider movement to professionalisation once the early nineteenth century gave energy to the identification and confrontation of otherness (quacks, irregular practitioners, female healers). However, in Britain it was not until the later nineteenth century (and later than other areas of Europe) that the need for formal qualifications and the professional oversight of doctoring activity reached parity with that which had been exercised by and over the apothecaries since 1815.[2] Even then, as Ingram's chapter and others in this volume demonstrate, medical professionalism continued to be organic. Against this backdrop, a false step or an inability to play the holistic role of the doctor led either to a failure to get established or to socio-economic ruin.[3]

Moneyed patients were certainly quick to criticise, as Scull's chapter conveys too. In letters to relatives, in diaries, through the press, and sometimes in written correspondence with doctors themselves, such people expressed their dissatisfaction with diagnosis, treatment, neglect of social duties and occasionally serious financial, medical or moral malpractice. The nineteenth-century correspondence of the Heywood family of Bolton (in the northern English county of Lancashire), for instance, contains more than 300 direct or indirect (broadly, it is pointless going to the doctor because he will do me no good) expressions of dissatisfaction with family doctors.[4] The scathing view of the efficacy of doctors and their remedies that opens Tobias Smollett's *The Expedition of Humphry Clinker* (1771):

> The pills are good for nothing – I might as well swallow snow balls to cool my veins – I have told you over and over, how hard I am to move; and at this time of day, I ought to know something of my own constitution. Why will you be so positive? Prithee send me another prescription . . .[5]

has vibrant resonance in contemporary letters. Writing from Bath, the English spa town, where he had repaired suffering from gout, the Reverend John Penrose noted:

> I am now to take the Water from the Cross Bath at 7 and 8 o'clock mornings, and from the King's Bath at 12, quarter of a Pint each time. Everyone who comes in tells me this exactness as to Time and Quantity is a mere farce, notwithstanding the Doctors so gravely prescribe.[6]

In turn, the ease with which a reputation, and hence an economic niche among moneyed patients like these, could be lost – explicit in such novels as George Eliot's *Middlemarch* (1874) – does much to explain the explosion of self-improvement, emphasis on training, and accumulation of local positions by doctors in the nineteenth century.[7] These broad outlines are clear. Much less work has been done on the relationship between doctors and their patient base among the labouring and dependent poor. As Digby and Crowther have persuasively pointed out, from the later eighteenth century, doctors came to play an ever greater role in the medical lives of the labouring sick, both inside and outside institutions.[8] Contracting a doctor for a fixed period rapidly became the norm among the parochial authorities (who were responsible for administering welfare) from the early nineteenth century, such that dependency was increasingly pathologised and brought under a medical ambit. The proportion of total poor law spending absorbed by medical relief increased consistently and strongly from the early 1800s. In turn, the implicit assumption in much of the secondary literature has been that formalised medicine was imposed, with more or sometimes less acceptance, on the poorest sections of society. Medicine was 'done to' this group, and historians of the poor law and of medicine have in particular concentrated upon the workhouse and hospital scandals that emerged from this dependency.[9] The evolution of patient rights and the duties of doctors were played out on the very bodies of the poor in the absence of formal regulation from the 1850s.

This chapter takes up the theme of the agency of the poor in their engagement with doctors. In particular, it deals with patients outside socio-medical institutions, enhancing the role of this volume in complicating assumptions about theatres of medical care and complaint, chronology, class and power. Rule-based rights and duties, of the sort inscribed into the daily routines of voluntary hospitals or the contracts signed by doctors to provide their services free of charge to workhouses, hospitals and medical charities, had a powerful effect in setting minimum standards, the breaching of which created colourful scandals throughout the period considered here.[10] On the other hand, admission to such institutions inevitably involved the sacrifice of some rights, aspects of agency and (crucially) a voice. In this sense, institutional scandals mask as much as they reveal.[11] In any case, the vast majority of medical encounters for most of the poor over most of their life cycle took place outside any institutional context; it is on this wider canvas that the medical agency of the poor needs to be drawn – an ideal manifest within this chapter and in those of Newsom Kerr, Thompson and León-Sanz, among others.

The sources for such an exercise are surprisingly common. They range from ego-documents such as autobiographies and pauper letters, through the expectations of doctors in their engagements with poor patients framed by third-party narratives, and to cases played out in legal and coronial courts, through which local expectations appear to have been forcefully shaped. This chapter focuses deliberately on the period from just before the first attempts at medical regulation of the apothecaries (the lowest rung of a formal medical hierarchy in England which had physicians at the top) until the 1870s. At the latter date an increasingly organised and regulated medical profession dominated by the surgeon-apothecary had begun to make real inroads into the power of other providers (chemists, quacks, informal practitioners) in the medical marketplace. It is in this period, in the absence of effective regulation of the doctor–patient relationship, that we most need to understand how the rights of patients and the duties of doctors were established, maintained and modified. Drawing on some 12,000 pauper letters and items of third-party correspondence, a small selection of autobiographies, vestry minutes and more than 30,000 coronial inquests for the English Midland circuit (the counties of Northamptonshire, Leicestershire, Lincolnshire, Warwickshire and Rutland), this chapter argues that through the use of third-party complaints, via direct engagement with doctors and those who commissioned healthcare, or using weapons such as rumour, the dependent and labouring poor actively shaped their perceived healthcare rights and the analogous duties for the doctors who increasingly treated their needs. They did not have healthcare 'done to them', but rather shaped its intensity and character, suggesting a wider need to rethink the nature and direction of power in the English and Welsh welfare system.

Rights, duties and third parties

The biggest conduit of medical care for the dependent and marginal poor was the poor law.[12] Even with the advent of the New Poor Law in 1834 and the incremental addition of infirmaries to workhouses that successive waves of building in poor law unions stimulated, most medical services for the poor were provided in their own homes. While the quality of those medical services has sometimes been questioned,[13] the sense that poverty was an increasingly medicalised condition in the period considered here is inescapable. Against this backdrop, it is important to understand that overseers under the Old Poor Law and Boards of Guardians under the New were finely attuned to the need to balance economy in the treatment of pauper patients with the setting of clear expectations and minimum standards in their engagement with providers of medical care. Such officials did not as a default position simply accept the lowest price with no thought as to what this meant for paupers. The explicit expectation-setting inscribed in doctoring contracts under the Old Poor Law has been well analysed for the county of Bedfordshire.[14] Jumping to a wider canvas suggests that at the same time as doctors across the country were increasingly successful between the 1790s and 1830s in establishing and renewing contracts with parochial authorities, so officials were increasingly successful in setting minimum standards. Contractual discussions recorded in the Memorandum Book for the Northamptonshire parish of Crick in 1830–31 are absolutely typical of the more than 500 such documents analysed for this chapter, and reflect discussions of economy and duty found in Price's and other chapters. Bargaining with Dr Thomas Osborne Walker for a renewal of contract, officials stipulated that if at any time Walker was unable to attend the poor, his assistant must do it at Walker's expense. Moreover, in return for a salary of £18 (dropping from the £22 agreed in 1826) the doctor had to consent to reduce the number of conditions excluded from the contract, increase the area over which he would travel and guarantee a minimum call-out time within the community itself.[15] While these contractual changes did not inevitably result in better treatment of the poor, the episode demonstrates well the balancing of the needs for economy on the one hand and supporting sick paupers on the other.

More widely, the dismissal of doctors or the failure to renew contracts where the standards expected by the parish had not been met was surprisingly common. A combined dataset of vestry minutes and overseers' correspondence for the counties of Northamptonshire, Berkshire and Wiltshire over the period 1800–34 identifies 127 cases of dismissal during a contract (for faults as varied as sexual or financial misconduct, failing to attend when called, and treating without authority) or of non-renewal because of inadequate performance. Parochial officials were, in other words, a major and active arbiter of basic standards of medical care for the dependent and marginal poor. It is important also to understand that the debates over doctoring contracts were played out in the public forum of the vestry and through the gossip networks of communities. It is simply inconceivable that dismissals or non-renewals of contract – in effect debates about minimum standards, the rights of patients and the duties of doctors – did not filter into the expectations of the dependent and marginal poor.

In turn, large-scale comparative work on parochial archives – particularly correspondence by or about the poor – has begun to reveal the surprising susceptibility of these parochial officials to complaints, illustrating the lineage of the negotiations found in Thompson's and León-Sanz's chapters in this volume. The agency of the poor themselves is considered in the next section of this chapter, but two other avenues seem to have been particularly important in indirect (via complaints about the action or inaction of officials) and direct (via complaints about the action or inaction of doctors) pressure for the evolution of minimum standards under the Old Poor Law. The first was official correspondence. Stretching to more than 4,000 items in the corpus underpinning this chapter, letters between local officials and between officials and third parties, such as magistrates, constitute the last great untapped resource for understanding both the Old Poor Law and the experience of the poor. Within this corpus, overseers and other officials were surprisingly sharp with each other and never more so than when there was a perception that minimal standards of medical treatment or attendance were not being met.

The case of Mary Tyrrell is an emblematic example of this process. Examined before the magistrate Oliver Craven on 13 September 1819, she noted that her husband and child had been taken ill while travelling between Cardiff and London, stopping their journey in Marlborough. Mr May, the overseer of the Parish of St Peters Marlborough, was called and 'said to informant [Mrs Tyrrell] this is a fine job to have such trouble on the Parish'. After failing to send a doctor, Mr May attempted to put the family on a wagon destined for their 'home' parish of Hungerford in Berkshire, but 'her Husband told her several times he thought he should die upon the Road, and beg'd her to go to the Overseer and ask him leave to stay till he was better'.[16] Refused, Mrs Tyrrell

> took her child to Mr Washbourne's the Parish Doctor and his assistant or apprentice examined the Child's tongue which at that time was very green, and he told informant her Child was Better Informant answered that her Child was not better but was much worse.[17]

With no further consideration the family were placed on the wagon and sent to Hungerford. The fact that Tyrrell questioned the judgement of the parish doctor points to the sort of agency explored in more depth later in this chapter. For now, it is important to observe that both the magistrate who took the examination and the overseer of Hungerford objected strongly to the actions of officials and doctors in Marlborough. The latter official sent a letter to his counterpart in Marlborough upon the death of Tyrrell's child in November 1819 pointing out that had their own parish doctor behaved 'as I would have expected of a medical man in this position', the child might have lived.[18] Trust, he observed, was the lifeblood of inter-parochial relationships and he regretted that in future medical cases he could 'trust no more'.[19]

Understanding the relationship between incidents such as this, the development of doctoring duties and the formation of parochial and pauper expectations is a complex matter. Three clear feedback loops can, however, be identified. First, and as in the case of Mrs Tyrrell above, the sharing of expectations of doctors and medical provision implicit in complaints of this sort fed directly into the authorial intent of those who drew up doctoring contracts. These became more precise and more prone to set minimum standards of attendance over the latter stages of the Old Poor Law, and nowhere more so than in Marlborough. Second, the underlying corpus provides evidence that officials did not construct their correspondence without reference to paupers themselves. At the very least, interviews were required to establish the medical and other facts of cases that prompted inter-parochial complaint.

Some records also suggest that officials wrote the complaint in the presence of the paupers, checked it with a representative of the family or individual, or even read it to the person concerned. Thus Eliza Wickes added a short paragraph to the letter sent by William Hughes, overseer of Rothersthorpe in Northamptonshire to his counterpart in Reading. Hughes's letter complained about the treatment of Widow Danbridge (Wickes' mother) in a recent bout of sickness, observing that money sent by the daughter to provide medicine had been used for other purposes and that the widow would have been better treated 'at home' had the overseer of Reading just conveyed her. Wickes added archly, 'We knows wot good docturin is and this us far from it'.[20] It is a short step from these observations to an accreting communal sense of what appropriate medical interventions looked like. Finally, it is important to understand that these incoming letters and complaints were not simply received and filed by the overseers of the poor. Some – as at Thrapston in Northamptonshire – copied all correspondence into a copy letter book which was passed between overseers as they entered and exited office, a rendering of collective memory on poor law and medical policy. Where a vestry or select vestry existed, as was increasingly the case in the period post-1790, the letters would have been public documents, for reading out and consideration at the meetings of ratepayers. Even where such oversight did not exist, medical cases were invariably expensive and necessitated the overseer consulting others in the community. There was, in other words, a collectivisation of the inter-parochial complaint which probably shaped both current and future practice.

In turn, these observations apply even more powerfully to a second conduit prompting the development of patient rights and doctoring duties: the correspondence of the epistolary advocates of the poor. This group – landlords, doctors, neighbours, family members, employers, clergy and even the odd aristocrat – wrote in support of claims for help with paying rent and in cases of unemployment. Above all other motives in the 1,200 letters of this sort in the underlying corpus, however, was sickness. While such epistolary advocates were unlikely to launch into complaint on the first occasion of writing, actions such as partial payment, not responding, or a refusal by officials to consider relief invariably occasioned such complaints. These might in turn stretch over a series of letters, providing an important window both onto embedded community expectations of doctors and officials and onto the process by which standards were raised and extended. William Hackworth, the sometime employer of John Bond, wrote from Box in Wiltshire to Chard in Somerset after an initial letter had gone unanswered to say that he was surprised that the overseer there had not had the good grace to order the doctor for Bond. 'It would be normal', he observed, for the doctor to visit regularly and for the parish to pay for salves, bandages and compresses as needed for the ulcer on Bond's leg.[21] Failure to comply with his request, Hackworth warned, would result in a complaint to the magistrates.[22]

Since the vast majority of all epistolary advocates were the social equals or (often) social superiors of the officials with whom they corresponded, sharp complaints were likely to have carried particular weight in shaping current practice and future standards. Of course, some officials and vestries railed against being lectured by people who were often outside the parish and had a poor grasp of the pressure on local ratepayers, nowhere more so than when English parishes wrote to their Welsh counterparts, but the spur to change provided by such correspondence is clear in most cases. After Hackworth's stinging letter, for instance, the parish of Box both drew up its first doctoring contract and enacted a policy of engaging doctors for the out-parish poor. The feedback loops to the expectations of the poor were fostered particularly strongly by the fact that few of these epistolary advocates wrote without referring to the paupers themselves, generating a common stock of knowledge about what the social and economic elites of communities thought of as acceptable medical care.[23]

The impact of the New Poor Law on the medical care of the poor is often seen to have been very negative, at least in the 1830s and 1840s.[24] More widely, there are reasons to expect a dwindling of the role of welfare officials in shaping the duties of doctors and the expectations of their poor and marginal patients. The formation of poor law unions and Boards of Guardians took decisions about the medical dimensions of pauper care to an extra-local level at the same time that the process reduced the need for correspondence between parishes and officials. Central directives on the personnel to be employed left less scope for the differences of practice that led to third-party complaints about standards of care. The emergence of roughly standard contracts for medical officers took several decades, but the existence of such contracts and models, allied with the greater circulation of information about welfare spending, might have been expected to lead to the definition, rather than creeping negotiation, of doctoring duties and patient rights. Moreover, the locus of complaint changed from parish and individual official to the union and central authorities. This changing situation is often assumed to have reduced the agency of the poor and their sponsors, allowing guardians to hide behind the administrative power of central authorities. Certainly, Elizabeth Hurren has shown that the late-Victorian authorities exhibited a systemic tendency to mute the voices of the poor.[25] On top of these changes, workhouse infirmaries and a resurgent voluntary and specialist hospital movement sucked some of the most difficult and contentious cases – those most likely perhaps to be the subject of complaint and of the associated setting of standards – out of the direct ambit of local officials. Even when there were medical 'scandals' in individual poor law unions, Kim Price has demonstrated beyond doubt that many of them were politically inspired and thus not likely to be vehicles for standard-setting.[26]

While there is much to commend this picture, however, it is far from complete. Complaints from paupers themselves and from their sponsors did not in fact dry up. Rather, the range of recipients of such communications expanded from two (parish; official) to seven (local official; medical or other officer; vestry; Board of Guardians; newspapers; central authorities; other local people), and the failure to constellate these different sources of information has generated a misleading picture of the extent of agency within the post-1834 welfare system. Indeed, there is evidence to suggest that the intensity of letter writing by epistolary advocates on behalf of the poor *increased* under the New Poor Law and actually gathered pace across the mid-Victorian period. A survey of third-party correspondence in local and national archives for the counties of Northamptonshire, Berkshire and Leicestershire shows that, while the number of letters sent (absolutely and per capita on the pauper population) by paupers themselves fell under the New Poor Law, third-party correspondence increased in every decade until the coming of poor law democracy in the 1890s. There are several potential readings of these observations, but the one preferred here is that doctoring duties and patient expectations continued to be negotiated for the poor at local level even after the 1858 Medical Act had set the foundation stones for professional regulation. The fact of this negotiation, I suggest, explains why the poor law medical system generated so *few* scandals and neglect cases when it could have generated so many.

Agency and expectation

Third-party complaints were just one way in which the boundaries between doctoring duties and patient rights and expectations for the poor were located and refined. Their extent suggests that the late twentieth-century patient groups discussed in Mold's chapter in this volume were born from collective memory and not just from high market capitalism. However, and notwithstanding an ingrained sense that poorer patients were relatively powerless in the doctor–patient relationship, the poor had gained and maintained considerable agency in shaping and constraining the actions of doctors in other ways too. One avenue was through the systematic appropriation of custom. In 1776, Anthony Fothergill warned his young protégé, James Woodforde, about engaging with paupers: 'If you set apart 2 hours every day in prescribing for paupers', he noted, 'they will not fail to spread your fame and bring in opulent farmers and by degrees the neighbouring gentry'.[27] Yet while this might be a good thing for a young doctor seeking his way in the world, Fothergill warned that

> to do this [you] must sit down resolutely bent to continue, for if the slightest hint escapes you of a design to relinquish, it will at once destroy the interest you have made and damp all future hopes of establishing among them.[28]

At the other end of the period covered by this chapter, the doctor and (later) author Arthur Conan Doyle fictionalised his own similar experiences of the poor in Portsmouth appropriating acts of charity and goodwill to create rights. In the *Stark Munro Letters*, the protagonist outlines the need to give his time free to the poor because 'it may be a nucleus for cases', and then goes on to lament the fact that 'Cases came dribbling in from day to day – all very poor people, and able to pay very poor fees', but acknowledges them as essential if he is to build up his practice.[29] Skirmishes between doctors – who largely seem to have felt the imperative to offer free or reduced-cost services to the poorest – and the poor – who clearly assumed that doctors had a moral duty to them over and above the time remunerated by the poor laws or paid for from their own pockets – are consistently and substantially evidenced in the material analysed for this chapter. Assumptions and assertions that a local doctor would treat sudden or potentially mortal illness 'kindly' (that is to say for free) are to be found in many hundreds of pauper letters. Local officials also elaborated a sense that sudden illness imposed different duties on local doctors, often making a point to their counterparts in other parishes that the bills they enclosed did not include remuneration for medical attendance and remedies. Even under the New Poor Law, as the case of Conan Doyle illustrates, doctors were unable to prevent individual acts of humanity becoming part of the customary collective duty of medical men.

The poor might also appropriate the authority (rather than simply the voices or words) of third parties in seeking to establish and maintain rights or to enforce doctoring duties. This was particularly so in the case of informal practitioners, who were by no means exempt from the sense that there were minimum – and enforceable – standards of care. In March 1817, Samuel Bamford and his friend Joseph Healey were on the run as the government sought to suppress radical agitation in north-west England. Healey was a cow doctor, learning his trade in the rural industrial areas north of Manchester, but he 'also dabbled a little in medicines for the human frame, and was successful in most of the cases which he undertook'.[30] His father had been a supernatural healer. After the latter's death, Healey was apprenticed in cotton weaving, married and came to Bamford's village of Middleton where he 'began by selling simple drugs'.[31] Book-learning allowed him to venture into compounding and prescribing medicines, 'breathing a vein', and eventually dentistry.[32] In his own view, he was a 'general practitioner of the surgical art' and was 'thankful, he needed not turn his back on any of his neighbours in the same line', even if he was deficient in obstetrics.[33] By the time he went on the run with Bamford in 1817, he was 32 years of age and of shabby appearance. His undercoat, 'by his almost incessant occupation in "the laboratory", preparing ointments, salves and lotions, had become smooth and shining as a duck's wing, and almost as impervious to wet'.[34] Entering a pub not long into their journey, the two men encountered a mother buying ale for a daughter with toothache. Healey intervened to offer his services. The woman was sceptical because of his 'unctuous clothes', but he 'pulled out a case of lancets and his tooth-drawing instrument', suggesting that to draw the tooth would be a 'mere flea bite'.[35] The pulling did not go well. There was a scream and crashing as the patient lashed out at Healey and two teeth rather than one came out, along with copious amounts of blood. A distraught mother quickly returned with a constable and an overseer. 'That little devil', she insisted, 'pretended to be a docthur', and the two officials duly decided to bring Healey and Bamford before the magistrates.[36] Seeking to avoid further public fuss, Bamford negotiated compensation of sixpence, and the two men were allowed on their way.

The involvement of non-familial third parties in the doctor–patient relationship was simultaneously a confirmation that basic patient rights existed or were thought to exist, a vehicle for locating the boundaries of those rights and analogous duties, and a way of reinforcing and publicising them. The fact that Healey was detained for pretending to be a doctor suggests that both the mother and the officials understood the way that a 'real' doctor should operate. In turn, and just as the mother had appropriated the authority of a constable and overseer, the underlying corpus of data is replete with instances where paupers sought to use third parties to derive rights or impose duties. This might involve invocation of a history of patronage by prominent local people, quotation from prescriptions or even medical textbooks, getting local doctors to endorse appeals for medical aid, writing to local newspapers, and even the engagement of solicitors to write letters to parochial authorities.

Sometimes, the involvement of a third party had consequences for rights and duties that resonated on the regional or even the national stage. Nowhere is this clearer than in the activities of coroners and their juries. Convened for cases of unexplained deaths, coronial juries had wide investigative powers and could send cases to higher courts for criminal prosecution. Their narrative verdicts, widely reported in the regional press, also had the power to affirm or establish basic standards of behaviour, to test the boundaries of rights and duties and to establish new rights; these sorts of influence are retained by coroners today and are shared by the criminal, professional and public hearings examined in the chapters in this volume by McHale and by Jones and Shanks. What this meant for *doctors* is explored in the next section, but in the meantime, it is clear that the coroner played an important part in regulating the practice and establishing the duties of *irregular* practitioners who did not claim to be doctors. The cases of the Midland circuit (reported in newspapers or preserved in coronial records) between 1800 and 1870 cover everything from suspected suicides to infanticides and accidents. They contain witness testimony, the deliberative processes of the jury and associated evidence, which might run from love letters to bottles of medicine. A consistent theme in these records is the activity of irregular providers of medicine – herbalists, quacks, chemists and others – and their periodic role in unexplained deaths. Whether for incorrect dosages, improper or inadequate guidance, active deceit or pretending to be more than they were, irregular practitioners found themselves in the coronial court with striking regularity. Sometimes, the cases themselves were initiated by paupers literally dragging the offending party into court. While cases were rarely referred on for criminal prosecution, no less than 533 resulted in narratives admonishing aspects of practice. Ultimately, one cannot know how these third-party judgements affected the rights of poor patients or the perceived duties of irregular practitioners, but the fact that they were widely reported and in multiple newspapers would suggest the potential for a wider disciplinary mechanism.

A third avenue for exerting agency was via direct complaints. It is becoming increasingly clear that workhouse and asylum inmates actively questioned the conditions there.[37] Complaints in and from other institutions, such as hospitals, have attracted rather less attention, a reflection perhaps of the sense from much of the literature on voluntary hospitals that the poor and their sponsors actively sought admission to medical institutions. Instances of paupers and labouring people refusing medical treatment or admission to institutions, however, are not uncommon. Retrospective complaints about the standard of treatment in medical institutions are also to be found, as for instance in the case of John Dorney of Rothersthorpe who complained to the parochial vestry that he 'was treated no better than a dog' when admitted to a hospital in Northampton suffering from gout.[38] Less is known about the agency of the poor within medical institutions at the time they were patients, a reflection of ingrained assumptions that rules on behaviour, visiting and the rights of doctors and their administrators in such institutions nullified pauper agency. Yet, and as the Introduction to this volume shows, there had been internal complaint mechanisms in such places as hospitals and asylums since the 1700s. Moreover, there are cases such as that of William Daniel who wrote in June 1828 from his bed at Stafford Infirmary to complain to the overseer of the Northamptonshire parish of Welton that:

> The docturs here are little more than quacks and treet a respektable man without the dignity due to Him Little more than purges which I could get myself if Wanted Consider Gent'n but would you subject yourself to those startin out and without the Qualerfurcations much needed for a corse such as Mine.[39]

While it is difficult to reconstruct the wider impact of such complaints, the local effect is clear in the sense that Welton cancelled its annual subscription to the Infirmary.

If the data for agency in relation to institutions is relatively thin, for the outdoor poor there is a much stronger sense that people had both a good understanding of their rights as patients and a determination to exercise them. Sometimes such rights were rhetoricised and operationalised through collective action, such as riots.[40] More widely, collective action against doctors who were seen to have contravened the norms of behaviour is surprisingly common prior to the twentieth century when looked for. John Paley of Carlisle – known disparagingly as 'Carver Paley' because of his proclivity to operate – was run out of town in 1838 by a mob incensed that he was rumoured to be experimenting on the poor.[41]

Cases such as this generated wide publicity and it is inconceivable that such public commentary did not impact the boundaries between patient rights and doctoring duties. It was, however, an ongoing and vocal assertion and defence of rights by the poor at the individual level which really shaped the nature of local medical practice. The underlying corpus of pauper letters contains narratives ranging from those that reflect on the failure of local doctors to cure the complaint which necessitated the pauper writing (thus costing ratepayers rather more), through those that questioned the competence of one doctor by comparing them to another, and to those which actively contested the knowledge, techniques or professionalisation of the doctor. When Jacob Curchin wrote a series of letters from Wisbech (Cambridgeshire) to Thrapston (Northamptonshire) claiming variously that 'Dr Metcalfe has dun me no good'; that Curchin had 'been passed off with some Julep and not a proper thing'; that 'I am worse than ever but wuld be better if I could just get a proper doctur'; and that 'he [Dr Metcalfe] never comes when called and dus not stay when asked', he was reflecting the tone, sentiment and content of more than 1,600 other letters in which paupers complained about medical care.[42]

It is easy to read these letters as narrow, inward-looking documents that would have had a minimal impact in terms of establishing or defending the rights of poor patients. This would be incorrect. It is clear from vestry minutes up and down the country that pauper letters were routinely read to public meetings by officials. The sense that paupers knew the letters they wrote would inevitably become public documents and public narratives, with potentially wide-ranging consequences for doctors and others named is illustrated by the case of Mary Ward. She wrote from London to Caversham in Berkshire and warned the overseer that she knew what had been said at the last vestry; 'I knows from common raport that others have a strong claim on you' and 'you will hablige me in making sure this letter is read at the vestry so that all the Gentlmn might no my case'.[43] The critiques discussed in the Introduction to this volume did not necessarily need widespread publication but merely local dissemination to have a significant impact on questioning practice gone wrong. Moreover, the fact that doctors often claimed a right of reply to the assertions in letters, or even wrote unprompted, suggests both that such men could garner knowledge of pauper complaints *and* that they were alive to their damaging nature.

Rights, duties and maintaining a reputation

The idea that doctors were consistently concerned about their reputations and standing is clear from the wider literature. The fragility of such reputation, both at the individual and at collective local or regional level, is less readily appreciated. In particular, reputations were susceptible to scandal and scandal was in its turn an important variable, shaping the boundaries between the rights of poorer patients and the duties of the doctors who attended them. While most scandals are subject to multiple potential readings in terms of cause and effect, there can be no doubt of their wider disciplinary and discipline-shaping nature. By way of example, the *Northampton Herald* newspaper on 14 July 1841 reported a legal case for damages brought by the father of Charlotte Roddiss who, it was alleged, had been seduced by a Northampton surgeon, Mr Faircloth.[44] The court heard that Charlotte was 27 years of age and got to know Faircloth when he was a pupil at the Infirmary. She 'kept company' until 1834 when he left for training in London. Faircloth returned in 1836; they courted and then parted when Roddiss thought that he was keeping company elsewhere. Faircloth then wrote to her in December 1838 seeking reconciliation. A year later, she went to his house for the first time and had sex, continuing in this vein to July 1840 when she found herself pregnant. In the ordinary course of events, this would have remained a simple breach-of-promise case.[45] But in response to her pregnancy, Faircloth asked Charlotte to take 'some drops [presumably an abortificant]' with 'an injunction of secrecy'.[46] This evidence, and the doctor's claim that he had never seen Roddiss except in a professional capacity, reinvented the case as one bound up with the proper behaviour of doctors on the one hand and the proper practitioner–patient relationship on the other.

The plaintiff, Mr Roddiss, claimed that when Charlotte refused to take the medicine, Faircloth began sending anonymous letters to her friends and family making accusations of sexual freedom. Confronted, Faircloth denied sending the letters but, asked to defend Charlotte, he simply claimed that he could not know whether the accusations were true because he was not always with her. In October 1840, Faircloth confirmed that he planned to deny any involvement and simply wrote Charlotte a note asking her father to pay 10s 6d for personal attendance and a dose of steel drops. Outraged, Charlotte gave him the money herself and he took it. Engaged subsequently by Mr Roddiss, Faircloth claimed in writing that he had only ever attended Charlotte professionally and that she had recently called to pay his bill. The child was born 13 March 1841. In court, Faircloth claimed not to have seen Roddiss for the two years before the birth and his counsel hinged Faircloth's defence on whether anyone had seen Roddiss either with Faircloth in public or going into and out of his house. No one had, and this was an important point in the case. Another was the 'most unprofessional prescription' for abortificants.[47] The judge – Baron Gurney – was clearly sceptical, reminding the jury that there was no evidence that the anonymous letters were written by Faircloth, that no promise of marriage had been broken, that Roddiss was not very young (i.e. she should have been worldly-wise) and that her father and mother had not taken due care and attention. Notwithstanding such direction, the jury found for the Roddiss family after a 'brief' consultation and awarded £80 damages plus costs.[48] At the core of this case, then, was the singular question of the boundaries of familiarity implicit in the doctor–patient relationship, itself keying into wider concerns of the time with the qualifications and deportment of irregular practitioners. The case and the censuring of the conduct of Faircloth that followed were reported in newspapers from Bristol and Cardiff to London (where the case was dissected in detail by the *Morning Post*), Truro and Glasgow. Of course, reporting and reception are two very different things, but it would seem likely that such scandals had at least a cautionary impact on other doctors.

Mr Roddiss was a butcher, and although this did not entirely lift him out of the threat of poverty, he sat at the top of the social group with which this chapter is concerned. The very poorest might also highlight and precipitate scandal, as anonymous letters to newspapers, poor law guardians or prominent local figures testify. For this group, however, another tool served even more effectively to generalise and enforce rights – the creation of rumour. The impact of a middle-class rumour mill on the career of Dr Tertius Lydgate in *Middlemarch* is well known.[49] The frequency and ferocity of such rumour by and relating to the poor is more opaque. But the corpus of coronial records analysed here is replete with cases where the coroner took it upon himself to investigate suspicious, or even not so suspicious, deaths in which doctors or other providers had involvement. Rumours might imply failure to attend, under- or over-dosing, neglect of family and friends, attempted cover-up, sexual irregularity, experimentation, misdiagnosis and over-charging. Thus, on 19 September 1817, an inquest was held into the death of March Racalous from Dowsby in Lincolnshire. She had been 'under the care of the medical gentleman who attends the poor of the parish' and, upon her death, a rumour swiftly circulated that his prescriptions had killed the patient.[50] The death of the child James MacGregor, also at Dowsby, on 2 July 1828, led to a rumour that the doctor had prescribed a fatal sublimate of mercury rather than the tonic he had talked to the child's mother about.[51] When Elizabeth Hutchinson, a pauper of Crowle in Lincolnshire, died on 16 June 1812, a persistent rumour that the parish doctor had failed to attend her prompted a long inquest with 16 witnesses.[52] Ann Rowston's death at Billinghay, Lincolnshire, on 9 September 1813 necessitated that a jury be 'summoned in consequence of a report having become prevalent in the neighbourhood that the death of the deceased had been caused by certain medicines administered to her by a travelling quack'.[53] These examples, chosen at random from a wider sample of 576 cases, point to the ease with which rumours about medical men could start, and the evidence points persuasively to the number of rumours increasing across the period considered in this chapter. Nor was the twentieth century immune, as Jones and Shanks' chapter in this volume suggests.

The coroner rarely found rumours of doctoring incompetence or malfeasance proven. In the case of March Racalous, she was deemed to have mixed the prescription of the doctor with 'laudanum and opium in such quantities as her weak frame was unable to bear';[54] for Elizabeth Hutchinson, the jury concluded that she had 'labored under a disease of the body for these last three months' and had died by a Visitation of God 'and not by any neglect of the said parish';[55] Ann Rowston's inquest yielded no evidence that 'the death of the unfortunate woman could be attributed to the said quack';[56] James MacGregor was killed by an error of the mother, who used medicine she had procured elsewhere, rather than 'a powder of medicine she had procured from a medical practitioner'.[57] Nonetheless, the length of the evidence usually presented, extensive cross-examination of the doctor and the number of witnesses called in these cases, allied with the fact that the perpetrator of the rumour was rarely identified, points to the power of rumour as a weapon of the weak, a de facto substitute for complaint on the part of the poor.

Conclusion

At the core of our understanding of the way that the poor experienced medicine and doctors is the implicit idea that medicine was 'done' to this group. There may have been resistance – as for instance with anti-vaccination riots – but the figure of the sick pauper desperately seeking admission to hospitals in nineteenth-century England has been a powerful coda to these instances. The evidence employed here suggests that it is time to rethink this underlying assumption. In practice, as we have seen, paupers were active in shaping the incidence, intensity and character of the medical care they received. Bringing together the largest corpus of pauper letters, overseers' correspondence, advocate letters and coronial records ever assembled allows us to see patterns otherwise hidden from the gaze of medical and welfare historians. Re-instituting those patterns suggests that the poor seeking medical aid could systematically appropriate the authority of third parties, the customary practice of doctors and the voices of advocates to push forward their cause. They could and did also complain directly, to parochial authorities, boards of guardians, government officials and doctors themselves, and we have seen evidence that the commissioners and providers of healthcare were sensitive to those complaints. The rise of the nineteenth-century information state both reinforced traditional avenues and destinations for complaint and opened up new ones. And if direct complaint did not work, then rumour might, given the extraordinary reputational and opportunity costs associated with repeated inquests into otherwise unexplained deaths. The poor complaining about medicine was thus an integral, and arguably a growing, part of the landscape of medical agency during the nineteenth century, and a key way in which the rights of poor patients and the analogous duties of doctors were established and navigated in a framework of non-existent or light professional and central regulation.

Notes

1 On patient narrative, see R. Porter, 'The Patient in England 1660–1800', in A. Wear (ed.), *Medicine in Society: Historical Essays* (Cambridge, 1992), pp. 91–118; M. Fissell, 'The Disappearance of the Patient Narrative and the Invention of Hospital Medicine', in R. French and A. Wear (eds), *British Medicine in an Age of Reform* (London, 1991), pp. 48–74; W. Wild, *Medicine-by-Post: The Changing Voice of Illness in Eighteenth-Century British Consultation Letters and Literature* (Amsterdam, 2006).

2 A. Morrice, 'Should the Doctor Tell? Medical Secrecy in Early Twentieth-century Britain', in S. Sturdy (ed.), *Medicine, Health and the Public Sphere in Britain, 1600–2000* (London, 2002), pp. 60–82; P. Corfield, 'From Poison Pedlars to Civic Worthies: The Education of the Apothecaries in Georgian England', *Social History of Medicine*, 22 (2009), pp. 1–21; M. Brown, *Performing Medicine: Medical Culture and Identity in Provincial England, c.1760–1850* (Manchester, 2011); A. Tomkins, 'Who were his Peers? The Social and Professional Milieu of the Provincial Surgeon-apothecary in the Late Eighteenth Century', *Journal of Social History*, 44 (2011), pp. 915–935.

3 I am grateful to Alannah Tomkins for sharing findings of her ongoing project which show the striking number of doctors enmeshed in bankruptcy or committing suicide when facing ruin.

4 Bolton Record Office, Heywood family papers, 1791–1869, ZHE/1–66. See also uncatalogued later deposits.

5 T. Smollett, *The Expedition of Humphry Clinker by the Author of Roderick Random*, volume 1 (London, 1820), p. 1.

6 B. Mitchell and H. Penrose (eds), *Letters from Bath, 1766–1767: Rev. John Penrose* (Stroud, 1983), 15 April 1766, p. 78.

7 H. Barker, 'Medical Advertising and Trust in Late Georgian England', *Urban History*, 36 (2009), pp. 379–398; Wild, *Medicine-by-Post*.

8 A. Digby, *Making a Medical Living: Doctors and Patients in the English Market for Medicine, 1720–1911* (Cambridge, 1994); A. Digby, *The Evolution of British General Practice 1850–1948* (Oxford, 1999); M. Crowther, 'Health Care and Poor Relief in Provincial England', in O. Grell, A. Cunningham and R. Jütte (eds), *Health Care and Poor Relief in Eighteenth and Nineteenth Century Northern Europe* (Aldershot, 2002), pp. 203–219.

9 See, for instance, S. Shave, '"Immediate Death or a Life of Torture are the Consequences of the System": The Bridgwater Union Scandal and Policy Change',

in J. Reinarz and L. Schwarz (eds), *Medicine and the Workhouse* (Rochester, NY, 2013), pp. 164–191.

10 See, for instance, K. Price, '"Where is the Fault?" The Starvation of Edward Cooper at the Isle of Wight Workhouse in 1877', *Social History of Medicine*, 26 (2013), pp. 21–37.

11 For the view that institutions are characterised by a 'thin' form of trust which stands in contradistinction to the 'thick' form of trust generated in personal and face-to-face relationships, see R. Putman, *Bowling Alone: The Collapse and Renewal of American Community* (New York, 2000).

12 For a survey, see S. A. King, 'Poverty, Medicine and the Workhouse in the Eighteenth and Nineteenth Centuries', in J. Reinarz and L. Schwarz (eds), *Medicine and the Workhouse* (Rochester, NY, 2013), pp. 228–251.

13 See Crowther, 'Health Care', pp. 210–213.

14 S. Williams, 'Practitioners' Income and Provision for the Poor: Parish Doctors in the Late Eighteenth and Early Nineteenth Centuries', *Social History of Medicine*, 18 (2005), pp. 159–186.

15 Northamptonshire Record Office (hereafter NRO), Crick memorandum book, 92P/117, p. 3.

16 Berkshire Record Office (hereafter BRO), examination, DP 71/13/1/23.

17 BRO, examination, DP 71/13/1/23.

18 BRO, loose letter, DP/71/13/1.

19 BRO, loose letter, DP/71/13/1.

20 Rothersthorpe Parish Chest (hereafter RPC), letter, accessed October 1997.

21 Somerset Record Office (hereafter SRO), letter, SP/13/12/1.

22 SRO, letter, SP/13/12/1.

23 For a particularly good example of a doctor writing on behalf of and with the assent of Thomas Jump, see S. King, T. Nutt and A. Tomkins, *Narratives of the Poor in Eighteenth-Century Britain* (London, 2006), pp. 229–260.

24 Digby, *Making a Medical Living*, pp. 142–144.

25 E. Hurren, *Protesting About Pauperism: Poverty, Politics and Poor Relief in Late-Victorian England, 1870–1900* (Woodbridge, 2007).

26 K. Price, 'A Regional, Quantitative and Qualitative Study of the Employment, Disciplining and Discharging of Workhouse Medical Officers of the New Poor Law throughout Nineteenth-century England and Wales' (PhD Thesis, Oxford Brookes University, 2008).

27 C. Lawrence, P. Lucier and C. Booth (eds), *"Take Time by the Forelock": The Letters of Anthony Fothergill to James Woodforde, 1789–1813* (London, 1997), p. 84.

28 Lawrence, Lucier and Booth, *"Take time by the forelock"*.

29 A. Conan Doyle, *The Stark Munro Letters* (London, 1895), pp. 23–24.

30 S. Bamford, *Passages in the Life of a Radical* (Oxford, 1984), p. 42.

31 Bamford, *Passages in the Life*.

32 Ibid.

33 Ibid.

34 Ibid., p. 43.

35 Ibid., p. 48.

36 Ibid., p. 49.

37 See, for instance, D. Green, 'Pauper Protests: Power and Resistance in Early Nineteenth-century London Workhouses', *Social History*, 31 (2006), pp. 137–159.

38 RPC, letter, accessed October 1997.

39 NRO, letter, 356P/6.
40 E. Hurren, *Dying for Victorian Medicine: English Anatomy and its Trade in the Dead Poor, c.1834–1929* (Basingstoke, 2012), pp. 124–136.
41 For this case, see *Carlisle and District Chronicle* (15 June 1838) at Carlisle Local Studies Library.
42 NRO, letter book, 152P/16.
43 BRO, letters, D/P 91/18/18/2–8.
44 *Northampton Herald* (14 July 1841).
45 J. Bailey, *Unquiet Lives: Marriage and Marriage Breakdown in England, 1660–1800* (Cambridge, 2003).
46 *Northampton Herald* (14 July 1841).
47 Ibid.
48 Ibid.
49 M. Pelling, 'Scenes from Professional Life: Medicine, Moral Conduct, and Interconnectedness in *Middlemarch*', in P. Ghosh and L. Goldman (eds), *Politics and Culture in Victorian Britain: Essays in Memory of Colin Matthew* (Oxford, 2006), pp. 220–236.
50 *Lincolnshire, Rutland and Stamford Mercury* (hereafter *LRSM*) (19 September 1817).
51 Lincolnshire Record Office (hereafter LRO), Kesteven Quarter Sessions, KQS/C1.
52 LRO, Lincolnshire Quarter Sessions, A/1/387/80–88.
53 *LRSM* (24 September 1813).
54 *LRSM* (19 September 1817).
55 LRO, Lincolnshire Quarter Sessions, A/1/387/80–88.
56 *LRSM* (24 September 1813).
57 LRO, Kesteven Quarter Sessions, KQS/C1.

8 Complaining in the age of consumption

Patients, consumers or citizens?

Alex Mold

In January 1984, a patient named Michael was taken seriously ill with kidney failure. Following dialysis, he developed an infection that required treatment with antibiotics. Michael told the doctor treating him that in the past he had reacted badly to penicillin, but he was prescribed the drug nonetheless. Michael developed what he called 'the mother and father of all rashes', which kept him in hospital for a further five weeks. Michael reported that:

> Afterwards, I asked, 'I said that I was sensitive to penicillin; why did you give it to me?' The answer was, 'Oh well, old boy, it was the best antibiotic for your particular infection and we thought that we could take the chance.' Whose chance? Whose life? Whose body? Who is the sufferer? What is the compensation? What is the complaints procedure? There appears to be no such procedure. The patient is just the fall guy who is in the hands of doctors who think that they know better than the patient.[1]

Michael's compliant might have fallen on deaf ears were it not for the fact the he was Michael McNair-Wilson, Conservative MP for Newbury, England. Though he was unfortunate to have been so unwell, in 1985 McNair-Wilson was lucky enough to have his name drawn in a parliamentary procedure known as the 'members' ballot', allowing him the opportunity to put forward a piece of legislation. McNair-Wilson took up the issue of patient rights, and the right to complain in particular. His draft Hospital Complaints Procedure Bill proposed that all hospitals be required to establish a complaints procedure. The Bill was discussed in the House of Commons in February 1985. The Under-Secretary of State for Health, John Patten, responded favourably to the Bill, stating that 'It should make a real contribution towards the provision of a more consumer-responsive NHS.'[2] Such a statement suggested that the ability to complain was being linked to the development of a more consumer-orientated NHS, but to what extent was complaining about medicine different in an age of consumption?

Complaining about healthcare, as the chapters in this volume demonstrate, was nothing new. People probably always have been and always will be dissatisfied with aspects of their medical treatment and wanting to make this dissatisfaction known. As described in this volume, this was achieved through the types of internal procedures outlined in the Introduction and by Thompson and León-Sanz; through the peri-public spaces of Price and King; the courtrooms and inquiries of Wall and McHale; the debates and critiques of Ingram and of Scull and Cook; and the media attention discussed by Newsom Kerr and throughout this collection. Yet, from the late 1960s onwards, the re-imagining of the patient as a consumer changed ideas about medical complaints. The ability to complain was a crucial issue both in the construction of the patient as a consumer and in the development of patient-consumer activism. This chapter will explore the ways in which complaining about medicine was different in Britain during the second half of the twentieth century. This period was an age of consumption, where consumerist ideas and approaches were applied to all spheres of life, including public services such as healthcare. The implications of such a development for the issue of complaining about medicine can be observed in three areas: first, the centrality of complaint to the notion of the patient-consumer; second, the conceptualisation of complaining as a right; and finally, the development of formal complaints procedures. This chapter will suggest that complaining played a crucial part in the construction of the patient as consumer, but that complaining was a somewhat ineffective tool for groups aiming to represent the patient-consumer. Difficulties around establishing complaint as a right, and the long delay surrounding the introduction of formal complaints procedures, point to much more fundamental issues with the whole notion of the patient as consumer.

Complaint and the patient-consumer

Although patients could be said to have operated as 'consumers' in the medical marketplace in Britain that predated the establishment of the National Health Service (NHS) in 1948, and patients were afforded some say in the way medical services were managed through mechanisms such as contributory schemes – as highlighted by Thompson and León-Sanz's chapters – this kind of patient involvement was not generally referred to in the language of consumption.[3] Specific engagement with the idea that patients were 'consumers' of healthcare only began to occur in the latter half of the twentieth century, as the proliferation of consumer goods and the development of the organised consumer movement started to have an impact on the delivery of public services. In the early 1960s, a handful of health economists such as D. S. Lees began to use the term 'consumer' in connection with health, as did think tanks and consumer groups such as Political and Economic Planning (PEP) and the Research Institute for Consumer Affairs.[4] An editorial in the *Lancet* in 1961 was moderately supportive, noting that:

'Emphasising the "consumer point of view" can be very valuable because undoubtedly patients have suffered in the past from having no means of judging the medical services and little or no means of addressing them.'[5]

The language of consumption was able to enter the healthcare arena partly because consumerist principles were beginning to proliferate within public services more widely. In the early twentieth century, consumer identity was tied to the development of welfare politics and social citizenship, but by the middle of the century, the 'citizen consumer' and the 'rational consumer' came into being.[6] During the 1950s, the development of an organised consumer movement concerned with consumers' rights and comparative testing moved consumption 'beyond things', to consider public, as well as private, goods and services.[7] Moreover, consumerism offered a tool for activists to right the wrongs of contemporary healthcare as they saw them.[8] Although satisfaction with the NHS at this time was still high – in 1961 PEP found that 86 per cent of families were satisfied with the attention given to them by their GP – medical care was not seen as infallible. Waning faith in the ability of biomedicine to conquer all ills and a series of high-profile scandals, such as that around thalidomide and the human guinea pig revelations about experiments being conducted on NHS patients, along with a host of other controversies outlined in the Introduction to this volume, undermined confidence in medicine and the medical profession.[9]

Patient-consumer organisations were set up with the aim, at least in part, to improve the situation around patient complaints. Helping patients to complain, informing people of the correct procedures and dealing with specific complaints, as well as campaigning for improvements in complaints mechanisms, were key areas of activity for such groups. A specific complaint – about the use of patients in NHS hospitals in research without their knowledge or consent – was the motivation behind the creation of the Patients Association (PA) in 1962. Helen Hodgson, a teacher, was moved to set up the organisation by 'reports on thalidomide babies, wrong patient operations and tests on patients'.[10] The association, however, rapidly found itself dealing with a broad range of issues relating to complaints. In its first 18 months of existence, the PA received 525 complaints from patients.[11] The PA did not take up individual complaints, but they did advise people on whether they were likely to have a case and how to negotiate the various levels of complaints procedure.

The Community Health Councils (CHCs) performed a similar function. Created in 1974 through the reorganisation of the NHS, 207 CHCs were established at the local level to be the 'voice of the consumer' within the health service.[12] One of their statutory roles was to act as the 'patient's friend' and assist patients in making complaints. Although all CHCs received complaints, the volume of complaints that they dealt with varied widely from council to council and changed over time. For its first three months of existence, one CHC reported receiving 22 complaints, while others reported 'minimal' complaints in their early years.[13] Yet, by the 1980s, South Birmingham CHC reported that complaints work took up about a quarter of the Council's time, and a study of CHCs by a firm of management consultants in the 1990s found that councils spent 50 per cent of their time dealing with complaints.[14]

Although complaints work was time-consuming, complaints were a useful source of information for patient-consumer organisations about the state of the NHS. Some attempt was made to analyse the complaints received by such groups as the PA and the CHCs in order to point to wider failings in NHS care. In 1964, the PA reported that of the complaints they had received, 21 per cent were about negligence, but over a third concerned what Helen Hodgson termed 'attitude to patients', including bad organisation, lack of communication, 'inhumanity' and discourtesy.[15] The PA tried to conduct a more formal analysis of complaints in the mid-1970s with the help of the Consumers' Association (CA), but this project never got off the ground.[16] As Glen O'Hara points out, in the 1960s and 1970s there was a lack of information about complaints and their handling. Little work had been done on categorising different types of complaint or using these to determine broader patterns.[17] One CHC examined the complaints that it had received in its first year of activity and found that these could be placed in three categories. In language reminiscent of Klein's classic study and picked up on in Clarke's Afterword to this volume,[18] the first was 'grumbles, comments and suggestions'; these required no specific action. The second was 'expressions of distress and dissatisfaction'; these were usually dealt with informally. Finally, there were 'protests, grievances or accusations'; these were more formal complaints that required referral to the relevant authority.[19]

Analysing complaints, even in this rather crude way, demonstrated to patient-consumer organisations the significance and value of complaints at both an individual and a collective level. In their 1974 handbook for CHCs, Jack Hallas and Bernadette Fallon argued that helping patients with complaints was 'one of the most important aspects of community health council work'. Aiding individuals who were less able to make their dissatisfaction known, whom they termed 'submerged groups', was particularly vital. In this way, Hallas and Fallon suggested, CHCs could act as an 'early warning system', bringing the Area Health Authority's attention to potential causes for dissatisfaction.[20] Patient-consumer groups were well aware that formal complaints were only the tip of 'the iceberg'.[21] Elizabeth Stanton, writing in the National Consumer Council's magazine, the *Clapham Omnibus*, stated that 'Most patients are grateful for any good done to them by the National Health Service, and are reluctant to complain formally if things go wrong'. But, she noted, 'consumer activists have realised for some years that this "gratitude barrier" is unhealthy not only for patients and their families but also for the medical profession and the NHS itself'.[22]

Complaints, patient-consumer groups suggested, operated as indicators of the quality of services being provided. Jean Robinson of the PA urged the CHCs to use complaints to 'make rational assessments of the quality of care'.[23] According to the editor of *CHC News*, Ruth Levitt, complaints were rarely isolated incidents; it was possible to generalise from specific misfortune and so advocate for wider change.[24] This was a view later echoed by the 1979 Royal Commission on the NHS, which established that there was a 'need to develop an effective role for CHCs, not simply as an aid to complainants, but on the much wider front of influencing health service provision to meet the needs of patients'.[25]

By the mid-1970s, it was evident that patient-consumer organisations had two key roles with respect to complaints. The first consisted of assisting patients to make complaints and offering practical support and guidance on complaints procedures. The second was about using complaints in a broader sense as a means to highlight deficiencies in the NHS and to campaign for improvements. To perform both of these roles more effectively, patient-consumer groups marshalled the language of patients' rights in order to campaign for the establishment of a formal right to complain.

The 'right' to complain

Three distinct, but overlapping, visions of health rights were articulated in Britain during the second half of the twentieth century: health as a human right, as a citizen's right, and as a consumer's right. The notion that health is a fundamental human right – that it is a right that individuals possess simply by being born – is almost as old as the notion of human rights itself. Most commentators place the 'invention' of human rights in the eighteenth century, and although the right to health was not among the initial rights established by the French National Assembly, it was added to the list of the state's obligations to its citizens by the Constituent Assembly in 1791.[26] In Britain, there was no such bargain between the state and citizen, and it was not until the United Nations Universal Declaration of Human Rights in 1948 that the right to health was contemplated on a global level. The UN Declaration asserted that 'Everyone has the right to a standard of living adequate for health and well-being of himself and his family, including food, clothing, housing and medical care.'[27] The right 'to the enjoyment of the highest attainable standard of physical and mental health' was also central to the establishment of the World Health Organization in 1946, and was enshrined in international law through the International Covenant on Economic, Social and Cultural Rights, which came into effect for member countries in 1976.[28] During the 1970s, the idea that health was a fundamental human right received added impetus from the Alma Ata Declaration on Primary Care in 1978, and through the international public health movement.[29] Health as a human right became linked to development goals in the 1980s, and since the 1990s to combating HIV/AIDS.[30]

Although the notion of health as a human right was significant at the transnational level, in the UK the notion of rights in health took a rather different trajectory over this period. Instead of being concerned primarily with human rights, the rights discourse in Britain seemed to focus more on the rights of citizens. This could be partly explained by long-running discussions about individual rights within healthcare in the UK. In the medical marketplace that predated the NHS, patients had contractual and common-law rights relating to healthcare, as with other goods and services.[31] Entitlement also lay at the heart of the gradual development of state-sponsored healthcare in Britain up to and including the establishment of the NHS. The 1911 National Health Insurance Act introduced compulsory health insurance for manual workers. In return for their financial contribution, members received benefit when sick and access to medical care without additional payment. Although, as Thompson points out elsewhere in this volume, such mechanisms could lead to friction, subscribers to hospital contributory schemes were entitled to some say in the way in which the institution was managed through representatives on hospital management committees.[32]

The coming of a collective system in the form of the NHS implied a more unified view of rights with respect to health. While the National Health Service Act (1946) was framed around the *duty* of the Minister of Health to provide a comprehensive service and not the *right* of the patient to receive this, the message that reached the public emphasised universal entitlement.[33] A leaflet distributed to all homes in 1948 asserted that the new service would 'provide you with all medical, dental and nursing care. Everyone – rich or poor, man, woman or child – can use it or any part of it.'[34] Underpinning such promises was the notion of social rights. For the sociologist T. H. Marshall, social rights permitted the citizen access to a minimum supply of essential social goods and services (such as medical attention, shelter and education), to be provided by the state.[35] The NHS, and the other achievements of the 'classic' era of the British welfare state (1945 to 1975), appeared to offer a kind of social citizenship based on collective rights.[36]

Interwoven with ideas about the health rights of citizens was another set of expectations: the rights that individuals could demand as consumers. The relationship between citizenship and consumption has been the subject of much research in recent years, and the activities of citizen-consumers can be detected as far back as the nineteenth century and beyond.[37] But by the middle of the twentieth century, citizen and consumer identities were becoming welded together more tightly. As discussed above, by the 1960s and 1970s, this approach had found purchase inside government. Organisations such as the National Consumer Council (NCC) were created (in the NCC's case in 1975) to represent the consumer within public services. State-provided amenities from housing to healthcare were being discussed in increasingly consumerist terms.[38] Consumer representation within the health service (in the form of the CHCs) was in line with the general trend towards the improvement of citizen-consumer representation, but here a particular language of entitlement around bodily autonomy was also in evidence. Although patients were supposed to give their consent to participate in medical trials (following the 1947 Nuremberg Code), this principle was widely ignored both in the UK and in the US.[39] For Hodgson, founder of the PA, the key issue was that 'Patients are not told if they are receiving new or orthodox treatment. I maintain that they *should* be told.'[40] The patient, she asserted, 'is entitled to know what treatment, if any, he is receiving'.[41] The PA was therefore keen to establish the right of the patient to give or withhold consent to all treatment, whether experimental or not.

The demand for bodily autonomy made by the PA echoed the kinds of rights claims made by the new social movements of this period. As the feminist historian Sheila Rowbotham commented, 'Rights were not abstract or about politics alone, they were active and about sex as well as economics.'[42] This wider conception of rights was crucial for dealing with the problems of 'quality of life, equality, individual self-realization, participation and human rights', representative, for German philosopher and sociologist Jürgen Habermas, of a 'new' form of politics.[43] The rights claims of the 1960s and 1970s were thus a different kind of rights claim from that of the past, rooted not in transactional contracts and the market place, or in the social contract between state and citizen, but in the politics of everyday life. Rights discourse became a way in which groups claiming to speak on the behalf of patients could articulate new demands about bodily autonomy and individual self-determination.

Rights claims were essential to the work of a number of groups that attempted to represent the patient as consumer in the latter half of the twentieth century. During the 1970s and 1980s, health consumer groups produced a range of guides to patients' rights. Publications included the Patients Association's *Can I Insist?* (1974), the *Which? Guide to Your Rights* (1980), a joint Consumers' Association/Patients Association publication, *A Patients' Guide to the NHS* (1983); the National Consumer Council's, *Patients' Rights* (1983); and the Association of Community Health Councils in England and Wales (ACHCEW), *Patients' Charter* (1986).[44] Such a proliferation of documents listing patients' rights can be read in two ways. On the one hand, the abundance of charters points to the importance of the language of rights for patient groups, but on the other hand, the apparent need for these rights to be stated and re-stated in multiple publications would suggest that there was widespread ignorance about patients' rights.

In some ways, the large number of charters produced by patient organisations hinted at the fragility and dubious legality of many of the rights proposed. Despite claiming to be comprehensive guides to the rights that patients held, many of these publications confessed to confusion and uncertainty about the nature and legitimacy of patient's rights. The NCC stated that 'It is difficult to say precisely what healthcare patients are entitled to expect of the National Health Service (NHS). There are clues, but most of them are open to different interpretations, and circumstances greatly affect cases.'[45] This was partly because, as the CA observed in their guide to consumers' rights across a range of different services (both public and private):

> There is no comprehensive list of rights which you can consult, nor is there any specific area of law that deals with them. Your rights are scattered among hundreds, perhaps thousands, of Acts of Parliament and secondary pieces of legislation. . . . Sometimes your rights are not written down at all. They may exist because of custom and tradition, or merely because there is nothing saying that they are absent.[46]

Indeed, most of the rights listed in the various guides and charters had no, or little, legal basis. Patients' rights claims lacked a solid foundation: they needed procedures and changes in law and practice in order to establish this.

The development of complaints procedures

Opportunities to create a right to complain arrived in the 1970s and 1980s as attempts were made to introduce a unified complaints procedure in all hospitals. Systems were in place to deal with patient dissatisfaction (as discussed in the Introduction to this volume), but a number of developments contributed towards a sense that these were inadequate. Patients were able to complain about an individual doctor's conduct to the General Medical Council (GMC), but the GMC was not primarily a machine to handle patients' complaints; it was instead a regulatory body for doctors.[47] There was a process in place to deal with complaints made against General Practitioners (GPs): patients could complain to the Executive Councils, later Family Practitioner Committees, and have their case heard by the local Medical Service Committee, which acted as a judicial tribunal.[48] However, there was no single system in place for complaints about treatment in hospital. Until 1966, when a Ministry of Health circular was issued, there was no official guidance on the establishment of hospital complaints procedures, and as a result these varied significantly from hospital to hospital. Even after the circular, much was left to local discretion: doctors handled complaints about other doctors, there was little or no external oversight, and the complaint procedures themselves were not binding.

Despite these difficulties, patients seemed to be becoming more willing to complain. The total number of written complaints investigated by hospital authorities in England and Wales rose from 7,984 in 1967 to 9,614 in 1971. This represented a slight rise from 1.59 complaints per 1,000 discharges in 1967 to 1.75 complaints per 1,000 discharges in 1971.[49] Furthermore, written complaints were likely to represent just a fraction of the total number of complaints made. Research in Scotland found that 25 per cent of patients interviewed in hospital claimed to have made some sort of suggestion about 'desired improvements'.[50]

The fact that few of these criticisms translated into formal complaints thus says rather more about hospital complaints procedures than about unwillingness on the part of patients to complain.

The issue of patient complaints was given added impetus in the wake of a series of medical scandals in the late 1960s and early 1970s, which exposed not only poor-quality care but also the inadequacy of complaints procedures. The publication of *Sans Everything: A Case to Answer* by Barbara Robb and the organisation Aid for the Elderly in Government Institutions presented a number of case studies of mistreatment of the elderly in NHS hospitals, but it also pointed to the unsatisfactory state of complaints procedures.[51] In 1969, a Council of Tribunals report into the allegations made by Robb echoed her criticism of complaints procedures and called for 'radical revision' of the complaints investigation machinery.[52]

The need for reform of complaints procedures was further underscored by the report on the Ely Hospital scandal, which was also released in 1969. Two years earlier, the British newspaper *News of the World* had printed allegations made by a nurse at Ely Hospital in Cardiff (a psychiatric institution) pointing to the mistreatment of patients but also to the suppression of complaints made by staff and patients' relatives and the victimisation of staff who did complain. The Ely report determined that the nurse's allegations were well-founded, and that a culture had been created at the hospital in which 'members of the nursing staff had been persuaded that it was useless, if not positively hazardous, to complain of matters which disturbed them'.[53] The report recommended that existing complaints procedures be reconsidered, and called for the establishment of an inspectorate for long-stay hospitals.[54] The Ely scandal was followed quickly by another, this time in a hospital for the 'mentally handicapped', in Dorset. Once again, the subsequent report into conditions at the Farleigh Hospital (published in 1971) found that complaints were handled poorly, and the report's authors asserted that the existing system for dealing with complaints within the NHS was inadequate.[55] A year later, yet another inquiry, this time into conditions at the Whittingham psychiatric hospital in Lancashire, discovered that complaints by staff were suppressed and that there was a failure to investigate other complaints. The report recommended that procedures for dealing with complaints from staff and patients be improved.[56] Taken together, these reports demonstrated that existing complaints procedures were in need of radical overhaul. Although many of the scandals centred on the difficulties experienced by staff wishing to speak out about conditions, they also shone a light on the whole issue of complaints. The problem, it seemed, was not confined only to long-stay hospitals. A co-ordinated, fair, open system for making complaints was required.

The task of providing guidance on the establishment of a complaints procedure was given to a governmental committee chaired by Sir Michael Davies, a barrister and later High Court judge. Established in 1971, the Davies Committee was made up of individuals from a diverse array of professional backgrounds, but what was particularly significant about the committee's membership was that doctors and other health professionals were in a minority: of the 17 committee members just three were doctors. This mixed membership suggested a real willingness to investigate the complaints issue not just from the point of view of the doctor but also from the perspective of the patient. This can also be seen in the way in which the Davies Committee conducted their investigation. They did hear from the various professional bodies and royal colleges, but the committee also sought the views of a number of patient groups, including the PA and the National Association for the Welfare of Children in Hospital.[57]

The opinions of these organisations were reflected in the committee's final report. The Davies Committee was keen to place their findings within the context of growing consumerism. The report commented:

> This is an age in which the legitimate interests of the consumer, who in the hospital service is the patient, are rightly receiving increased protection in many fields. . . . We see no reason why these general principles should not apply to the hospital service.

Moreover, the Davies Committee contended, 'Few [patients] have any serious grievances. But those who do have the legitimate right – no less – to have their dissatisfaction fully and fairly investigated.'[58] Such a strong statement suggested that complaints procedures would be strengthened considerably. Yet the fate of the report tells a rather different story. Overall, the Davies Committee made 82 separate recommendations and proposed a complex and legalistic complaints procedure based on a tribunal system. They also separated out clinical and non-clinical complaints, leaving doctors to investigate allegations about medical mistakes. Despite this concession to professional self-regulation, the report was not well received among the medical community. The joint Medico-Legal Sub-committee of the Central Committee for Hospital Medical Services of the British Medical Association (BMA) and the Joint Consultants Committee (JCC) argued that the report implied that 'every encouragement be given to all citizens . . . to make a suggestion or complaint, not only when it is reasonable, but on any occasion, however trivial'. The effect of this atmosphere of complaining, they contended, would be 'to damage the service profoundly and to the detriment rather than to the advantage of the community in which it exists to serve'.[59] The Council of the BMA and the JCC told Sir Henry Yellowlees (the Chief Medical Officer) that 'no part of the proposals put forward by the Davies Committee can be considered as acceptable to the medical profession until the considered view of the Association has been submitted'.[60]

Despite the fact that the BMA had given evidence to the Davies Committee, doctors were obviously unhappy with its findings. In contrast, patient groups were broadly supportive. For example, the PA 'welcome[d] the constructive nature of the report and its sympathetic approach to the anxieties and preoccupations of patients'.[61] But the reception given to the Davies report illustrated the relative lack of power of patient groups when compared to professional groups. The report, according to the sociologist Margaret Stacey, was met with 'thundering silence' and long delay.[62] A draft code on hospital complaints procedure was produced in 1976, and this was followed by another consultation document in 1978. In 1981, a Department of Health circular was issued to all hospitals, but the complaints procedure was still a draft and not compulsory. It was not until 1985 and the passing of the Hospital Procedure Complaints Act, 12 years after Davies reported, that hospitals were actually required to have any sort of complaints procedure in place.

Moreover, even the creation of this piece of legislation was due to serendipity as much as design. As mentioned in the introduction to this chapter, the origins of the Hospital Complaints Procedure Act lay in a private member's bill, not a specific attempt by the government to introduce legislation on this issue. Most MPs, when given the chance to get their name on the statute books through the members' ballot, opted to put forward a technical piece of legislation that the government wished to see passed but that was not significant enough to be included in the main legislative programme.[63] Much important legislation was passed through private members' bills, particularly on social and moral issues, such as the Abortion Act (1967), but most of these bills resulted from pressure-group lobbying. However, this does not appear to have been the case with the Hospital Complaints Procedure Act: patient-consumer groups had no direct involvement in the creation of the Act. Instead, McNair-Wilson acted alone. Following months of hospitalisation and a number of medical mishaps, McNair-Wilson published a 'Patient's Charter' which he hoped would redress the power imbalance between doctors and patients 'by laying down certain basic patients' rights which will apply to every person'.[64] According to Linda Mulcahy, who interviewed McNair-Wilson before he died in 1993, the MP had wanted to use his bill to get his entire charter made into legislation, but the Secretary of State for Health told him that he would only get government backing if he selected just one clause from the charter to form a bill.[65] McNair-Wilson chose the introduction of a complaints procedure; this was duly translated into legislation, and passed unopposed in February 1985.[66] The Hospital Complaints Procedure Act required health authorities in England and Wales and health boards in Scotland to establish a complaints procedure and draw this to the attention of patients.[67] The Department of Health drafted further guidelines on the complaints procedure, and this was finally issued to all hospitals in 1988.[68]

Conclusions

What does this tell us about complaints, rights, consumerism and the relationship between these? It might have been largely due to chance that the Hospital Complaints Procedure Act entered the statute books, but it is possible to argue that without the broader discussions about patient rights and complaining, and specifically the work of patient groups in producing patient guides and supporting complainants, McNair-Wilson would not have written his charter. Patient consumer groups helped to produce a language of patients' rights that was then taken up by politicians, as can be seen in the later establishment of the *Patient's Charter* by the Department of Health in 1991 and the *NHS Constitution* in 2009, both of which feature the right to complain as a 'long established' patient right.[69]

Consumerism provided a discourse that drew attention to the rights of the individual and also, to some extent, of the collective with respect to medical services. Being able to complain was a key facet of consumer identity, and as patients began to be seen as consumers, so the importance attached to complaints increased. But this language only took patient-consumers so far. As the fate of the Davies report and the long-winded attempts to establish an organised hospital complaints procedure demonstrated, the tools provided by consumerism were insufficient in the face of more entrenched interests and powerful actors. The continued dominance of the medical profession, and the relative weakness of patient-consumer organisations when compared to professional groups, undermined attempts to introduce complaints procedures and strengthen patients' rights in this area.

Furthermore, issues remained around the effectiveness of rights claims. Even if we take the Hospital Complaints Procedure Act as giving the patient the right to complain, many patients continued (and continue) to find it difficult to complain. In 2008, a survey conducted by the PA revealed an NHS complaints system that, they said, was cumbersome and variable and took too long.[70] Recent scandals over poor care within the NHS, such as at Stafford Hospital, demonstrate that complaining about medicine continues to be a highly contentious area. Even in the age of consumption, complaining about healthcare or treatment upsets what has been widely understood as the traditional doctor–patient relationship and power balance. By no longer being 'passive recipients', patient-consumers were challenging deep-seated assumptions about the contract formed between doctor and patient.[71]

Such a tension raises more fundamental questions about the meaning of consumption and the patient-consumer within a collective system such as the NHS. As patients lacked what historian Roy Porter called the 'power of the purse', complaining and the wider discourse around patients' rights was one of the few tools available to patient groups.[72] Rights held considerable rhetorical power, but they lacked legal or practical purchase. Underpinning this absence of applicability was a deeper level of uncertainty about who was complaining: was it the patient, citizen or consumer? This also had an impact on the nature of the rights that were being exercised: were these human rights, citizens' rights or consumers' rights? This was important, because different types of rights laid claim to different things and were treated in slightly different ways. For example, as a citizen, a patient might assert his or her right to *receive* a certain service, but as a consumer, he or she might instead assert his or her right to *choose* a certain service. Without a clear basis for or understanding of what kind of rights were being asserted, patients' rights claims were weak, sometimes conflicting, and left open to co-option by other actors.

Since the 1990s, the patients' rights agenda and the interests of the patient-consumer have been taken on by a succession of governments that have tended to focus on the desires of the individual patient-consumer rather than the needs of patient-consumers plural. Gradual, but persistent, marketisation of the NHS under the Conservative, Labour and Coalition governments has resulted in the prioritisation of one right above all others: the right to choose. The difficulties surrounding choice in health have been much examined, but it is the coupling of rights and choice that would seem to have the most significant implications for a collective health system such as the NHS.[73] Indeed, if the right to choose has replaced the right to receive, then complaining about medicine would become more, not less important. Complaint may still have potential value as a collective tool, not just an individual one, as it could provide a way for patient-consumers to make their views heard. The possibilities offered by mechanisms such as the 'super-complaint', a sort of class action by complainants, and trialled in 2001 by the CA in the healthcare arena with respect to private dentistry, might provide ways to effect change on a grander scale.[74] Perhaps, then, to really make a difference we should all moan less and complain more.

Notes

1 House of Commons Debates, 22 February 1985, vol. 73, cc1370–86.

2 Ibid.

3 M. Jenner and P. Wallis (eds), *Medicine and the Market in England and its Colonies, c.1450–c.1850* (Basingstoke, 2007); R. Porter, 'The Patient's View: Doing Medical History from Below', *Theory and Society*, 14, 2 (1985), pp. 175–198; M. Gorsky, 'Community Involvement in Hospital Governance in Britain: Evidence from Before the National Health Service', *International Journal of Health Services*, 38, 4 (2008), pp. 751–771; M. Gorsky and J. Mohan with T. Willis, *Mutualism and Health Care: Hospital Contributory Schemes in Twentieth Century Britain* (Manchester, 2006).

4 D. S. Lees, *Health Through Choice: An Economic Study of the British National Health Service* (London, 1961); Political and Economic Planning, *Family Needs and the Social Services* (London, 1961); Research Institute for Consumer Affairs, *General Practice a Consumer Commentary* (London, 1963).

5 Anon, 'Patients as Consumers: Wants and Needs', *The Lancet*, 277, 7183 (1961), pp. 927–928.

6 F. Trentmann, 'The Modern Genealogy of the Consumer: Meanings, Identities and Political Synapses', in F. Trentmann and J. Brewer (eds), *Consuming Cultures, Global Perspectives: Historical Trajectories, Transnational Exchanges* (Oxford, 2006), pp. 19–69; M. Hilton and M. Daunton, 'Material Politics: An Introduction', in M. Daunton and M. Hilton (eds), *The Politics of Consumption: Material Culture and Citizenship in Europe and America* (Oxford, 2001), pp. 1–32.

7 M. Hilton, *Consumerism in Twentieth Century Britain: The Search for a Historical Movement* (Cambridge, 2003).

8 Similar developments were occurring in other countries at the same time. For the US, see N. Tomes, 'Patients or Health-care Consumers? Why the History of Contested Terms Matters', in R. A. Stephens, C. E. Rosenberg and L. R. Burns (eds), *History and Health Policy in the United States: Putting the Past Back In* (New Brunswick, 2006), pp. 83–110.

9 M. Pappworth, 'Human Guinea Pigs: A Warning', *Twentieth Century*, 171 (1962), pp. 67–75; M. Pappworth, *Human Guinea Pigs: Experimentation on Man* (London, 1967). For an historical account of these revelations, see J. Hazelgrove, 'The Old Faith and the New Science: The Nuremberg Code and Human Experimentation Ethics in Britain, 1946–73', *Social History of Medicine*, 15, 1 (2002), pp. 109–135.

10 Contemporary Medical Archives Centre, Wellcome Library, London (hereafter CMAC), SA/PAT/H/1, press cuttings November 1962–November 1963, letter to the *Sunday Times* from Helen Hodgson (25 November 1962).

11 '525 Complaints on the NHS: Need for Change of Staff Attitude', *Guardian* (4 September 1964), p. 5.

12 Health Minister Keith Joseph in the House of Commons, *House of Commons Debates*,19 June 1973, vol. 858, col. 380.

13 Association of Community Health Councils in England and Wales [hereafter ACHCEW] CD-ROM, vol. 2, *CHC News* (January 1976), p. 8.

14 'Joining the Queue for Good Health', March 1987, press release on South Birmingham CHC Annual Report, inserted into 1984–86 Annual Report; M. Gerrard, *A Stifled Voice: Community Health Councils in England, 1974–2003* (Brighton, 2006), p. 174.

15 CMAC, SA/PAT/H/3, 'Patients Complain', *New Society* (10 September 1964); letter from Helen Hodgson to the *Sunday Telegraph* (7 February 1965).

16 CMAC, SA/PAT/D/13/1, patient complaints – Patients Association Complaints Analysis Project 1976–1983.

17 G. O'Hara, 'The Complexities of "Consumerism": Choice, Collectivism and Participation within Britain's National Health Service, *c.*1961–*c.*1979', *Social History of Medicine*, advance access: first published online 4 October 2012, p. 10, http://shm.oxfordjournals.org/content/early/2012/10/04/shm.hks062.full, accessed 5 April 2014.

18 R. Klein, *Complaints against Doctors: A Study in Professional Accountability* (London, 1973).

19 ACHCEW CD-ROM, vol. 2, *CHC News* (January 1976), p. 8.

20 J. Hallas and B. Fallon, *Mounting the Health Guard: A Handbook for Community Health Council Members* (Oxford, 1974), p. 31.

21 Klein, *Complaints against Doctors*, p. 104.

22 CMAC SA/PAT/A/1/6, E. Stanton, 'Patients' Rights and Responsibilities', *The Clapham Omnibus*, 11 (Winter 1981).

23 ACHCEW CD-ROM, vol. 2, *CHC News* (May 1976), p. 1.

24 Levitt quoted in Gerrard, *A Stifled Voice*, p. 229.
25 Cmnd 7615, Royal Commission on the National Health Service Report (London, 1979), p. 155.
26 L. Hunt, *Inventing Human Rights: A History* (New York, 2007); M. R. Ishay, *The History of Human Rights: From Ancient Times to the Globalization Era* (Berkeley, 2004); D. Porter, *Health Civilization and the State: A History of Public Health From Ancient to Modern Times* (London, 1999), p. 57. See also John Clarke's Afterword in this volume.
27 United Nations, *Universal Declaration of Human Rights*, Article 25 (1948).
28 World Health Organization, *Constitution of the World Health Organization* (1946), www.who.int/governance/eb/who_constitution_en.pdf, accessed 15 July 2011. United Nations, *International Covenant on Economic, Social and Cultural Rights* (1966/1976), www2.ohchr.org/english/law/pdf/cescr.pdf, accessed 15 July 2011.
29 *Declaration of Alma Ata: International Conference on Primary Health Care*, USSR, September 1978.
30 A.-E. Birn, 'Special Section – Health and Human Rights: Historical Perspectives and Political Challenges', *Journal of Public Health Policy*, 29 (2008), pp. 32–41; D. Tarantola, 'A Perspective on the History of Health and Human Rights: From the Cold War to the Gold War', *Journal of Public Health Policy*, 29 (2008), pp. 42–53; S. P. Marks, 'The Evolving Field of Health and Human Rights: Issues and Methods', *Journal of Law, Medicine and Ethics*, 30 (2002), pp. 732–754; K. Cmiel, 'The Recent History of Human Rights', *American Historical Review*, 109, 1 (2004), pp. 117–135.
31 See, for example, C. Crawford, 'Patients' Rights and the Law of Contract in Eighteenth Century England', *Social History of Medicine*, 13, 3 (2000), pp. 381–410.
32 Gorsky, 'Community Involvement'.
33 National Health Service Act, 1946, Chapter 81 (London, 1946).
34 *The New National Health Service*, 1948. Quoted in C. Webster, *The National Health Service: A Political History* (Oxford, 2002), p. 24.
35 T. H. Marshall, 'Citizenship and Social Class', in T. H. Marshall and T. Bottomore (eds), *Citizenship and Social Class* (London, 1992), pp. 3–51.
36 On the 'classic' welfare state, see R. Lowe, *The Welfare State in Britain since 1945* (Basingstoke, 2005).
37 See, for example, F. Trentmann, 'Citizenship and Consumption', *Journal of Consumer Culture*, 7, 2 (2007), pp. 147–158; F. Trentmann and V. Taylor, 'From Users to Consumers: Water Politics in Nineteenth-Century London', in F. Trentmann (ed.), *The Making of the Consumer: Knowledge, Power and Identity in the Modern World* (Oxford, 2005), pp. 53–79.
38 On consumerism and housing, see P. Shapely, 'Tenants Arise! Consumerism, Tenants and the Challenge to Council Authority in Manchester, 1968–92', *Social History*, 31, 1 (2006), pp. 60–78.
39 Hazelgrove, 'The Old Faith and the New Science'; D. J. Rothman, *Strangers at the Bedside: A History of How Law and Bioethics Transformed Medical Decision Making* (New York, 1991), pp. 61–63.
40 Hodgson quoted in 'Now a Voice for Patients', *The Times* (17 June 1963), p. 15.
41 H. Hodgson, 'Medical Ethics and Controlled Trials', letter to the *British Medical Journal* (18 May 1963), pp. 1339–1340.
42 S. Rowbotham, 'Introduction', in H. Curtis and M. Sanderson, *The Unsung Sixties: Memoirs of Social Innovation* (London, 2004), pp. ix–xii, p. xi.
43 J. Habermas, 'New Social Movements', *Telos*, 49 (1981), pp. 33–37.
44 Patients Association, *Can I Insist?* (London, 1974); Consumers' Association, *The*

Which? Guide to Your Rights (London, 1980); Consumers' Association/Patients Association, *A Guide to the National Health Service* (London, 1983); National Consumer Council [hereafter NCC], *Patients' Rights: A Guide for NHS Patients and Doctors* (London, 1983); ACHCEW, *Patients' Charter: Guidelines for Good Practice* (London, 1986).
45 NCC, *Patients' Rights*, p. 5.
46 Consumers' Association, *The Which? Guide to Your Rights*, p. 9.
47 M. Stacey, *Regulating British Medicine: The General Medical Council* (Chichester, 1992), p. 56.
48 Klein, *Complaints Against Doctors*, 16–21.
49 Stacey, *Regulating British Medicine*, p. 17.
50 Department of Health and Social Security [hereafter DHSS], *Report of the Committee on Hospital Complaints Procedure* (London, 1973), p. 7.
51 B. Robb, *Sans Everything: A Case to Answer* (London, 1967).
52 Council on Tribunals, *The Annual Report of the Council on Tribunals 1968* (London, 1969), p. 10.
53 Cmnd. [Command Paper] 3975, *Report of the Committee of Inquiry into Allegations of Ill-Treatment of Patients and Other Irregularities at the Ely Hospital, Cardiff* (London, 1969), p. 73.
54 *Report of the Committee of Inquiry into Allegations of Ill-Treatment*, p. 132.
55 Cmnd. 4557, *Report of the Farleigh Hospital Committee of Inquiry* (London, 1971), p. 23.
56 Cmnd. 4861, *Report of the Committee of Inquiry into Whittingham Hospital* (London, 1972), p. 42.
57 DHSS, *Report of the Committee on Hospital Complaints.*
58 Ibid., p. 4.
59 National Archives [hereafter NA], MH 159/281, Hospital Complaints Procedure: The Report of the Davies Committee – Report of the Joint Medico-Legal Subcommittee to the CCHMS and JCC, [April 1974].
60 NA, MH 159/281, Elston Grey-Turner, Deputy Secretary of the BMA to Dr H Yellowlees (CMO), 25 April 1974.
61 NA, MH 159/281, The Patients Association: Comment on Report of the Committee on Hospitals Complaints Procedure, March 1974.
62 Modern Records Centre, University of Warwick, MSS.184 Box 2: 'The NHS Complaints Procedure Three Years On: Opening Address by Meg Stacey'.
63 D. Marsh and M. Read, *Private Members' Bills* (Cambridge, 1988), p. 42.
64 McNair-Wilson's charter was published by ACHCEW. See ACHCEW Health News Briefing, 19 November 1984, *The Patient's Charter*. From the CD-ROM 'The Golden Age of Patient and Public Involvement: Celebrating the Work of Community Health Councils, 1974–2003, Vol. 2', available from the Wellcome Library, London.
65 L. Mulcahy, *Disputing Doctors: The Socio-legal Dynamics of Complaints about Medical Care* (Maidenhead, 2003), p. 41.
66 See *House of Commons Debates*, 22 February 1985, vol. 73, cc. 1370–86.
67 Hospital Complaints Procedure Act, 1985, Chapter 42 (London, 1985).
68 Mulcahy, *Disputing Doctors*, p. 41.
69 Department of Health, *Patient's Charter* (London, 1991); Department of Health, *The NHS Constitution* (London, 2009).
70 Patients Association, *NHS Complaints: Who Cares? Who can Make it Better?* (London, 2008).
71 See, for example, discussions of the implications of the Francis Report on the conditions at Stafford Hospital and what this means for patient complaint mechanisms,

such as A. O'Dowd, 'BMJ Round Table: After Francis, What Next for the NHS?', *British Medical Journal* (10 April 2013), 346, f.2074, pp. 1–3.

72 Porter, 'The Patient's View', p. 189.

73 See, for example, J. Clarke, N. Smith and E. Vidler, 'The Indeterminacy of Choice: Political, Policy and Organisational Implications', *Social Policy and Society*, 5, 3 (2006), pp. 327–336; J. Appleby, A. Harrison and N. Devlin, *What is the Real Cost of More Patient Choice?* (London: King's Fund, 2003); Which?, *Which Choice? Health* (London, 2005).

74 C. Hall, 'Super Complaint on Private Dentists', *The Daily Telegraph*, 30 October 2001, www.telegraph.co.uk/news/uknews/1360904/Super-complaint-on-private-dentists.html, accessed 5 April 2014.

9 Complaining about typhoid in 1930s Britain

Rosemary Wall[1]

In 1938, the British newspaper the *Manchester Guardian* commented that the Croydon typhoid epidemic of 1937 was 'distinctive' because of the

> intense public interest it aroused, in that it provoked the formation of a Typhoid Outbreak Committee of residents determined to probe all the circumstances before the onset of the disease, and in the decision of the [central government's] Ministry of Health that a full inquiry . . . was needed to establish the cause of the epidemic.[2]

Yet this was not the only outcome that was particularly unusual among the major epidemics of typhoid that struck three very different English towns in the 'Hungry Thirties': Malton, North Yorkshire (1932); Bournemouth, Hampshire (1936); and Croydon, Surrey (1937).

Typhoid is a bacterial disease, transmitted faecal-orally. Epidemics often began as a result of healthy carriers of the disease contaminating water or milk supplies.[3] Complaints about typhoid from the local residents in Croydon included a deputation to Whitehall, the seat of British governmental administration in London, in order to present a petition for the inquiry. Even before this, the epidemic was unusual in receiving significant national news coverage when it was in its earliest stages, and as such supports other chapters in this collection by emphasising the centrality of the media in revealing and shaping complaint. From 4 November 1937, there were reports of 10 people being unwell in Croydon in the major national newspapers, including the *Daily Telegraph*, *Daily Herald*, *Daily Express* and *The Times*, and even the Scottish *Glasgow Herald*.[4] Following the inquiry, local residents successfully campaigned for the mass compensation of 260 sufferers from the disease, arguing that the local authority had been negligent. A test case resulted in the payment of a total sum of £92,000 (the equivalent of approximately £3 million today) in damages and costs.[5] With the test case occurring in November 1938, a year after the epidemic, a Bill had to be passed in Parliament to extend the usual time limit for payments allowed under the Public Authorities Protection Act,

1893. The change in the law resulting from the Bill led to a much wider discussion in the House of Commons regarding patients' right to complain, with several earlier cases discussed. The limitation for claims was changed from six to 12 months after an incident. The limit was already 12 months for fatalities.[6] Indeed, this chapter may be considered the prelude not only to Mold's discussion of patient groups in this volume but also to McHale's assessment of the impact of complaints in pushing forward the legal framework for complaining about medicine.

This sequence of events and the number of successful claims in Croydon are unique in British history and, considering the difficulties in claiming for such epidemics, the Croydon test case should be iconic in demonstrating how a successful compensation claim can be made for an epidemic.[7] At the time, the *Modern Law Review* reported that it was 'rare for the circumstances giving rise to an action to have effects as far-reaching and, ultimately, as beneficial as in this case'.[8] The importance of the case for environmental law has been recognised.[9] However, in her discussion of disease and compensation, legal historian Jane Stapleton argues that the use of test cases for class actions are only a 'remote possibility' in Britain, in contrast to the US, where they have been used for pharmaceutical and environmental contamination litigation. For infectious disease,

> it is unclear how far courts would hold the party responsible for the initial contagion or contamination liable for the catastrophic results. Even though the courts might want to avoid the potential multiplication of litigation recognition [that] such a duty might entail, in practice they might be swayed by compensatory policies in those few cases where medical causation could be traced and proven.[10]

How did such an unlikely outcome occur in Croydon?

The Croydon epidemic was not unique in terms of the numbers of people suffering and dying from the disease during outbreaks in the 1930s. The epidemic in the town, located 10 miles south of London, had resulted in 297 cases (43 fatalities) from a population of 40,000 who consumed the contaminated water supply in South Croydon. In Malton, a country town near York in northern England, there were 249 cases (including 23 deaths) from a population of 4,500, but a total of 270 cases and 24 deaths as a result of associated illness further afield.[11] In the southern seaside resort of Bournemouth, and the neighbouring towns of Poole and Christchurch, 718 people suffered from typhoid in 1936, 200 of whom were visitors; 51 people died. This epidemic was the result of milk indirectly contaminated by a typhoid carrier.[12] Indeed, in November 1937 the *Manchester Guardian* remarked that the Croydon epidemic was not yet as notable in terms of the proportion of cases among the community as the epidemics in Malton and Bournemouth.[13] Yet although the number of cases in comparison to the population was less significant, the case mortality rate was much higher.

Each of these epidemics resulted in a response from the central government in terms of a report from a representative of the Ministry of Health, a normal response to significant epidemics.[14] The Malton epidemic was followed by a local public inquiry regarding the building of a new water supply and the Bournemouth epidemic resulted in a local inquiry held 'in camera' (in private) several months after the outbreak, with a report of the inquiry issued in April 1937. Subsequently there were a couple of individual lawsuits.[15] Yet the Croydon epidemic resulted in an inquiry led by the Ministry of Health while the epidemic was still in full flow and in the aforementioned test case at the High Court in London.[16] This chapter examines the different responses to these epidemics in order to unpack why the residents of Croydon made such a heightened and successful complaint.

Studying typhoid is a particularly useful device for looking at complaints about public health, as it is one of several diseases which have been seen as 'a recognized marker of civilization – or the lack of it'.[17] Typhoid epidemics provide a tool to examine community and class reactions to crises and to analyse popular arguments as to whom to blame. Typhoid was indiscriminate of class: Prince Albert died from the disease in 1861. As with epidemics more generally, the outbreaks of typhoid studied within this chapter unfold in 'dramaturgic form', with burgeoning tension, 'crisis of individual and collective character', and finally 'closure'.[18] However, despite suffering from the same disease, communities' responses were not uniform and in the 1930s people reacted to their experience and grief in increasingly litigious ways. Therefore, this chapter seeks to situate these epidemics within the 'unity of place and time' which define each episode.[19]

Not only were the geographical locations and demographics different, but the epidemics occurred at different stages of the economic depression and recovery of the 1930s. Britain was suffering from the effects of the Wall Street crash of October 1929 and the subsequent collapse of world trade, in addition to the decline of staple industries in the face of international competition. Severe unemployment of around 25 per cent of the working population began to be reduced only as Britain prepared for another world war in the latter years of the decade.[20] However, the effect of the economic depression was uneven, being particularly concentrated in the industrial areas of the North, Scotland and Wales, hence apparently having less effect on the locations featured within this chapter.[21]

Complaints about illness were not new to this interwar context. As the Introduction and King's chapter in this volume suggest, patients had claimed rights in relation to healthcare, in terms of contracts and common law, since the eighteenth century, and as a regulator, the General Medical Council provided a body to complain to about particular doctors from its establishment in 1858.[22] An Act authorising tort actions regarding death by negligence was instituted in 1846.[23] In September 1897, an epidemic of typhoid in Maidstone, Kent, in south-eastern England, resulted in over 1,300 cases and a cash settlement for sufferers.[24] In March 1898, residents decided to bring a combined action against the Water

Company at the High Court. Although the company offered £3,000 if the group did not take the case to court, this sum was refused.[25] However, by April, the *Kent Messenger* reported that a grant of £3,000 had been given to campaigning sufferers by the Water Company through 'generosity', not through acceptance of responsibility.[26] Before there was any litigation in court resulting in a mass award of compensation in Britain, a typhoid epidemic in Olean, New York (US), in 1928 resulted in a claim for $425,000 following 248 cases and 25 deaths. Payments were awarded to cover medical and nursing expenses, loss of earnings, deaths and incapacity, in addition to funds to somewhat compensate people who became typhoid carriers.[27] The pleas for compensation in 1930s Britain should also be contextualised in existing law, which highlighted the idea of compensation for bacterial disease; the Workmen's Compensation Act (1906) permitted claims for anthrax.[28] People have therefore been seeking compensation for infectious disease for a considerable time.

This chapter seeks to discover why a mass compensation claim was launched and succeeded in Croydon in 1938. What was different about Croydon compared to the origins, complaints and reporting of the earlier epidemics? Did the way in which medicine was financed in the 1930s lead to a change in the public's response between 1932 and 1937, and did the response differ because of the locations of the epidemics?

Malton, 1932

Malton's water supply was polluted by excreta from a typhoid patient at Spring Hall Hospital due to faulty drainage, caused by the vibrations of heavy traffic.[29] Generally, there was a charitable reaction to the epidemic. The Typhoid Relief Fund collected £8,700 locally and nationally to help those in hardship, including from damage to trade.[30] Not only did the local community organise financial aid, but people volunteered their time, undertaking activities such as producing and issuing bulletins about disease transmission, canvassing residents about milk suppliers, volunteering at the hospital, collecting infected bedding (despite the risk) and donating blood. Dances and a nativity play raised additional funds, and the Archbishop of York kicked off a charity football match.[31]

Although the people of Malton were less litigious than the inhabitants of Maidstone in 1897, or even Croydon in 1937, complaints arose, many from a local hairdresser, L. Verron. His complaints included writing to the Prime Minister about a doctor charging him for inoculating his family (although the Medical Officer of Health (MOH) – an official appointed locally to be responsible for local public health – stated that he could inoculate for free), letters to the local newspaper regarding the cost of the epidemic to the local ratepayers in terms of trade and nursing care, and a demand for a Parliamentary inquiry.[32] Another correspondent to the local press complained that the epidemic had been kept secret and about the retention of a patient with typhoid within the ‘Poor Law Institution’ (as the local residents still called Spring Hall Hospital, which had been Malton’s workhouse until 1930). However, in contrast to the demands of Verron and to the residents of Croydon five years later, this correspondent argued that an inquiry would be a distraction from dealing with the epidemic and probably would not prove anything, and another letter argued that the cost of an inquiry would add to the costs of the epidemic for the ratepayers.[33]

At the local inquiry regarding the water supply, Verron argued that the Ministry of Health should have provided a grant rather than a loan to assist Malton in the aftermath of the epidemic.[34] This suggestion follows a complaint made by the MOH, L.C. Walker. According to the local press, Walker placed more responsibility with the Ministry than the local government at the Urban Council meeting at which he responded to the Ministry of Health report; he accused the Ministry of not passing on knowledge gained from inspections which revealed problems with the water supply in Malton. There was conflict between local and central government, with Walker disputing the content of the report in general as he claimed that it misrepresented his decisions regarding the inpatient at Spring Hall and that Dr Vernon Shaw from the Ministry took the credit for actions which he had already ordered.[35]

Tensions were also expressed through the language of ‘compensation’, which was used frequently in correspondence between the mother of a nurse who contracted typhoid and the organisers of the Relief Fund.[36] Further to this, when a man wrote to the committee requesting ‘more liberal compensation’ for a ‘needy’ woman, he was advised that the aim was not to ‘compensate victims of Typhoid’, but to help people avoid ‘financial hardship’.[37] Additional complaints included the alleged unfair distribution of funds, and queries included the ‘principle of “compensation”’ with regard to the lost earnings of deceased children.[38]

Although failings in the supply of water were highlighted within the local and Ministry reports, Malton residents expressed relatively little anger towards the medical profession or the local Council administration, unlike the residents of Croydon five years later. Perhaps this was because George Parkin, a general practitioner in Malton and the Deputy MOH, had died after assisting many patients during the epidemic.[39] Also, despite accusations of secrecy, the MOH very publicly issued warnings about boiling water and milk, by way of a town crier, the day after the first case of the disease was officially reported.[40]

Bournemouth, 1936

Despite the charitable spirit evident in Malton, there is no mention of a typhoid relief fund for the Bournemouth epidemic in the local and regional newspapers, the *Bournemouth Echo* and the *Western Gazette*. The epidemic became apparent from early August as a result of a typhoid carrier unwittingly infecting a milk supply.[41]

Effluent from the carrier's home was reported to have discharged into a stream from which Arthur Newman's cows drank in nearby Wimborne.[42] Newman produced milk for a dairy which received milk from 37 farms, thereby contaminating the whole supply.[43]

More than a month after the epidemic commenced, an Anti-Typhoid League was established by local residents, meeting for the first time on 25 September. A public meeting attended by a thousand people was held on 23 October, at which the announcement was made that the local government and the League had agreed to hold an inquiry 'in camera' with no further public discussions. The final decision regarding any culpability would be presented in a report written by a judge who would be appointed by representatives from both sides. In addition, donations were called for in order to assist the League's work.[44] Although the epidemic arose from a dairy's contaminated milk, the local residents involved in the League tried to implicate the local government. They complained that the epidemic was concealed in order to avoid damage to trade and tourism, a common criticism during epidemics, and one which arose in Malton.[45] However, following the local inquiry, Judge D. Cotes-Preedy, K.C., dismissed this complaint as lacking a 'scintilla of evidence'.[46]

The epidemic led to a claim for damages in May 1937 by a household comprising a family of four, two relatives and a governess, who spent their holiday in Bournemouth. The mother, May Square, had become a 'semi-invalid' after suffering from typhoid. Their allegation was that 'an express or implied warranty of purity in the sale of milk' had been breached in August 1936 as the product sold was infected with the 'typhoid germ'. One of the plaintiffs, the solicitor Alwyn Square, had received a letter from Model Farm Dairies which offered to supply 'pure, rich, clean milk twice daily'. Further allegations were 'breach of statutory duty' and 'misrepresentation'. One of the key complaints highlighted that the milk was sourced and 'bulked' from 37 farms. As a result, should one of these supplies have been infected, the whole tank would be contaminated.[47]

Satisfied this was not a case of fraud as the plaintiffs alleged, Mr Justice Lewis invited evidence regarding the accusation of negligence.[48] As Peter Atkins has discussed, the law regarding responsibility for impure milk was complicated, especially in relation to mixed milk supplies, and the concept of warranties developed from the late nineteenth century in order to protect wholesalers and retailers from farmers.[49] On the fifth and final day of the case, Lewis awarded damages on the basis of 'breach of warranty' and 'breach of statutory duty', with £400 awarded to Alwyn Square, £250 to May, £50 and £60 to their son and daughter, respectively, and £60 and £105 for one of the relatives and for the governess. Yet Lewis also spoke of the consequences of the epidemic for the defendants; although W. B. Long, the owner of the dairy, was an 'apostle of clean milk', and had won two certificates of merit from the county of Dorset, his dairy had been forced into liquidation. Lewis exonerated Newman, who could not have suspected the contamination of the stream and because his utensils, sheds and animals were clean. The case was not closed, however, as a stay of execution was granted to allow for an appeal.[50]

In 1938, the appeal resulted in the decision regarding breach of statutory duty being revoked, as there was no evidence that the defendants knew that the claims in the dairy's publicity material were untrue and the brochure did not act as insurance that no contamination could occur. According to Norman Birkett, acting on behalf of the plaintiffs, if this decision had been upheld, 100 other claimants would have mounted claims. Despite remaining well during the epidemic, Alwyn Square retained his £400 for breach of warranty, as the leaflet had stated the milk was pure; Model Farm Dairies had not contested this at the appeal. The five members of the household who had been unwell had no grounds for damages. The dairy was defended by the eminent barrister Sir Walter Monckton, advisor to King Edward VIII during his abdication, who was becoming an expert on typhoid, having represented Croydon during the 1937 inquiry.[51] Legal proceedings involving the epidemic arose again in the 1940s, when Long, the dairy's owner, decided to take action against the typhoid carrier. The carrier was a Conservative Party MP from 1910 to 1922 and again from 1937 to 1945; he was friends with Winston Churchill and was protected from the media by being left unnamed in all press reports. After a year-long case, Long was denied compensation.[52]

Croydon, 1937

Meanwhile, the outbreak in Croydon in 1937 was determined to have been caused by a typhoid carrier working on a well. The recent Bournemouth epidemic initially influenced Croydon's MOH, Oscar Holden, to focus his inspections on milk as well as water, and this led to subsequent criticism: the Ministry of Health report concluded that Holden was ignorant of the fact that water was the most common cause of transmission.[53]

In contrast to the previous epidemics, the first difference was that a local citizen spotted an epidemic in its very early stages. Charles Rimington was an employee of the Bank of England. His son was one of the first residents to contract typhoid and Rimington's immediate response to Richard's diagnosis on 29 October 1937 was to interview people who were unwell among his local community, determining that the water supply was the only common factor. He urged Holden and the Borough Engineer, Charles Boast, to investigate the source of bad smells and whether roadworks were contaminating the water supply.[54] Next, he organised a meeting for 40 local residents on 31 October to which Holden and Boast were invited.[55] The local residents discussed the cause of the epidemic and the prevention of the disease.[56] However, the tone soon changed to complaining as a result of the attendees' distrust of Holden's expertise. For example, Ronald Moss, a local resident, was 'amazed' that Holden apparently thought that it was 'inconceivable' that water was the means of transmission, as the water was tested once a month; Moss knew about typhoid transmission from time spent living in India.[57] The citizens were also annoyed about the lack of precautions disseminated to the people of Croydon.[58]

Within a few days of this meeting, a group of lay citizens formed the South Croydon Typhoid Outbreak Committee (SCTOC) with Rimington as chair. They met every night for a month working on publicity regarding the epidemic.[59] From 12 November, the Committee grew even more critical of the local government, with Rimington leading a deputation to the alderman responsible for the Croydon Water Committee. They wrote to the Ministry of Health on 17 November, petitioning for an inquiry, and on the following day, Rimington led a deputation to the Ministry.[60] The timing of the inquiry, which began in mid-December, is one of the most unusual aspects of the community's challenge to the local authority and gave the members of the SCTOC ample opportunity to convey their opinions. Over the 16 days of the inquiry, many expert witnesses were called and the assessors and experts visited the well. Indeed, Holden subsequently complained that the inquiry placed an additional burden on him while fighting the epidemic.[61]

The uniqueness of the reaction to the Croydon outbreak may be explained by Rimington's disruption of the dramaturgy of epidemics which has been described by historian Charles Rosenberg. In comparison to the League in Bournemouth, the residents organised to combat and complain about the epidemic after a matter of days in contrast to over a month. Therefore, whereas Rosenberg describes the usual response of a doctor realising an epidemic was brewing and reporting suspicions to the local authority, in Croydon an intelligent lay citizen noted the epidemic and instilled a heightened response from the community and the national press at a particularly early stage.[62] Whereas the 'first act' of the story of the epidemic usually ended in an 'increasingly ominous mood', the Croydon epidemic was immediately threatening among the local community.[63]

The press revealed the dangers of the epidemic to the nation. Holden had no option to keep panic at bay while the cause of the epidemic was investigated. He made a public statement which was relayed in the major national papers during the first few days of the epidemic.[64] The *Manchester Guardian*, which largely represented Liberal Party views in this period, and the *Daily Worker*, founded by the Communist Party, focused on the 1932 and 1936 epidemics in detail, criticising the parsimony of the coalition government which was perceived to have led to declining standards in public health. In contrast, the Croydon epidemic was thoroughly reported over the entire political spectrum of the press, as revealed in the extensive scrapbooks of newspaper articles compiled in 17 volumes by Croydon Corporation and the lawyer Walter Monckton.[65] For example, the right-leaning *Daily Sketch* regularly portrayed Croydon as a dangerous and frightening place to be in 1937, yet the newspaper only mentioned the Malton epidemic twice in 'Rest of the News' and once more when Parkin, the local doctor, died.[66] The newspaper reported typhoid in Bournemouth in a very cursory fashion and with a relatively positive spin.[67]

The lack of reports on the epidemics within the *Daily Sketch* (circulation of 750,000 in 1935) in the early 1930s illustrates the escapism that newspapers offered during a difficult decade through 'gossip, entertainment and human interest stories', depicting society as 'unified and stable' rather than dwelling on unemployment.[68] The post of Press Secretary to the Prime Minister was established in 1931, which led to the press accepting restrictions on their reporting in exchange for information from Whitehall. Yet in 1937, the Croydon Chamber of Commerce campaigned against sensationalist newspaper reports, hiring a news agency on 24 November. Importantly, the BBC was used to publicise its viewpoint; three-quarters of the British population had a wireless set in their household by the late 1930s.[69] Indeed, Lesley Diack and David Smith have explained how critical the role and management of the media could be for tackling infectious disease with the example of the 1964 Aberdeen typhoid epidemic.[70] The response within the newspapers presumably made a difference to public and political reactions to the Croydon epidemic, locally and in Whitehall, particularly in affecting the demand for an early inquiry.

The report which followed the inquiry substantiated the SCTOC's complaints of negligence. The chief assessor, Harold Murphy, argued that better communication was needed regarding the cessation of chlorination of the water supply which had occurred during the work on the well. In addition, considering that the work on the well was not urgent, medical examination of the workers could have been carried out and Widal tests used to detect typhoid carriers. Murphy also criticised the limitations of Holden's communication with local doctors.[71] In response, the Water Committee offered to resign, but the members of Croydon's local government decided that prevention of a future incident was more important than punishment.[72] Rimington reacted with eight demands to Croydon Corporation, which were reported across the national press on 2 March 1938. These included daily bacteriological examination of the water and reorganisation of local management of water and public health, together with urging for those found responsible to resign and for compensation to be considered.[73]

Within a month, writs began to be issued to the Corporation. A test case, *Read* v. *Croydon Corporation*, was prepared and heard in the High Court in December 1938. The case resolved that payments would be made for medical expenses and 'pain and suffering and general inconvenience caused by [the plaintiff's] illness'.[74] There were limits to what qualified as 'inconvenience'. For example, this did not include charges for the luxurious Langham Hotel used by the plaintiff and his daughter while away from a 13-room house which was judged big enough for them to reside in safely with unwell members of their family.[75] Yet the case was not decided in terms of a consumerist contract as in *Square* v. *Model Farm Dairies*, for a contract could not apply between the local authority and a ratepayer. In this instance, the ratepayer was eligible to action under 'breach of statutory duty' according to the Waterworks Clauses Act 1847, not merely the residents of the house. However, Read's daughter was eligible to claim under common law negligence.[76]

In contrast to the epidemic of typhoid in Malton, which was also caused by a faulty water supply, the residents of Croydon successfully claimed compensation instead of relying on charitable donations. However, in *The Times*, Rimington appealed to the nation for donations to help the SCTOC with their legal expenses, with any surplus promised to the Croydon General Hospital.[77] This Relief Fund had only raised about £300 by March 1938, nowhere near the £8,700 collected by the Malton Typhoid Relief Fund. This may have been due to the way in which Rimington advertised the fund, or because of the mentality towards healthcare financing at the time, especially as the Bournemouth epidemic does not seem to have generated a fund like that held in Malton. Yet limited philanthropy still existed to aid typhoid victims at this time; for a smaller epidemic in four villages in Somerset in January 1938, £235 had been collected through a national appeal by mid-February to provide food for 42 sufferers of typhoid and their dependants.[78] The next section analyses whether changes in healthcare financing affected responses to these typhoid epidemics between the Malton epidemic of 1932 and the Bournemouth and Croydon epidemics in 1936–37, leading to complaints, consumerism and expectations of compensation in lieu of charity.

From charity to compensation

The increasing role of the state in medical care may have hindered charitable efforts by the late 1930s, leading to an expectation of support from local authorities or central government rather than charitable relief funds. By the time of the Aberdeen epidemic in 1964, after the 1948 establishment of the National Health Service, a motion calling for a relief fund for sufferers was simply rejected.[79] Manual workers' healthcare had been funded through compulsory contributions since the National Health Insurance Act (1911).[80] Isolation hospitals were already run by local authorities and many poor law infirmaries became municipal hospitals in 1930. Nick Hayes and Barry Doyle have argued that charitable funding of voluntary hospitals came from a broader demographic during the interwar period. While middle-class and church donations based on prestige or altruism generally declined, community-based fundraising activities (such as galas and dances, like those used to raise money for the Malton epidemic) increased. As the decade advanced, the middle classes continued supporting hospitals through employer contributions and may therefore have thought that they were already contributing to healthcare expenses; for almost half of hospitals, charitable donations increased between 1926 and 1938.[81] Indeed, in Bournemouth, the *Echo* Shilling Fund had raised almost £38,000 by October 1936; the target was £70,000, with funds intended for scientific equipment, extensions to hospitals and establishing homes for the care of older people, for example.[82] Considering the decline in amounts raised after the Malton epidemic, it appears that communities deemed that specific typhoid relief funds were no longer as appropriate by the second half of the 1930s.

Additionally, expectation of local authority financial support was allied towards attitudes of blame and retribution. Smith *et al.*'s study of typhoid in Aberdeen in 1964 reveals the legacy of the Croydon compensation claims. The community attempted to gain compensation for typhoid caused by canned corned beef from Argentina, which was probably contaminated as a result of unchlorinated water entering damaged cans during the cooling process. The British treasury stated that a compensation claim was difficult and unlikely to succeed in comparison to the Croydon case, as Aberdeen's local government had not been negligent.[83] Therefore, the failure of the call for compensation in 1964 was not necessarily because the financing of healthcare had changed with the arrival of the NHS, but because the local authority and the local water supply were not involved. As Mold discusses in this volume, complaining was actually becoming more formalised in the 1960s with new organisations such as the Patients Association providing advice on how to complain.[84] Therefore, the outcome of the complaints might have been very different in Aberdeen had the epidemic been caused by a polluted water supply within Britain.

The complaints in Croydon were even more pioneering considering that they preceded the development of the Consumers' Association in 1956, which pushed consumer activism 'beyond things' to include public services.[85] Frank Trentmann and Vanessa Taylor have argued that consumer rights in general began with complaints about water, but their study of Victorian London focused on the value, supply and increasing need for water for personal hygiene, not on complaints about water carrying disease.[86] With water in Croydon, people took these consumerist complaints to a new level to complain successfully in court about the quality of water. During the inquiry, Holden was questioned about the way in which the public could complain about water quality. Murphy proposed that as water had to be paid for and there were penal consequences for non-payments, how could it be that if 'somebody is selling you water that is full of *bacillus typhosus*, that person is under no penal consequences at all?' Holden replied, 'That is how I see it.'[87] The public acted as consumers in Croydon decades before associations such as the National Consumer Council were established in 1975 in order to 'represent the consumer within public services'.[88] They wanted to know why the local authorities had failed in their duty of care to supply clean water and to stem the epidemic.

Place and complaining

In contrast to these reactions in a substantial town near London, the response of fundraising more than complaining in Malton may have been a result of small-town culture. P. J. Waller has argued that the best of the 'traditional and modern' were blended in the idea of the country town and that the appeal of 'neighbourliness' led to the attraction and idealism regarding these towns; 'civic-mindedness fed from deep wells of continuity and convention'.[89] The community of the North Yorkshire town of Malton may have been predisposed to respond by offering assistance to each other. However, 'village-like social structures' can also emerge in urban areas, for example the streets around St Augustine's Avenue in Croydon, where the SCTOC was based.[90]

Another key difference between Croydon and the other two locations was its proximity to Whitehall. Rimington was easily able to physically lead a deputation to the Ministry of Health. Furthermore, the threat of the Croydon epidemic to Londoners may have affected the press's reaction. For example, one of the articles printed by the *Daily Express* announced that a girl from Croydon had been taken ill at Lloyds in the financial City district of London. The article began by highlighting that Croydon was only 10 miles away from the capital city.[91] Within this volume, Matthew Newsom Kerr highlights the role of NIMBYism in complaints about the risk of infectious disease.[92] NIMBYism may well have led to the heightened response from the London-based national press and to the quick decision by the Ministry of Health to organise an inquiry.

Disrupting traditional 'dramaturgies'

The public interest in the Croydon epidemic was 'intense'.[93] This may have been because of the location's proximity to London but also because of the actions of one individual, Charles Rimington, who highlighted the epidemic at an unusually early stage. Like Erin Brockovitz, famous for challenging Pacific Gas and Electric for polluting the water supply in Hinkley, California, in 1996, and Julie Bailey, who established the campaign group Cure the NHS in 2008 as a result of the sub-standard care of patients at Stafford Hospital in the UK, Rimington was an 'ordinary hero' carrying out his own research.[94] Probably driven partly by grief, but initially starting his campaign while his son was sick rather than deceased, Rimington triggered and chaired the community organisation and was the face of the campaign in the press. His social class and power presumably affected his success in complaining; whereas Verron, a hairdresser, did not succeed with his grievances about the water supply in Malton, Rimington, an employee of the Bank of England, gained a following among the commuter middle class of Croydon and was able to travel easily to London in order to complain to central government. Class was also important in the Bournemouth case; the

Anti-Typhoid League was composed of 15 people with 'business interests and property' in the three boroughs and Alwyn Square, a solicitor, was suitably educated and possessed an adequate income to bring the suit regarding the dairy.[95]

For the relief fund to have attracted so few charitable donations compared with Malton suggests that the changing provision of hospital finance had a part to play in the increasing litigation concerning typhoid. However, it may have been the way the campaign was marketed as a means to raise funds to cover legal expenses. A combination of the changing response of the breadth of the national press to typhoid epidemics, the accumulation of epidemics in the 1930s, the location of the epidemic, and the persistence of a local community advocate led to Croydon's compensation case being extraordinary.

One of the major reasons for the public, political and press reaction to the Croydon epidemic stems from it being the third large-scale epidemic in the 1930s – an echo of social scientists Ian Butler and Mark Drakeford's 'scandal inflation'.[96] Historian Anne Hardy has argued that English approaches to the disease were led by 'a mix of resignation and complacency'.[97] Could the press and the Ministry of Health no longer ignore these recurring epidemics?

The threat of a large-scale typhoid outbreak affecting the water or milk supply has now diminished. In response to the last of these three epidemics, chlorination of water was used for most public water supplies.[98] Compulsory pasteurisation of milk eventually occurred from 1949.[99] The discovery of the antibiotic chloromycetin for tackling typhoid in 1948, and the development of chloramphenicol in 1950, largely removed the deadly risk of the disease; no-one died as a result of typhoid in Aberdeen in 1964.[100] Therefore, the events of 1937–39 and the complaints about the Croydon epidemic are likely to remain unique in British history.

Notes

1 This chapter is derived from research which was first undertaken for my PhD, funded by the Arts and Humanities Research Council (award number 103736). It furthers research presented in R. Wall, *Bacteria in Britain, 1880–1939* (London: Pickering & Chatto, 2013), where many more details regarding the biomedical aspects of these epidemics can be found. I am very grateful for Jonathan Reinarz's and Rebecca Wynter's comments on my drafts, and to Lindsay Moir, Stefan Ramsden, Douglas Reid and Joseph Wall for their advice. However, any misinterpretations within the chapter are my own.

2 'The Typhoid Report', *Manchester Guardian* (15 February 1938), p. 10.

3 See Wall, *Bacteria in Britain*, pp. 125–176.

4 Croydon Local Studies Library and Archives Service [hereafter CLSLAS], Sir Walter Monckton, KC, 'Outbreak of Typhoid in Croydon, November 1937, Press Cuttings November 4–25, Local Papers November 26–7, Volume 1, Town Clerk Croydon', fs70 (614.4) CRO, pp. 1–2.

5 CLSLAS, Report of the Finance Committee, Meetings held on 20 June 1938 and 30 October 1939, Finance Committee Minute Book, 1 November 1937 to 31 October

1939, CBC; 2005 sum based on £92,000 in 1935 and 1940, 'Currency Converter', www.nationalarchives.gov.uk/currency/, accessed 25 April 2014.

6 Clause 21 – Limitation of Actions against Public Authorities, HC Deb 3 May 1939, *Hansard*, 346 cc1954–2027; Message from the Lords, HC Deb 11 May 1939, *Hansard*, 347 cc. 691–92.

7 However, the Croydon case is briefly mentioned in terms of breach of statutory duties, for example J. Goldring, L. Maher, J. McKeough and G. Pearson, *Consumer Protection Law* (Sydney, 1998), p. 135; and in terms of the lack of contract between a ratepayer and local authority, H. Street, *Governmental Liability: A Comparative Study* (Cambridge, 1953), pp. 108–109. S. Deakin, A. Johnston and B. Markesinis, *Markesinis and Deakin's Tort Law* (Oxford, 2007) discusses compensation for economic loss for the father, but does not acknowledge the child's right to action, p. 303.

8 'Notes of Cases: Breach of Control – Breach of Statutory Duty – Negligence', *Modern Law Review*, 2, 4 (March 1939), p. 310.

9 J. McLoughlin, *The Law Relating to Pollution* (Manchester, 1972), pp. 42–43; S. Bell, D. McGillivray and O. W. Pedersen, *Environmental Law* (Oxford, 2013), pp. 376 and 640.

10 J. Stapleton, *Disease and the Compensation Debate* (Oxford, 1986), pp. 33–34, 38, 50 and 60–68.

11 North Riding of Yorkshire County Council, *Annual Report of the County Medical Officer of Health for the Year 1932* (York, 1933), pp. 1 and 34.

12 M. Graham, *The Typhoid Epidemic in Bournemouth, Poole and Christchurch 1936* (Christchurch, 1997); D. F. Smith and H. L. Diack with T. H. Pennington and E. M. Russell, *Food Poisoning, Policy and Politics: Corned Beef and Typhoid in Britain in the 1960s* (Woodbridge, 2005), p. 11.

13 'Our London Correspondence', *Manchester Guardian* (23 November 1937), p. 10.

14 W. Vernon Shaw, 'Report on Outbreak of Enteric Fever in the Malton Urban District', *Reports on Public Health and Medical Subjects*, 69 (London, 1933); W. Vernon Shaw, 'Report on an Outbreak of Enteric Fever in the County Borough of Bournemouth and in the Boroughs of Poole and Christchurch', *Reports on Public Health and Medical Subjects*, 81 (London, 1937); Ministry of Health, *Report on a Public Local Inquiry into an Outbreak of Typhoid Fever at Croydon in October and November 1937* (London, 1938).

15 North Yorkshire Record Office, Typhoid Relief Fund (hereafter NYRO, TRF), 'Proposed Water Scheme for Malton: Public Enquiry', unlabelled newspaper (22 July 1933), Water File, ZPB; 'Health Authorities and the Fever Outbreak', *Bournemouth Echo* (6 April 1937), p. 1; Graham, *Typhoid Epidemic*, pp. 8 and 27.

16 CLSLAS, Test Action, *A. and P. R. Read* v. *Croydon Corporation*, November 1938, CLSLAS, fs70 (614.4) CRO.

17 A. Hardy, 'Scientific Strategy and Ad Hoc Response: The Problem of Typhoid in America and England, *c.*1910–50', *Journal of the History of Medicine and Allied Sciences*, 69, 1 (2014), p. 4.

18 See C. Rosenberg, *Explaining Epidemics and Other Studies in the History of Medicine* (Cambridge, 1992), p. 279.

19 For 'unity of place and time', see Rosenberg, *Explaining Epidemics*, p. 279.

20 K. Laybourn, *Britain on the Breadline: A Social and Political History of Britain Between the Wars* (Gloucester, 1990), pp. 7–9.

21 K. Williams, 'The Devil's Decade and Modern Mass Communication: The

Development of the British Media during the Inter-war Years', in B. Moore and H. van Nierop (eds), *Twentieth-Century Mass Society in Britain and the Netherlands* (Oxford, 2006), pp. 93–114, p. 93.

22 A. Mold, 'Patients' Rights and the National Health Service in Britain, 1960s–1980s', *American Journal of Public Health*, 102, 11 (2012), pp. 2031 and 2034; C. Crawford, 'Patients' Rights and the Law of Contract in Eighteenth Century England', *Social History of Medicine*, 13, 3 (2000), pp. 381–410.

23 J. F. Witt, *Lessons from History: State Constitutions, American Tort Law, and the Medical Malpractice Crisis*, The Project on Medical Liability in Pennsylvania funded by the Pew Charitable Trust, 2004, at www.pewtrusts.org/uploadedFiles/wwwpewtrustsorg/Reports/Medical_liability/medical_malpractice_witt_030904.pdf, accessed 18 May 2012).

24 Local Government Board, *Twenty-Seventh Annual Report of the Local Government Board, 1897–98* (London, 1898), Appendix B, p. 70.

25 'Private Meeting', *Kent Messenger* (5 March 1898), p. 5.

26 '£3,000 Grant', *Kent Messenger* (16 April 1897).

27 Hardy, 'Scientific Strategy', p. 20.

28 Wall, *Bacteria in Britain*, p. 67.

29 North Riding, *Annual Report of the County Medical Officer of Health, 1932*, p. 34; NYRO TRF, 'The Typhoid Report – and After', unlabelled newspaper (17 March 1933), Press Cuttings, ZPB.

30 NYRO TRF, letter from Relief Committee to North Riding Lieutenancy, 6 January 1933, Box 1, ZPB.

31 NYRO, TRF, Report of the Typhoid Relief Committee (Efforts of the Committee), File of Administrative Papers; letter from Violet Chomley to Captain Gibson, 9 December 1932, Box 1, ZPB; NYRO, TRF, 'Our Relief Fund Now Totals £1,388', *Yorkshire Herald* (12 December 1932); 'Our Malton Fund £2,180', *Yorkshire Herald* (24 December 1932), press cuttings, ZPB.

32 NYRO, TRF, 'Sixty Typhoid Cases', *Yorkshire Gazette* (28 October 1933); 'Letter to the Editor: The Typhoid Disaster', *Malton Messenger* (31 December 1932), press cuttings, ZPB; NYRO, TRF, 'Letter to the Editor', *Malton Messenger*, letter written 2 January 1933, Box 3; NYRO, TRF, 'Proposed Water Scheme for Malton: Public Enquiry', unlabelled newspaper (22 July 1933), File on Water, ZPB.

33 NYRO, TRF, 'Letter to the Editor', unlabelled newspaper, letter dated 21 January 1933; 'Letter to the Editor from F. S. H. Ward', *Malton Messenger*, letter dated 21 December 1932, File on Water, ZPB.

34 NYRO, TRF, 'Proposed Water Scheme for Malton: Public Enquiry', no newspaper title (22 July 1933), Water File, ZPB.

35 NYRO, TRF, 'Complaints from the MOH', *Yorkshire Gazette* (31 March 1933), Box 3, ZPB.

36 NYRO, TRF, letters between Mrs A. and Mr E. and the Relief Committee, February to May 1933, Box 1, ZPB.

37 NYRO, TRF, letters between Mr S. and the Relief Committee, 21 and 22 February 1933, Box 1, ZPB.

38 NYRO, TRF, letter, February 1934, File of Administrative Papers, Box 1, ZPB.

39 NYRO, TRF, Malton and District Relief Fund Minute Book, 27 May 1933, ZPB.

40 NYRO, TRF, 'Dr L. C. Walker on the Epidemic', *Yorkshire Gazette*, 18 November 1932, File of Administrative Papers, Box 3, ZPB.

41 Graham, *Typhoid Epidemic*, p. 7.

42 A. S. MacNalty, 'Prefatory Note by the Chief Medical Officer' in W. V. Shaw, 'Report on an Outbreak of Enteric Fever in the County Borough of Bournemouth', pp. 3–4; 'Dairy Company's Defence', *Manchester Guardian* (6 May 1938), p. 16.
43 Graham, *Typhoid Epidemic*, pp. 1 and 6–7.
44 Graham, *Typhoid Epidemic*, p. 13; 'An Agreement Reached: Local Authorities and Typhoid Outbreak', *Bournemouth Echo* (24 October 1936), p. 12; 'Health Authorities and the Fever Outbreak', *Bournemouth Echo* (6 April 1937), p. 1.
45 Graham, *Typhoid Epidemic*, pp. 12–14; Rosenberg, *Explaining Epidemics*, p. 281; R. J. Evans, *Death in Hamburg: Society and Politics in the Cholera Years, 1830–1910* (Oxford, 1987), pp. 285, 290, 304–305 and 380; F. M. Snowden, *Naples in the Time of Cholera, 1884–1911* (Cambridge, 1995), pp. 2, 64, 246–267 and 333.
46 'Typhoid Outbreak Not Mishandled: Judge and Allegations', *Manchester Guardian* (7 April 1937), p. 4; Smith *et al.*, *Food Poisoning*, pp. 11–12.
47 'Claims Against Dairy after Typhoid Outbreak: Alleged Breach of Warranty', *Manchester Guardian* (4 May 1938), p. 13; '"Odious" Charge in Milk Case', *Manchester Guardian* (5 May 1938), p. 12; 'Court of Appeal. Typhoid Fever: Dairy Company's Appeal. Square v. Model Farm Dairies (Bournemouth), Limited', *The Times* (26 January 1936), p. 4.
48 'Dairy Company's Defence', *Manchester Guardian* (6 May 1938), p. 16.
49 P. Atkins, *Liquid Materialities: A History of Milk, Science and the Law* (Farnham, 2010), especially pp. 208–210.
50 'Claims against Dairy after Typhoid Outbreak: Alleged Breach of Warranty', *Manchester Guardian* (4 May 1938), p. 13; 'Typhoid From Milk', *Manchester Guardian* (11 May 1938), p. 12.
51 'Dairy Company Win their Appeals', *Bournemouth Echo* (26 January 1939), p. 3; 'Court of Appeal: Typhoid Fever', *The Times* (26 January 1939), p. 4.
52 Graham, *Typhoid Epidemic*, pp. 8 and 27.
53 Ministry of Health, *Report on a Public Local Inquiry*, pp. 4 and 14.
54 CLSLAS, Inquiry into the Outbreak of Typhoid Fever in October and November 1937, Minutes of Proceedings, Town Clerk, Croydon, CAS, CBC, fs70 (614.4) COR, M. Lyons, 6 January 1938, pp. 741–743; C. Rimington, 6 January 1938, pp. 743–744 and 752–754.
55 CLSLAS, Typhoid Inquiry, R. Moss, 5 January 1938, p. 683.
56 CLSLAS, Typhoid Inquiry, O. Holden, 22 December 1937, pp. 187–188; Moss, 5 January 1938, pp. 683–686; Rimington, 6 January 1938, p. 745; M. K. Humphreys, 6 January 1938, pp. 740–741; C. Green, 10 January 1938, p. 861.
57 CLSLAS, Typhoid Inquiry, Moss, 5 January 1938, p. 684; Rimington, 6 January 1938, p. 759.
58 CLSLAS, Typhoid Inquiry, Rimington, 6 January 1938, p. 759.
59 CLSLAS, Typhoid Inquiry, Moss, 5 January 1938, pp. 690–691.
60 CLSLAS, Typhoid Inquiry, Rimington, 6 January 1938, pp. 746, 747 and 756.
61 Smith *et al.*, *Food Poisoning*, p. 14, citing 'Croydon Epidemic of Typhoid', *British Medical Journal*, 2 (1938), p. 1059.
62 See Rosenberg, *Explaining Epidemics*, p. 281.
63 Rosenberg, *Explaining Epidemics*, p. 282.
64 CLSLAS, Monckton, press cuttings, Volume 1, pp. 1–2.
65 Over 40 reports on the Malton epidemic appeared in the *Manchester Guardian*, for example, and reports in the *Daily Worker* were made almost daily between 16 November and 7 December 1932; CLSLAS, Monckton, press cuttings, Volumes

1–15; CLSLAS, Croydon Press Cuttings, Volumes 1–2, S70(614.4) CRO. Also see Graham, *Typhoid Epidemic*, p. 11. For discussion regarding the political approach of newspapers in the 1930s, see C. Seymour-Ure, 'The Press and the Party System between the Wars', in G. Peale and C. Cook (eds), *The Politics of Reappraisal, 1918–1939* (London, 1975), pp. 232–257.

66 For example, 'Croydon Fears Further Typhoid Cases', *Daily Sketch* (20 November 1937); 'Croydon's Typhoid War', *Daily Sketch* (27 November 1937); 'The Rest of the News', *Daily Sketch* (3 November 1932), p. 3, (5 November 1932), p. 3; 'Doctor Hero', *Daily Sketch* (5 December 1932), p. 5.

67 'Girl Guides Die of Typhoid: M.O.H. and Funeral Service Order', *Daily Sketch* (4 September 1936), p. 2 [the deaths refer to a holiday camp near Brighton, not Bournemouth]; 'Baby Born in Fever Hospital', *Daily Sketch* (10 September 1936), p. 2; 'You can Now Sit Back and Laugh at these Complaints', *Daily Sketch* (12 September 1936), p. 9.

68 Seymour-Ure, 'The Press and the Party System', p. 237; Williams, 'The Devil's Decade', p. 95.

69 CLSLAS, 'Croydon Typhoid Outbreak 1937' (Croydon: Croydon Local Studies Library, 1995), LS/95/590, S70 (614.4); Williams, 'The Devil's Decade', p. 95.

70 L. Diack and D. Smith, 'The Media and the Management of a Food Crisis: Aberdeen's Typhoid Outbreak in 1964', in V. Berridge and K. Loughlin (eds), *Medicine, the Market and the Mass Media: Producing Health in the Twentieth Century* (London, 2005), pp. 79–94, pp. 81–82.

71 Ministry of Health, *Report on a Public Local Inquiry*, pp. 9–11 and 16–17.

72 'Plain Speaking at Special Council Meeting', *Croydon Advertiser* (4 March 1938), Croydon press cuttings, Volume 2, pp. 147–150.

73 For example, 'Typhoid Demand – "Sack Committee"', *Daily Express*, 'Jeers at Typhoid Meeting', *Daily Herald*, 'Croydon Typhoid Outbreak: Residents' Demands to Council', *The Times*, 'Croydon Committee Offer to Resign', *Daily Sketch* (all 2 March 1938), CLSLAS, Monckton, press cuttings, Volume 15, no page numbers.

74 CLSLAS, Finance Committee Meeting, 8 December 1938.

75 CLSLAS, Test Action, 11 November 1938, H. J. Wallington, p. 90.

76 *Read* v. *Croydon Corporation* [1938] 4 All ER 631, *All England Law Reports*, www.lexisnexis.com, accessed 30 November 2013.

77 'Letter to the Editor', *The Times* (1 December 1937), p. 12.

78 'Somerset Typhoid Epidemic', *Aberdeen Press and Journal* (14 February 1938), p. 10; Ministry of Health, *Annual Report of the Ministry of Health 1937–38* (London, 1938), p. 30.

79 Smith and Diack *et al.*, *Food Poisoning*, p. 123.

80 A. Mold, 'Complaining in the Age of Consumption', in this volume.

81 N. Hayes and B. M. Doyle, 'Eggs, Rags and Whist Drives: Popular Munificence and the Development of Provincial Medical Voluntarism Between the Wars', *Historical Research*, 86 (2013), pp. 716–721.

82 'Will You Do Your Bit?', *Bournemouth Echo* (16 October 1936), p. 12.

83 Smith *et al.*, *Food Poisoning*, pp. 35, 77, 143–145 and 156.

84 A. Mold, 'Repositioning the Patient: Patient Organizations, Consumerism, and Autonomy in Britain during the 1960s and 1970s', *Bulletin of the History of Medicine*, 87 (2013), pp. 225–249; Mold, 'Complaining'.

85 Mold, 'Patients' Rights', p. 2032.

86 F. Trentmann and V. Taylor, 'Liquid Politics: Water and the Politics of Everyday Life in the Modern City', *Past and Present*, 211 (2011), pp. 199–241. Peter Atkins has discussed debates around consumerism and the quality and composition of milk from the 1870s; see Atkins, *Liquid Materialities*.
87 H. Murphy and O. Holden, Typhoid Inquiry, 29 December 1937, p. 396.
88 See Mold, 'Complaining', on consumerism in the 1970s.
89 P. J. Waller, *Town, City and Nation: England, 1850–1914* (Oxford, 1983), p. 214.
90 G. Day, *Community and Everyday Life* (Abingdon, 2006), p. 114.
91 'Social Life at Standstill in Town of 250,000', *Daily Express* (20 November 1937), Monckton, newspaper cuttings, Volume 1, p. 63.
92 See Kerr's chapter in this volume.
93 'The Typhoid Report', *Manchester Guardian* (15 February 1938), p. 10.
94 M. McCann and W. Haltom, 'Ordinary Heroes vs. Failed Lawyers: Public Interest Litigation in *Erin Brockovich* and Other Contemporary Films', *Law and Social Inquiry*, 33 (2008), pp. 1045–1070; 'About Cure the NHS', www.curethenhs.co.uk/about-cure-the-nhs/, accessed 30 November 2013.
95 'Letter to the Editor from D. E. Norman, Chairman of the Anti-Typhoid Committee', *Bournemouth Echo* (21 October 1936), p. 1.
96 I. Butler and M. Drakeford, *Scandal, Social Policy and Social Welfare*. Revised Second Edition (Bristol, 2003/2005).
97 Hardy, 'Scientific Strategy', p. 7.
98 D. J. Dawson and D. P. Sartory, 'Microbiological Safety of Water', *British Medical Bulletin*, 56 (2000), p. 75.
99 J. Phillips and M. French, 'State Regulation and the Hazards of Milk', *Social History of Medicine*, 12, 3 (1999), pp. 385–388.
100 Smith *et al.*, *Food Poisoning*, pp. 20 and 22.

Part IV

Public relations

10 Sites of complaint and complaining

Fever and smallpox hospitals in late-Victorian London

Matthew Newsom Kerr

Public protest over the siting of infectious disease hospitals was perhaps nowhere more forcefully and persistently expressed than in Victorian London. While widely understood from the 1870s onward to be a critical institution of professional public health, the isolation hospital was also seen as redistributing and reconstituting some of the most distressing dangers of urban modernity. Most Londoners, in fact, assumed that a 'fever and smallpox' hospital would necessarily reproduce and magnify the risk of disease to the neighbourhood in which it was located. It allegedly altered the perceived and lived experience of the unfortunate area in which it was located – and of course jeopardised the value of property and disrupted patterns of capital investment. Informed by these fears, opponents of local hospitals lodged complaints through mass demonstrations and marches, via lawsuits and petitions, and – as articulated elsewhere in this volume – in the press. A tense late-Victorian discourse about hospitals, this chapter argues, challenged conventional medical visions of urban terrain, meaning and practice. As echoed in Rosemary Wall's chapter, these were grievances toward medicine in which private and public harms were not easily disentangled and where the separation of self-interest and community interests was never completely straightforward. Indeed, shared public complaints were often organised around a complex sense of place. Hospitals were not only manufactories of local complaint but also themselves the sites of complaining.

Attention and anxiety in London centred mainly on the activities of the Metropolitan Asylums Board (MAB).[1] Established in 1867 as a rates-supported agency to gather together sick paupers from the various metropolitan workhouses, the MAB quickly grew into an extensive network of some of the largest hospitals on earth. During epidemic panics, the infectious sick from all social classes were swept up into hastily built establishments often accommodating over 500 patients. The MAB eventually assumed broader public health responsibilities for London: seeking ever more effective control over outbreaks by isolating known cases as they arose, as opposed to their erratic natural distribution in households, public spaces and general hospitals. Seeking to harmonise this goal of spatial separation

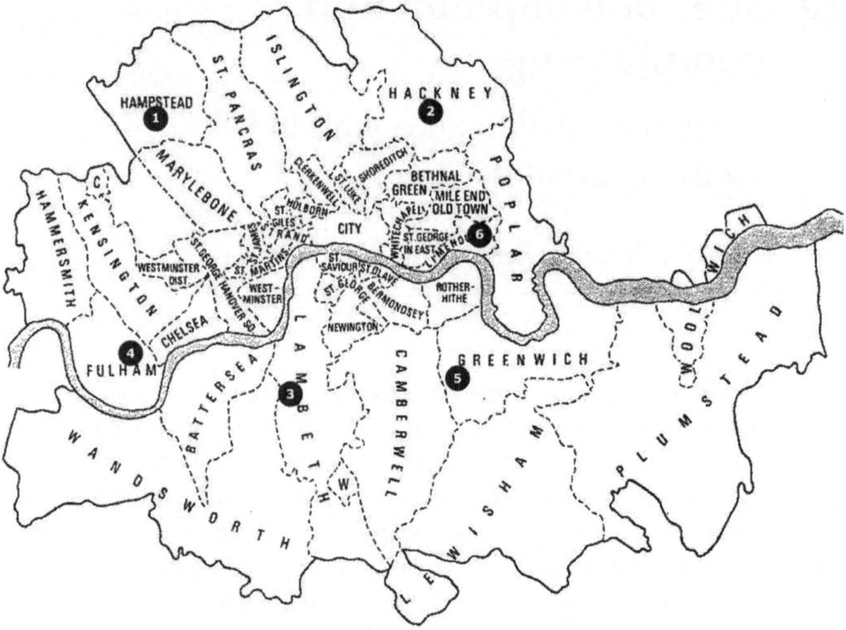

Figure 10.1 Metropolitan Asylum Board Hospital Sites, 1869–83.

Notes
1 Hampstead Hospital – opened 1869, renamed the North-Western Hospital in 1883.
2 Homerton Hospital – opened 1871, renamed the Eastern Hospital in 1883.
3 Stockwell Hospital – opened 1871, renamed the South-Western Hospital in 1883.
4 Fulham Hospital – opened 1877, renamed the Western Hospital in 1883.
5 Deptford Hospital – opened 1877, renamed the South-Eastern Hospital in 1883.
6 Limehouse Temporary Smallpox Hospital – January–March, 1877.

with the principle of geographic proximity, the MAB located isolation hospitals among the population served. In a telling gesture of central planning, a map of London was used to plot an equilateral triangle whose angles fell within three miles of any populated part of the metropolis. The first three hospitals (one opened in 1869 and the next two in 1871) were sited as close as possible to the apexes of this triangle. The next two hospitals (opened in 1877) completed a ring within the city (see Figure 10.1). So, while patients were isolated, the hospitals were not. It was an arrangement that 'preclude[d] the idea of escaping, even for a short time, from the environment of houses' – each of which would contain a likely complainant.[2]

It is safe to say that every neighbourhood chosen for a MAB hospital voiced opposition. Whether methodical and attention-grabbing or unruly and short-lived, expressions of public dissent were defined almost entirely through the lens of locality and often refracted through the local press. This immediately introduces the notion of NIMBYism in considering complaints about medicine –

especially as charges of the 'not in my backyard' sentiment in recent decades have been deployed to depict geographically defined complainers as self-serving. Yet, a host of scholars have criticised the NIMBY label, warning of how it fosters an impression that experts always represent rationality or that administrators necessarily seek the public good over private interests.[3] Not only do accusations of NIMBY tend to presume the legitimacy of controversial uses of space, they often portray local opposition as a species of territorial selfishness. While there is undoubtedly a great deal to be said about the self-serving nature of complaints such as those against the isolation hospitals, the NIMBY label unfortunately reifies a simplistic binary between civic interest and self interest. It also risks legitimising an authority-centred model of decision-making that takes credit for upholding the public good while at the same time obscurinig its own interestedness. The challenge, this chapter suggests, is not to deny the contestedness of place nor to yearn for a depoliticised (or indeed despatialised) public sphere, but rather to understand and critique how local complaints of this kind are historically moulded by unequal distributions of power, informed by symbolic appropriations of place, and redirected by scientific and medical technologies. Complaints about the location of hospitals, while easily dismissed in the vein of generalised 'NIMBY syndrome', should instead prompt serious consideration of the spatial interests of urban medical institutions such as the MAB. Doing so also requires thinking of these complaints as engaging with the complex discursive location of 'place' within medical authority.

Disputes over hospital sites in the 1870s and 1880s bear some passing similarity with another breed of organised complaints about the medicine of infectious disease: anti-vaccinationism.[4] As with that form of politicised complaining, anti-hospital agitations provide an opportunity to consider public health's relationship with the public sphere and the perception that medicine must carefully navigate invisible boundaries. Admittedly, complaints about the siting of hospitals were overwhelmingly episodic and situational – and therefore difficult to classify as 'movements' themselves or as parts of a cohesive 'movement' – but they nonetheless help to resituate the expression of medical knowledges and prompt us to recognise the often highly-contested processes in the medicalisation of the urban terrain. In this case, the act of complaining illustrates practices of spatial claim-making that not only reflect the social ecology of neighbourhoods (which may be likened to Pilar León-Sanz's notion of 'emotional community' in this volume) but also shape public health practice in important ways. This chapter will briefly review three epicentres for infectious hospital protest in London, stressing the symbolic and practical geographies of Hampstead, Limehouse and Fulham, the locations of which may be seen in the map in Figure 10.1. The chapter then considers common complaints about MAB hospitals in the 1870s as forms of participation in public health policy and in epidemiological discourse. The conclusion traces how local complaints were incorporated into metropolitan health strategy.

The MAB's first hospital for fever patients opened in 1869 at a relatively inconspicuous site in Hampstead between Haverstock Hill Road and Fleet Road (today occupied by the Royal Free Hospital). Victorian Hampstead was already 'the archetype of a high-class residential district',[5] boasting a conspicuous lack of congested roads, railway lines, fever nests, or high mortality rates. This suburban flavour, prized by private residents, was, due to its history and patterns of development, intimately tied to Hampstead's renown as a destination for mass recreation – in particular Hampstead Heath, a popular green space that attracted tens of thousands of Cockney holidayers seeking wholesome and rustic amusement. A well-funded and energetic indigenous campaign against the hospital periodically flared into action for over a decade after it opened, producing various committees, deputations and memorials, petitions, public meetings of indignation, demonstrations, and one solemn torch-lit procession through the parish. These protests succeeded in closing the hospital from 1872 to 1875, and again from 1879 to 1882 as result of a court injunction. The MAB's decision in 1884 to cease admitting smallpox patients at its town hospitals (more on this below) was cheered as a victory by Hampsteadians, but it essentially ensured that the Hampstead Hospital would continue as a depot for fever patients (which it did until 1948).

Although complaints about the Hampstead Hospital were organised primarily by local residents, the issue captured metropolis-wide attention. The district was consistently depicted as a chief 'lung of London' that would be spoiled by the accommodation of urban contagions. As one newspaper observed, 'a pest house in the midst of the people's play-ground and health resort does appear strange'.[6] A more alarming tone was captured by British weekly magazine *Punch*, whose cartoon on the controversy imagined unsuspecting day trippers shadowed by smallpox and fever (see Figure 10.2). This vision of 'a suburban play(gue)-ground' only vaguely references Hampstead as a site of privileged residence. In fact, the meaning of Victorian Hampstead was consistently mapped in relation to the metropolis's regions of civility and hygiene, which gave rise to a defensive suburban identity that complicates its reputation as a welcoming open space for all Londoners. For example, as critics suggested, designating a salubrious suburb as the site for aggregating the city's infectious sick – presumably from poor neighbourhoods – distracted from the more important task of sanitarily reforming the slums.[7] The Hampstead Hospital blurred the distinct and properly separate spaces of health and contamination; it both challenged and underscored the metropolitan topography of class. Recalling the colonial mapping of Australia as the destination of penal transportation, *The London Figaro* questioned: 'why should Hampstead be the sanitary Botany Bay?'[8]

The defensiveness of complaints about Hampstead Hospital, as the *Punch* cartoon suggests, was perfectly commensurate in many minds with an articulation of the common good. Hampsteadians, it should be noted, rarely failed to protest

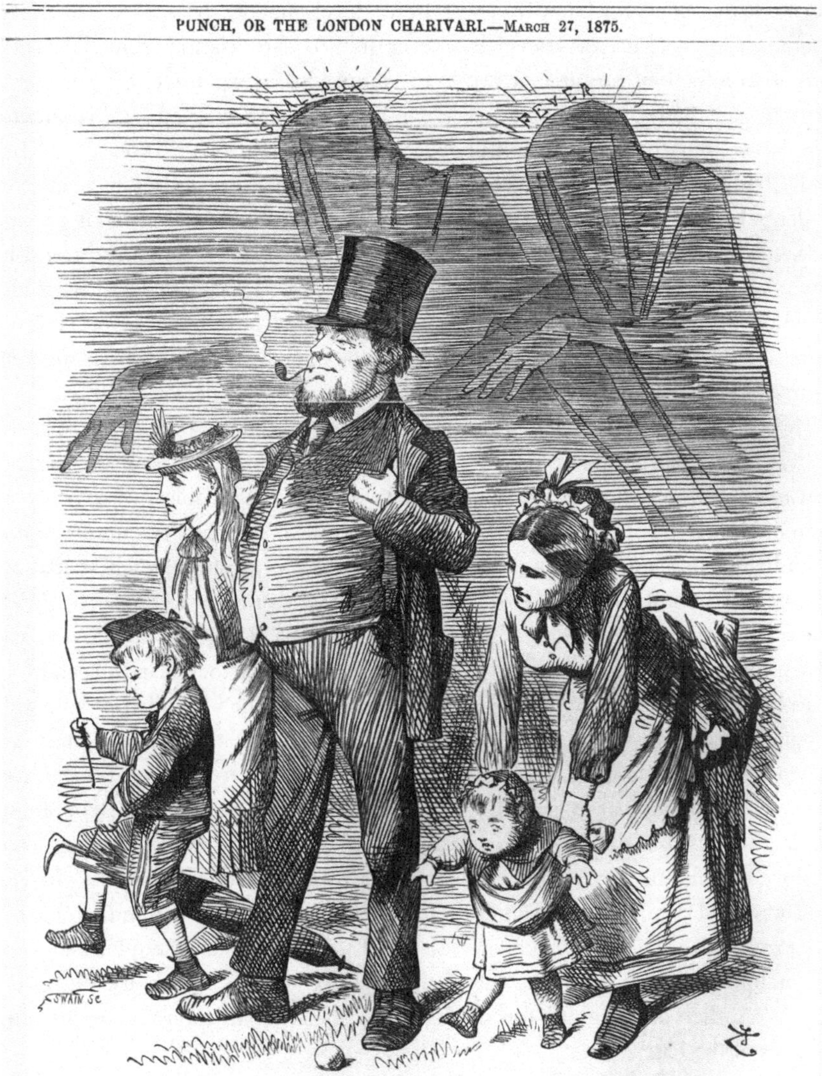
PUNCH, OR THE LONDON CHARIVARI.—MARCH 27, 1875.
SMALLPOX
FEVER
SWAIN SC
"HAPPY HAMPSTEAD!"
(A SUBURBAN PLAY(GUE) GROUND.)
SUNDAY-OUTER. "HA, MY DEAR! NOW THIS IS WHAT I CALL PLEASANT AND SALOOBRIOUS! DO THE YOUNG 'UNS NO END O' GOOD. LET'S GET ON TO THE 'EATH."

Figure 10.2 Hampstead Hospital creates a 'play(gue) ground', cartoon by John Tenniel (source: *Punch*, 27 March 1875).

that the hospital destroyed the value of property in the parish, which possessed enormous prospects for lucrative and tasteful development.[9] Hampstead, with its reputation for health, was especially susceptible to depreciation from the presence of an infectious hospital. It was even admitted that expensive suburbs were necessary for the health of London as a whole, as they encouraged local residents to preserve such naturally healthful spaces as the Heath for everyone.[10] To be candid, though, this argument was nearly inseparable from desires to preserve residential genteel Hampstead from the rude 'streetcar buildouts' advancing from decidedly less fashionable districts to the east, such as Camden Town and Kentish Town. Under the noxious shadow of the hospital, one local vestryman warned, the whole area 'would become the resort and residence of the very worst class of people'.[11] The hospital represented disease, of course, but also down-market infiltration – which to many minds was practically synonymous with contagion.

The protracted agitation in Hampstead contrasts with a short-lived controversy at Limehouse in the beginning of 1877. In many ways this East End parish at the centre of a desperate landscape of urban deterioration could not have been more dissimilar from Hampstead. A sharp outbreak of smallpox (combined with the difficulty of acquiring new hospital sites, thanks to agitations such as that at Hampstead) compelled the MAB to requisition a disused warehouse on Dod Street as a temporary hospital. Running alongside the Limehouse Cut, a canal known for the transport of offensive and injurious manufactory materials and for its accumulation of reeking sewage, Dod Street exemplified the district's horrid sanitary reputation. Local civic leaders characterised the immediate vicinity as 'the most stinking hole in any part of London'.[12] This depiction of Limehouse corresponds to popular imaginings of the East End as a font of metropolitan disease; its disagreeable hygienic mapping – significantly enough – was also employed by fearful locals to disqualify the parish as a medically suitable site. It also supported common complaints about the parish's situation within the metropolitan terrain of health and power. *The East End Observer*, for example, believed the smallpox hospital boldly exploited the nasty renown of Limehouse and presented 'another opportunity for the West to look down upon and revile the denizens of the East'.[13]

Limehouse experienced a convulsion of civic society during the seven weeks following the announcement of the hospital. A local watch committee organised several large public meetings, during which impassioned members of the audience periodically shouted threats to 'blow it up' or inflict harm upon specific officers of the MAB. At least one mass meeting nearly resulted in a violent attack on the hospital. Patients suddenly started arriving in ambulances on 30 January, sparking panic in the neighbourhood and a 'regular stampede' of workers from nearby factories.[14] Local organisers nonetheless kept up a constant schedule of demonstrations. Toward the end of February, Parliament was presented with a petition containing 16,300 signatures and the government quietly agreed to close the hospital as soon as possible, although it gave no indication that public protest had played any role in this decision.[15]

The local practice of complaining about the temporary smallpox hospital provides a glimpse into the area's purposeful geographic self-imagining. One demonstration consisted of a well-planned procession to Trafalgar Square by four to five thousand people from Limehouse, Stepney and Poplar. Marchers and vehicles of every description streamed behind the band of the Tower Hamlets Rifle Volunteers, the Loyal Order of Ancient Shepherds in full regalia and banner, and Dr Barnardo's Blackshoe Union Jack Brigade with banners and band. Many participants sported some sort of decoration denouncing the MAB and its hospital. One of them was a 'monster yellow banner' bearing in large black letters the words 'Small-Pox v. Peace'; another banner displayed a 'monster plan' of the hospital and its location in Limehouse. Marchers gave out loud groans at Cornhill when passing the business office of the warehouse owner who had leased his building to the MAB; they were equally enthusiastic in their cheers when in Queen Victoria Street and passing the house of a Limehouse factory owner who was active in denouncing the hospital. Despite torrential rain, tired and wet marchers trudged down the Embankment and filled Trafalgar Square. Opposition to the hospital, while responding to a grievous strike on the local sense of place, also mobilised deliberate reference to the placement of Limehouse in the social, economic and political topography of the metropolis. Complainants physically traversed the boundaries and distances that had come to define their subjection – demonstrating that the public sphere at many different levels was organised as a spatial performance. Furthermore, complaining about medicine, as complaining about any number of issues, would be deployed in the idiom of class-specific public theatricality.[16] Nonetheless, and perhaps because earnestness in the East End press did not easily translate into a wider impression of respectability, the emergency smallpox hospital failed to catch metropolitan attention as at Hampstead. Most Londoners – to the extent they noticed at all – tended to view the Limehouse controversy as a parochial matter.

As at Hampstead and Limehouse, public groups responding to the MAB's hospital in Fulham ordered their complaints within a set of local spatial practices and meanings. Fulham, a secluded spot of market-gardens and sparse habitation, was just starting to see development which would link it to the more established neighbourhoods of Kensington and Brompton. When it opened in 1877 the hospital was separated from the Brompton Cemetery by the West Junction Railway and flanked by sports grounds: to the north the Lillie Bridge Grounds (venue for the Amateur Athletics Association championships) and to the south the London Athletic Association (today Stamford Bridge, home of Chelsea Football Club). 'Monster meetings', as they were billed in the local press, denounced the hospital at the sports grounds in 1879 (no small irony, given that patients reportedly watched competitions from the windows).[17]

Irritation grew into outright panic at the beginning of 1881 with a return of the dreaded smallpox to the metropolis and a subsequent stream of 'unsightly ambulances' filling West End thoroughfares. A group of gentlemen opposing the Fulham Hospital convened at Edmund Tattersall's Subscription Rooms in Knightsbridge, a hallowed horse-trading venue that combined elite and popular spheres of assembly.[18] The proprietor of the Lillie Bridge Grounds claimed that since the 'plague spot was planted in our midst' the patrons of recreation and sport had avoided the district. Assuming a role common to local newspapers in such disputes, the *Westminster and Chelsea News* aggressively supported this public agitation and dolefully predicted that the 'reign of terror' visited on Fulham would rapidly transform it into a deserted village.[19] This position was supported by the parish medical officer for Brompton, Dr Francis Godrich, who brought forth evidence claiming to show a stubborn prevalence of smallpox near the hospital since it had opened. The intensity of local alarm and enthusiasm is suggested in the fate of the octogenarian Dr Godrich, who died of a heart attack in March 1881 while delivering a speech to a clamorous public assembly at the Chelsea Vestry Hall.[20] By this time, popular opinion had been conditioned by a legacy of complaints about MAB hospitals and, while this was not separated from acknowledgements about the depreciation of property, the London public generally concurred with increasingly dire warnings about their dangers.

One consistent theme in the Fulham complaints was a perception that the district had become the destination for all of London's smallpox and that residents bore an unequal share of the burden for metropolitan disease. Writing to *The Times*, Edmund Tattersall insisted that the people of west London did not object to providing for local victims of epidemics, but declined to being 'inundated' by patients from the likes of Limehouse and Whitechapel.[21] A deputation of residents suggested to the MAB that patients at Fulham Hospital be limited to persons residing in the Parliamentary borough of Chelsea (consisting of Kensington, Chelsea, Hammersmith and Fulham parishes). When this proposal was rejected, the residents' committee took the MAB to court and attained an injunction restricting admissions to smallpox patients residing within one mile of the hospital – a clear reminder that complaints about urban public health were regularly spatial, the politics of its implementation habitually geographic.[22]

Opponents of the MAB drew upon a range of thinking to support complaints that infectious hospitals imperilled health. Many of these concerns bore strong affinity to core themes of mid-century sanitary reform, especially the suspicion of hospitals as almost irredeemably unhygienic. Generations of city dwellers had been trained to think of epidemic disease through the language of environmental pollutants, foetid airs and miasmas. From the perspective of nearby residents, the MAB hospitals did not isolate these ingredients, but rather amalgamated, condensed and intensified them. The main litigant against the Hampstead Hospital, for example, claimed that disease had spread from it in a more virulent form and hypothesised that this was because patients had been 'aggregated together, just as hot cinders, when heaped together, made a raging fire, but, when separated, soon cooled down'.[23] These criticisms mirror the strong aversions to institutional crowding that had led Florence Nightingale and other hygienists to conceive of the ideal hospital as a giant aerating machine, which protected inmates and rendered noxious effluvia inert by 'oxygenating' it into the open atmosphere. A leading figure in the protests at Fulham, meanwhile, accused MAB hospitals of being 'badly situated, badly constructed, and above all, badly ventilated' – meaning that they were too freely ventilated.[24]

Complaints against the MAB highlight the contested medicalisations of Victorian urban space. Infectious hospitals and burial grounds according to one editorial were 'kindred centres of corruption',[25] showing that hospital opponents sought to take up the sanitary logic which in previous decades had closed the London churchyards. A memorial drafted by Hampstead residents proposed that this type of regulation, 'which is sound and reasonable with regard to infection from the dead, must be of infinitely greater importance as regards infection from the living'.[26] Many comparable complaints about infectious hospitals played upon fears of foetid effluvia that in previous decades had both guided the introduction of sanitary infrastructure and also generated new anxieties about interconnectedness by the common sewerage. The architect Sydney Smirke wondered if authorities had considered the effect of

> pouring, day and night, a constant current into the public drains of the outpouring of a great typhus hospital? The excreta of infectious patients formed a deadly, concentrated poison. This fluid ('thick and slab', like the witches hell-broth) would creep through the small brick drains which ramify, in a thousand branches, a foot or two only below the lower floor of every house in London.[27]

The infectious hospital, in other words, could become another target of misgivings already voiced about the position of pumping stations, outflows and sewer ventilation shafts. Both hospitals and sewerage works appeared to a wide variety of observers as dangerously incontinent, seeping or venting their contents to the outside world in disturbing ways.

Complaints about hospitals focused upon not only concentrating and broadcasting disease matter, but also organising the possibilities of dangerous contact between sick and healthy. Any one MAB hospital might accommodate patients from any part of the metropolis, and so each constituted a new crossroads of contagion. Ordinary hospital operations required a distressing movement of doctors, nurses, workmen, washerwomen, provisioners and friends visiting the sick. Rumours flew in Fulham of residents seeing nurses in their uniforms walking up and down Seagrave Road among neighbourhood children.[28] Hackney inhabitants resentfully claimed that hospital nurses would attend services at St Matthias' Church and sit among the congregation.[29] Furthermore, a seemingly alarming number of the infectious sick made their own way to the hospitals during the MAB's first decade of service. In 1872, a servant employed at a house in Hampstead was turned out upon falling ill of smallpox; not knowing where the hospital was located, she went door to door before she was conducted there.[30] Numerous stories told of similarly disoriented patients finding no vacancies at one hospital and traipsing to another (and then also perhaps another). Sometimes patients arrived at the hospitals in ordinary hackneys and omnibuses, and thereby fuelled long-standing apprehensions about the insalubrity of public conveyances.[31] One resident of Hampstead complained of discharged smallpox patients at the nearby railway station, 'the appearance of their faces striking terror into the lookers-on'.[32] Possibly more troubling were homeward-bound ex-patients or hospital visitors not visibly dangerous but still capable of infecting fellow passengers. The wife of a seriously ill patient in the Stockwell Hospital reportedly visited him twice a day and afterwards boarded an omnibus and train despite being warned against it by the hospital authorities.[33] Hampstead locals, meanwhile, never tired of relating their anxiety at being forced to 'run the gauntlet' of invisible infection saturating the streets around the hospital.[34]

The MAB hospitals also gathered together ambulances – at the time one of the most distressingly visible emblems of deadly disease. It is useful to recall that ambulances were completely novel to city dwellers of the 1870s, and in fact were introduced for civilian use as a means of transporting patients to the infectious hospitals.[35] Initially operated by over 40 separate London parishes and vestries, the first infectious ambulances rarely included nurses, or indeed any sort of medical attendant. Worse, drivers became infamous for stopping at pubs *en route* to hospital and leaving the vehicles and patients to be inspected by bystanders. These notoriously shabby disused hackneys were often crudely labelled with large red letters, causing 'a shudder to nervous people'.[36] Sir Rowland Hill – inventor of the penny post, famous Hampstead resident and miserably irate neighbour of the smallpox hospital – objected to having 'the whole sickening traffic . . . almost literally under my eye'.[37] Another correspondent in Hampstead related what he claimed was a common experience on the High Street: 'ladies would run into my counting house, and remain there until the hearse had passed out of sight, and nursemaids would come in with perambulators, stand there, and shudder for some time before they could go out'.[38] At other times, a rather different species of complaint was also lodged: that ambulances attracted inquisitive crowds. Groups of children reportedly made a game of riding the outside of the vehicles, peering through windows and counting pocks on patients' faces.[39] 'The transit of patients was in itself a source of contagion anywhere and everywhere', according to one opponent of the Fulham Hospital, 'but all the evils were centralised at the hospitals themselves'. Ambulances bringing patients from distant parts of London, he argued, facilitated a 'parade of the disease in the streets'.[40]

To many of their local critics, the MAB hospitals exhibited a porosity that confounded the presumed goal of isolation. Popular anecdotes told of smallpox patients sitting on the wall surrounding Hampstead Hospital, shaking hands with their friends and buying fruit or tobacco 'as freely as if no contagion could be communicated'.[41] Likewise, a Limehouse vestryman complained that convalescents at the emergency hospital were seen lolling out of windows and addressing unwanted comments to passers-by.[42] Such stories conveyed a sense of imperfect control over inmates but also amplified the impression of an ominously permeable barrier between the sick and healthy. The resident of an adjoining estate in Hampstead complained that patients occasionally strayed out of the hospital grounds and stole flowers from his garden.[43] Perhaps most alarming were stories of delirious patients wandering from hospital grounds – as in Hampstead, where a near-naked man was found wandering Linsmore Road and only with difficulty brought back to the hospital.[44] Similar stories centred on an impression of terrifyingly transparent hospital borders. Insufficiently high walls might allow a hospital's activities to be 'directly under the eye of the inhabitants of [nearby] houses', one physician explained. He 'constantly had complaints from the neighbours on that score' and saw to it that the windows were frosted so they 'might not be annoyed by being compelled to see what went on in the wards'.[45] Such concerns speak to a new sense of intolerance toward the visual compulsions imposed by urban life. Structural alterations to hospitals, however, usually emerged only out of a long process of protest about proximities and lines of sight. A higher wall had been promised at the Hampstead Hospital, but when this was not completed by the time of a smallpox epidemic in 1876, the MAB received a letter from Reverend Edward Buckler, director of the contiguous St Dominic's Priory and Girls Orphan School:

> When I sit in some rooms on our *ground* floor, I can see over the Hospital wall, right through the windows of the wards of the Hospital . . . [I]t seems so extremely wanton . . . [A]mongst others, I am full of anxiety and disappointment, and also full of indignation at the reckless way that a foul disease is thrown in our midst without precautions being first of all taken for our protection . . . I speak only of the lowness of the wall, because it is a standing visible danger, and the effects on my orphan children might be most disastrous.[46]

Notwithstanding the affected nature of some complaints, it is instructive to observe that these disputes over the siting of infectious hospitals also provided some of the first substantial public discussions of germ theory. At this point still a loose set of ideas popularised in England by such scientists as the charismatic John

Tyndall, the germ theory of disease proposed that epidemics could always be traced to infected individuals. 'Disease-germs' given off by the sick were believed at this time (reminiscent of theories of miasma) to float on the air as scabs, flakes and particles, to attach themselves to airborne dust, or to impregnate somehow the gases emitted from sewage. An editorial in *The Standard*, reviewing the several controversies over the location of MAB hospitals, concluded that 'the doctrine of fever germs is not comforting'.[47] Likewise, a Hampstead clergyman ventured that none could safely say whether the 'dry fever organisms' presumed to be emitted from a hospital would be safely diluted or otherwise rendered inert by the time they reached surrounding residents.[48] This admittedly rudimentary language of germs lent a degree of authority to anti-hospital agitations. As one editorial ran:

> In more ignorant times than these [an infectious hospital] would have excited little or no alarm, because little, almost nothing, was known as to the mode in which these dire diseases are propagated. But these are days when knowledge is widely diffused, and Professor Tyndall has but lately taught people a salutary fear of 'germs' of disease.[49]

Popular complaints such as these show that the spatial and visual understanding of 'germs' at this time better fitted anti-, not pro-, hospital arguments. It is important to recall that infectious disease hospitals had not originated in an effort to control germs per se – rather, they were intended as spatial management of the infectious sick, a technique of urban quarantine that predated the discovery of specific microbial pathogens.

The introduction of germ theory allowed for new articulations of long-standing medical fears and social anxieties – often very much in conflict with one another. Speaking out against the Fulham Hospital in 1881, the MP for Chelsea, J. B. Firth, complained that the health authorities had promised the isolation of the sick, 'But a great many people accepted the "germ" theory.' The surrounding neighbourhood was thickly populated and 'If the wind blew in a particular direction the germs might be conveyed to persons looking out of a window.'[50] Firth, it should be noted, placed this scenario of infection in a rather visual frame – one that connoted distance, yet also an inability to adequately perceive the source of danger. The prevalence of smallpox around the Fulham Hospital, he complained, was 'not brought about by persons who had embraced the patients, but by people who had resided as ordinary citizens in their own homes'.[51] Germs could acquit one of culpability, in other words, but they might also add to one's unsettling sense of invisible connections that could not be guarded against. Complaining about hospitals therefore became not only one of the first opportunities for the public to dwell upon the arcane urban hazards of germs, but also an occasion to employ cutting-edge scientific language against objectionable medical practices.

Local agitations against the infectious hospitals were seldom grounded in grand ideological principles and therefore bore little straightforward connection to systematic medical heresies such as anti-vaccination. Of course, some of the most outspoken critics of public hospitals also opposed vaccination. Yet just as many (and perhaps more) persons who protested the actions of the MAB also greatly supported vaccination, at times arguing that reliance upon hospitalising smallpox victims detracted from the more important task of vaccinating the susceptible.[52] Some stated that they were grateful that vaccine was available to neighbours of smallpox hospitals, but complained that no such protection existed for diseases such as scarlet fever or typhus.[53] It was not uncommon, on the other hand, for doctrinaire anti-vaccinationists to heartily endorse hospital isolation in preference to that invasive medical procedure. Scruples about the siting of hospitals lent themselves less to heterodox forms of complaining and more toward the somewhat prosaic distrust of specialisation and experimentation. For example, one concerned doctor in Hampstead condemned the unworried attitude of professional public health officers, as they were 'really experts, and did not have any practice among those who suffered'. Had you lived in the neighbourhood after the opening of the hospital, he pleaded in a letter to *The Lancet*, 'you would have seen, and therefore believed' that it radiated deadly disease.[54]

A crucial turning point regarding the fate of metropolitan fever and smallpox hospitals was reached by the early 1880s. Hampstead Hospital had been closed by court injunction, and the Fulham Hospital was now shut to all not living within one mile. While judges and juries were disposed to agree with local complainants, they declined to endorse any particular theory of how a hospital might pose an infectious danger to neighbourhoods. This was clearly not satisfactory for most health officials, who initially adopted a fully defensive posture. The medical press tended to regard hospital oppositions as guided by 'unenlightened selfishness'. According to the *British Medical Journal*, they provided clear instances of the 'battle between private interests and public needs' – the Victorian version of a NIMBY accusation.[55] Nevertheless, public administration had to consider the 'state of popular feeling', which was 'getting perilously near a point which will make the establishment of such hospitals, whether large or small, impossible'.[56] It was in this light that public health officials applauded the appointment of a Royal Commission in 1881 to inquire into the whole issue of metropolitan fever and smallpox hospitals. They were shocked, however, by one of its central findings: namely, that there was sufficient evidence showing higher rates of smallpox clustering in the vicinity of the Fulham Hospital and that smallpox hospitals must somehow necessarily pose a danger to surrounding populations.[57] Several health officials remained openly unconvinced (and indeed, in the next century, the distal aerial diffusion hypothesis of smallpox was found to be spurious). But in the meantime, the Government was obliged to accept the Royal Commission's judgments about deleterious 'hospital influences' during smallpox epidemics.

The official crisis of confidence in infectious hospitals, which had originated in public complaints and was now fuelled by professional debate, prompted the MAB to systematically rethink the spatial technologies of isolation. Activities of nurses came under greater scrutiny and control in subsequent years, as did the movements of doctors and other staff. Hospital superintendents imposed vigorous new rules so as 'to fence round the practice of visiting with every precaution consistent with humanity'.[58] Visitors were to submit themselves to special surveillance: donning a special body-length cloak in the wards, refraining from touching the patient, and washing hands with carbolic soap upon exiting. For the MAB, the question of visitation became a technical matter of policing compliance and maintaining oversight even after the visitor left the hospital.[59]

In order to improve the reputation of ambulances and suppress the contamination of ordinary hired vehicles, the MAB Chairman explained, it was imperative for a central authority to gain 'control of the patient from his door to the hospital'.[60] By the mid-1880s the Board had effectively assumed this undivided responsibility for removing and transporting all infectious patients in London. It established ambulance stations at the metropolitan infectious hospitals and staffed the vehicles with liveried drivers and trained nurses. Special telephone communication allowed an ambulance crew to start out at any moment of the day within three minutes of receiving a message from the central office. This quasi-military drill stressed constant readiness and efficiency, but also strict disinfection. The 'patent safety fever van', for example, acknowledged public anxieties by featuring ventilation shafts treated with germicide solution.[61] Apart from these measures, the central priority of the vehicles themselves was the management of mobility and visibility. This in effect required the MAB ambulances to maintain a deliberately low profile – their activities were 'of necessity as stealthy as those of the Fire Brigade are sensationally dramatic', one journalist noted.[62] Carriages were evidently marked, but not overtly conspicuous; a few resembled ordinary broughams and could be sent to 'good' neighbourhoods without much objection, while others were equipped with one-way glass to prevent the public from viewing patients.[63] By 1907 the MAB had completed nearly three-quarters of a million removals, but, through the policing of the multifarious elements of visibility, the ambulances also evidently became less noticeable and disappeared as a target of popular alarm and complaint.

The reassessment of isolation in the 1880s also led to structural alterations to the hospitals themselves. Higher walls were ordered, for example. Redesigned entrances enabled quicker admission of ambulances off the outside streets, and the purchase of additional land extended the buffer zone around hospitals. More radical architectural schemes included designs to arrange circular wards around large ventilating shafts that would send hospital air through furnaces before it was released into the atmosphere, but these were deemed far too expensive to be used on the large scale required in the metropolis.[64] Indeed, as the institutional treatment of 'infectious fevers' became practically routine by the mid-1890s, the MAB was regularly accommodating 20,000 patients yearly.[65] The Board addressed most local concerns about hospitals through a territorial strategy of managing the accumulation of infectious cases. First, it constructed a secondary ring of convalescent hospitals in outer London, which allowed it to decrease the number of acute fever inmates 'per acre' in town. Patients initially accommodated at the inner-ring hospitals were transferred to spacious extra-metropolitan grounds once they became suitable for transport. Second, smallpox hospitals were removed altogether from the urban landscape. After 1884, nearly all smallpox cases were immediately whisked away to a series of floating hospitals and a companion onshore encampment 17 miles downstream from central London. This remote location was serviced by a novel system of river ambulance steamers kept in constant readiness for the occasional case of smallpox.[66]

The remapping of sites and the increasing technical sophistication of hospitalisation illustrate the degree to which the problem of medical isolation had been professionally redefined. Indeed, it was not until the 1880s that the term 'isolation hospital' came into general use by health officials in preference to 'infectious disease hospital' – a rhetorical shift signifying how public health science had responded to public opposition. Another terminological change was just as significant. In 1883, the MAB ceased referring to the urban hospitals by the name of the neighbourhood or parish in which they were situated, and instead adopted the designations of the postal code – e.g. the Hampstead Hospital became the North-Western Hospital (see Figure 10.1). Large organised campaigns against the creation of new MAB hospitals continued into the next decade (at Tottenham in 1892–93, for example). But these were mostly perfunctory agitations and were mitigated by the fact that the institutional treatment of infectious disease had also been made less frightening from the patients' perspective. Undoubtedly, local objections were also increasingly counterbalanced by the more and more methodical and competent image projected by the MAB.

The typical MAB hospital was widely regarded by the end of the century as a site of highly regulated space, and this meant the shadow of its spatial policing falling well beyond the institution's boundaries. Public complaints of 'hospital influences' had become a central concern of medicine, subject to close examination and measurement, and henceforth deemed a specialty of public health science.[67] Local agitations against the siting of infectious disease hospitals, therefore, might have initially posed a challenge to the medical government of urban terrain, but ultimately prompted the further medicalisation of that region between hospital and community. Complaints, we may reasonably conclude, were incorporated largely to the benefit of institutionally-sited medicine. Viewed in a rather different light, though, mass hospitalisation clearly introduced difficult questions about the locations of public and private interest. Indeed, although municipal health managers were able to reconstruct new narratives about indispensable sanitary geographies, the hospitals themselves consistently problematised any clear distinction between civic good and self-centredness. The history of complaints against fever and smallpox hospitals, we may conclude, involves more than simple NIMBY attitudes toward unpopular land-use decisions. They provide a window into some of the complex spatial politics of medical science and practice. To be sure, the transformation of infectious hospitals into isolation hospitals at the end of the century may be traced to the political effectiveness of public protest – these were sites of medicine decisively moulded by their emergence as sites of complaint and complaining.

Notes

1 M. Gwendoline Ayers, *England's First State Hospitals and the Metropolitan Asylums Board* (Berkeley, CA, 1971).
2 *The Times* (30 November 1878), p. 9.
3 T. Gibson, 'NIMBY and the Social Good', *City and Community*, 4 (December 2005), pp. 381–401; M. Wolsink, 'Invalid Theory Impedes our Understanding: A Critique on the Persistence of Language of NIMBY', *Transactions of the Institute of British Geographers*, ns31 (2006), pp. 85–91.
4 N. Durbach, *Bodily Matters: The Anti-Vaccination Movement in England, 1853–1907* (Durham, NC, 2005).
5 F. M. L. Thompson, *Hampstead: Building a Borough, 1650–1964* (London: Routledge, 1974), p. 3. See also A. Farmer, *Hampstead Heath* (London, 1996).
6 *Borough of Marylebone Mercury* (4 November 1871), p. 2.
7 J. J. G. Wilkinson, *Small-Pox and Vaccination* (Providence, RI, 1892), p. 22.
8 Reprinted in *Hampstead and Highgate Express* [hereafter *HHE*] (12 December 1874), p. 5.
9 *Times* (11 December 1874), p. 6; *HHE* (12 December 1874), pp. 2–3.
10 P. Hill, *Report from the Select Committee on Hampstead Fever and Small Pox Hospital*, Sessional Papers, 363 (27 July 1875), p. 64.
11 W. J. Wetenhall, *Camden and Kentish Towns Gazette* (12 December 1874), 3.
12 *Lloyd's Weekly Newspaper* (21 January 1877).
13 *East London Observer* (24 February 1877), p. 5.
14 *East London Observer* (13 January 1877, p. 5; 27 January 1877, p. 6; 3 February 1877, p. 3).
15 *Hansard's Parliamentary Debates* (20 February 1877), col. 738–754; *East End News* (23 February 1877), p. 2.
16 See, for instance, E. Hadley, *Melodramatic Tactics: Theatricalized Dissent in the English Marketplace, 1800–1885* (Palo Alto, CA, 1995).
17 *West London Observer* (29 March 1879), pp. 2–3.
18 *Morning Post* (12 February 1881), p. 3; *Westminster and Chelsea News* [hereafter *WCN*] (12 February 1881).
19 *WCN* (19 February 1881; 26 February 1881).
20 *WCN* (22 May 1880; 5 June 1880; 12 March 1881).
21 *Times* (28 February 1881), p. 6.
22 *WCN* (26 February 1881; 27 August 1881).

23 P. Hill, *Transactions of the Sanitary Institute of Great Britain*, Volume III (1881–82), p. 61.
24 A. Godrich, *Globe and Traveller* (9 February 1882), p. 6.
25 *The Hour*, reprinted in *Camden and Kentish Towns Gazette* (9 January 1875), p. 2.
26 *HHE* (12 December 1874), pp. 2–3.
27 *Times* (12 February 1875), p. 12.
28 *Times* (25 March 1881), p. 8.
29 *Hackney Guardian* (10 May 1871), p. 1.
30 *HHE* (11 May 1872).
31 M. L. Newsom Kerr, '"Perambulating Fever Nests of Our London Streets": Cabs, Omnibuses, Ambulances, and Other "Pest Vehicles" in the Victorian Metropolis', *Journal of British Studies*, 49 (April 2010), pp. 283–310.
32 *HHE* (6 January 1877), p. 3.
33 *The Lancet* (1 December 1877, p. 827; 8 December 1877, p. 865).
34 'Letter from "L"', *HHE* (22 May 1875), p. 3.
35 Newsom Kerr, '"Perambulating Fever Nests"'.
36 *HHE* (5 January 1884), p. 3.
37 *Times* (15 March 1875), p. 9.
38 *HHE* (6 September 1884), p. 3.
39 Newsom Kerr, '"Perambulating Fever Nests"', pp. 302–306.
40 J. P. Bridgewater, *Transactions of the Sanitary Institute of Great Britain*, Volume III (1881–82), p. 57.
41 *HHE* (13 April 1872).
42 *East London Observer* (17 February 1877), p. 3.
43 Hill, *Report from the Select Committee on Hampstead*, p. 56.
44 *Camden and Kentish Towns Gazette* (13 May 1871), p. 3.
45 *British Medical Journal* (26 December 1874), p. 826.
46 London Metropolitan Archives, *MAB Minutes v.10* (2 December 1876), pp. 521–522.
47 *The Standard* (25 November 1874), p. 4.
48 T. Sadler, *A Few Words on the Hampstead Hospital Question* (London, 1875), p. 5.
49 *The Echo* (25 November 1874).
50 *Times* (9 March 1881), p. 7; *Lancet* (12 March 1881), p. 436.
51 *WCN* (26 February 1881), p. 8.
52 *WCN* (12 March 1881), p. 7.
53 *North Londoner* (28 November 1874), p. 6.
54 *North Londoner* (26 December 1874), p. 2; *Lancet* (2 January 1875), p. 27.
55 *London Medical Record* (23 December 1874), p. 800; *British Medical Journal* (27 May 1882), pp. 788–789.
56 *Lancet* (19 March 1881), p. 468.
57 *Royal Commission on Small-Pox and Fever Hospitals*, Sessional Papers, c.3314 (London, 1882).
58 *Report of Dr. Bridges, Inspector of the Local Government Board, on Small-pox in the Hospitals of the Metropolitan Asylums Board, from 1876 to 1878* (24 February 1880), p. 6.
59 G. Mooney, 'Infection and Citizenship: (Not) Visiting Hospitals in Mid-Victorian Britain', in G. Mooney and J. Reinarz (eds), *Permeable Walls: Historical Perspectives on Hospital and Asylum Visiting* (New York, 2009), pp. 147–173.
60 Sir E. Hay Currie in *Royal Commission on Small-Pox and Fever Hospitals*, p. 26.
61 *Lancet* (23 August 1884), p. 330.
62 *London Argus* (13 September 1901), p. 1.

63 Newsom Kerr, '"Perambulating Fever Nests"'.

64 'Memorandum on the Administration of Urban Hospitals for Small-Pox by Dr. J. Burdon Sanderson', *Royal Commission on Small-Pox and Fever Hospitals*, p. 315.

65 *Report for the Year 1897 of the Statistical Committee* (London, 1898), p. 12.

66 A. Hardy, *The Epidemic Streets* (Oxford, 1993), pp. 110–150; P. P. Mortimer, 'Ridding London of Smallpox: The Aerial Transmission Debate and the Evolution of a Precautionary Approach', *Epidemiology and Infection*, 136 (2008), pp. 1297–1305.

67 A key text here is W. H. Power, 'Report on Later Observation (1881 to 1884) of the Influence of Fulham Small-Pox Hospital on the Neighbourhood Surrounding it', Appendix A. No. 11, *Fourteenth Annual Report of the Local Government Board, 1884–85: Supplement Containing the Report of the Medical Officer for 1884* (London, 1885), pp. 55–89.

11 No defence?

Perceptions about five doctors accused of killing a patient (1957–2009)

June Jones and Andrew Shanks

Introduction

Perhaps the most serious medical complaint which could be made against a doctor is that they have killed a patient, either deliberately or negligently. Fortunately such cases remain rare, but when they do happen, media coverage is extensive. Very few doctors have been prosecuted for killing patients in the UK, and very few of these prosecutions have been successful. Perhaps the main reason for this is that a defence can exist against charges of murder: the doctrine of double effect (DDE). The doctrine was first described in the thirteenth century by St Thomas Aquinas, in his discussions about whether it was lawful to kill in self-defence.[1] The doctrine now forms part of international case law as providing a defence against a charge of murder in certain circumstances. There are four stated criteria within the DDE, all of which must be satisfied if a defence is to be proven:

1 The act must be good, or at least morally neutral (independent of its consequences).
2 The agent intends only the good effect. The bad effect can be foreseen, tolerated, and permitted, but it must not be intended.
3 The bad effect must not be a means to the good effect.
4 The good effect must outweigh the bad effect.[2]

Within medical practice, the doctrine allows for pain-relieving medication to be given, which may have the *side effect* of shortening a patient's life, providing that the *intention* is only to ease suffering. Intention is crucial to the defence. For a charge of murder to be proven in the criminal courts, the prosecution must show *beyond all reasonable doubt* that the defendant intended to cause the death of the patient (i.e. the patient did not die from natural causes). Take, for example, analgesic medication. The aim is to relieve pain, but it is also known that it may have the side effect of causing drowsiness, dizziness, even unconsciousness and breathing difficulties. Physicians are aware of the effects and side effects of the drugs they prescribe; they must be careful to give a sufficient amount of the drug for pain relief, but not enough to cause side effects likely to be fatal. Doctors who are accused of killing a patient by drug overdose may have a defence if they can prove that they gave a reasonable quantity of the necessary drug and were able to strike the balance between intended effects and side effects.

Medical practice in the UK is regulated by the General Medical Council (GMC). The Medical Act of 1858 introduced a statutory framework where doctors convicted of felonies or misdemeanours could be removed from the medical register and were therefore barred from practising.[3] The GMC remit includes a 'Fitness to Practise' assessment of physicians whenever the ability to practise according to professional standards is called into question. This chapter, like most others found in this collection, finds that complaining about medicine has incrementally drawn the boundaries of professional conduct by means of the press, official hearings, and the law.

In 2012, the GMC's assessment of professional standards work was formally set up as an operationally separate adjudication service, called the Medical Practitioner Tribunal Service.[4] Assessment of a doctor's suitability to practise has always been judged by fellow medical professionals, but with lay members included on the panel. It is notable that since the creation of the National Health Service (NHS) in 1948 only five doctors have attempted to use the DDE to provide a defence against a charge of murder:

- Dr John Bodkin Adams (1957)
- Dr John Carr (1986)
- Dr Thomas Lodwig (1990)
- Dr Nigel Cox (1992)
- Dr Michael Munro (2007)

This chapter examines these five British cases, in which doctors were accused of killing patients by drug overdose. The case of Harold Shipman, perhaps the most famous UK instance of a physician accused of murder, is not examined: he denied the criminal charges and DDE was not used as a defence at his trial in 1999–2000. He was a mass murderer who happened to be a doctor.

As part of the research for this chapter, we have used corpus linguistic analysis.[5] Language concordancing takes data in the form of words, and subjects this 'corpus' or body of text to computer analysis to investigate patterns of language use. This technique is now well-validated as a method for language analysis across various subject areas. Many leading dictionaries in the contemporary world are concordance based, and the method is widely used in forensic linguistics (e.g. to assess whether a document has been forged or to examine witness statements).[6] Corpus linguistics is useful to this study because, at a basic level, it exposes word frequency which presents the most common ways in which problems and issues are expressed.[7] In areas that have become polemicised (such as where doctors are accused of murder, but use a defence of merely intending to alleviate suffering), a picture can be gained of competing definitions and discourses through the number of their occurrences. When these frequencies change over time, they present important clues as to how public and professional opinion might have been shaped.

Analysis for this study began through the collection of a corpus of text about the five doctors. *The Times* and *The Guardian* were selected as broadsheet newspapers with differing political standpoints – the former associated with conservative views, the latter manifesting a left-leaning stance – and known for reporting cases of legal and professional interest. It became clear that the case of Bodkin Adams had attracted the most media attention, so an additional corpus was then constructed by examining all occurrences of 'Bodkin Adams' in six British newspapers available in electronic archives. Three of these were tabloid newspapers: the *Daily* and *Sunday Mirror*, the *Daily* and *Sunday Express*, and the *Daily* and *Sunday Mail*. The other three are considered broadsheet newspapers: the *(Manchester) Guardian*, the *Daily* and *Sunday Telegraph*, and *The Times*. These were principally chosen because the archives were readily accessible, but also they represent (and certainly represented in 1956–57) a broad spectrum of political opinions, were read by people across socio-economic categories and had wide readerships.[8]

In addition, we also examined the professional and academic literature on Bodkin Adams from 1957 onwards. Interestingly, some of the first academic articles to be published are found outside the context of the English legal system, namely from law reviews in the United States and Germany.[9] *The Report of the Tucker Committee*, published for the UK Parliament in July 1958, concerning, among other things, the effect of pre-trial publicity on jurors, was an early attempt at analysis of some of the aspects of the Bodkin Adams trial. In the UK's main medical research journals, the *British Medical Journal* and the *Lancet*, the case is reported contemporaneously with great brevity and with few facts presented.

We begin by presenting the five cases in turn, showing how the media reporting of each case often presented biased information to the public. We then provide thematic data and analysis of the corpus to show how the press have shaped the narrative around killing by physicians.

The five doctors

1 Dr John Bodkin Adams (1957)[10]

Rumours were circulating in Eastbourne that Dr Bodkin Adams was responsible for the deaths of a number of his rich private patients. Mrs Edith Alice Morrell suffered from cerebral arterial sclerosis, a hardening of the arteries supplying blood to the brain. Bodkin Adams was her private physician, treating her symptoms with morphine and heroin, an unusual choice, to say the least: heroin was normally used to control pain in terminal cancer. The two narcotics were closely restricted and monitored, primarily because they were known to have dangerous side effects and to be addictive; there was also a lucrative market in their illegal trade, so prescribers, dispensers and administrators were required to keep a register under the Dangerous Drugs Act, 1920.[11] Morrell's tolerance became evident, requiring increases of both drugs over the last months of her life. She died in November 1950, following the increasingly large doses being prescribed daily by Bodkin Adams in the last two weeks of her life.[12]

In 1956, another of Bodkin Adams' rich private patients died. Mrs Gertrude Hullett had been depressed following the death of her husband in March 1956. She was treated by Bodkin Adams with barbiturates to help her anxiety. She reportedly spent the last three days of her life in a coma and died on 23 July 1956. Bodkin Adams had contacted her solicitor on several occasions before her death, saying that she wanted to change her will to leave him her Rolls Royce. The will was changed nine days before her death. Bodkin Adams also presented a cheque she had made out to him for £1,000, asking for it to be specially cleared, just five days before her death. Hullett was cremated and, on 21 August, the coroner's inquest delivered a verdict of death by suicide.[13]

On 1 October 1956, Bodkin Adams told a local police officer in private conversation that he had expected legacies from Hullett and Morrell who had recently died, leaving substantial estates. The expected legacies had not materialised and he appeared disappointed. His disappointment, taken together with the rumours, prompted a police investigation. Later that month, he was arrested on the relatively minor charges of failure to keep a register of drugs used under the 1920 Act, making a false statement on a cremation form, and the forgery of NHS documentation. While the police were searching his home in his presence, he was observed by one of the officers to hide two ampoules of morphine in his pocket. When questioned, he produced the ampoules and confessed that he had not wanted the police to find them.[14] In an attempt to explain his patients' legacies, Bodkin Adams admitted that he had often asked private patients for gifts rather than payment for services in order to avoid paying income tax.[15] In December 1956, he was charged with the murder of Morrell. Hullett had been cremated, so there was no evidence available to establish a cause of death and he was not charged with her murder. Evidence of the care he gave to Hullett was, however, allowed as part of the preliminary hearing in Eastbourne, as the cases were similar. It was decided, in moving to the criminal court, that he would only be tried on the Morrell case, this being the stronger of the two based on evidence available at the time. Police testimony described Bodkin Adams' arrest for Morrell's murder; when the charge of murder was read out, he responded 'Murder, I did not think you could prove murder. She was dying in any event.' It was also claimed that he asked 'will there be any more charges of murder?'.[16] There appeared to be sufficient evidence to establish that Bodkin Adams was motivated by greed, and intended the deaths of his patients.

The evidence given at Bodkin Adams' trials at the lower Crown Court in Eastbourne and the highest criminal court in England, the Old Bailey, proved most interesting. Far from being unaware of the side effects of the drugs he was prescribing, it was revealed he had a postgraduate diploma in anaesthetics and was working for the NHS as a part-time anaesthetist at Princess Alice Hospital, Eastbourne. A colleague gave evidence that Bodkin Adams had asked about an antidote for barbiturate poisoning, claiming he was dealing with such a case in the community. The antidote had been dispensed to Bodkin Adams by the hospital pharmacist.[17] He asserted that he had given such an antidote to Hullet two days prior to her death, but the pathologist report following the post mortem revealed large quantities of barbiturates in her liver.[18] Atropine was given to reduce the amount of secretions Morrell had, making her final days more comfortable as she became drowsier, but it also acts as a mild antidote to morphine.[19] As a trained anaesthetist, Bodkin Adams would have used this drug as part of a general anaesthetic in his hospital practice, and would have known its effects and side effects. It remained unexplainable why a doctor intending to murder his patient would at the same time be giving an antidote to the drug he was using to cause death.

Much was made in the press reports about Bodkin Adams increasing the dose of morphine and heroin during the last weeks of Morrell's life. While this was true, it is far from the whole story. Bodkin Adams was in practice with three other partners. While he was away on holiday, a Dr Harris cared for Morrell. He noted that she was becoming more agitated and her health was deteriorating. In order to control her anxiety and cerebral irritation, Harris increased the dose of morphine, adding another morphine compound to her prescription list.[20] When Bodkin Adams returned from holiday, he continued with the new regime, and increased it as he deemed necessary. In addition, at trial Harris was asked whether he continued giving the daily 'special injections'. He had, claiming they were vitamin injections.[21] The media portrayed Bodkin Adams as acting alone, but this was not borne out by the facts of the trial. One of his own partners was involved with her care and was the physician who instigated the escalation of morphine at the end of her life. His use of atropine and the fact that his colleague was the one to escalate the morphine prescription cast sufficient doubt about Bodkin Adams' intentions, crucial to his defence under the DDE. The prosecution case had centred on the dose of the drugs, claiming that each successive dose was sufficient to kill the patient, thus trying to establish his intention to kill. The defence was able to cast doubt on this claim, arguing that if each successive 'lethal' dose was sufficient to kill the patient, it did not explain why Morrell had survived the administration of such 'lethal' doses for weeks. The prosecution claimed that she had developed a tolerance to high doses of addictive drugs, and that the drugs had a cumulative effect, producing death which must have been intended due to the quantity of the doses being prescribed. The defence openly admitted that Bodkin Adams' clinical care fell far below the expected standard of the profession, but argued that this, in itself, was not proof of murder.[22]

During the Old Bailey trial for the murder of Morrell, the judge told the jury:

> you may think it is significant and sinister that for the period that he was prescribing very large quantities of morphia and heroin Bodkin Adams was concerning himself so much about her will, telephoning the solicitor, trying to get a codicil executed in his favour.[23]

The press were quick to report a pattern: both Hullett and Morrell had made changes to their wills, just before their deaths, in Bodkin Adams' favour. Besides being left Hullett's Rolls Royce, he also claimed that Morrell wanted her will changed, and on this occasion, the press reported that he was left another Rolls Royce, a chest of silver, and jewellery which was kept in a safe box in the bank. It became clear during the trial, however, that this was not the case. The codicil that the physician had tried to arrange with the solicitor had never been enacted. He *was* given the Rolls Royce, but not through the will. Rather, her son gave it to him after her death in recognition of his kindness to his mother and the fact that it was well known in the family that she wanted him to have it.[24] Additionally, the value of the silver chest which he was bequeathed was valued by her solicitor as £276. Her chauffeur was left £1,000, the gardener £500 and all the dahlia plants, and the nurses £300 each.[25] Bodkin Adams received less from her estate than any other employee in her household. These facts do not affect the argument about the physician's motive, but they do create and promote the public impression of a doctor who seeks to influence estates in his favour.

Also crucial to the defence case were several private nurses who had cared for Morrell in her home, and their nursing notes, which were submitted as evidence. It became apparent that the nurses had spoken to each other during train journeys to and from the trial, colluding on evidence they would give.[26] A total of four nurses who cared for Morrell at the time of her death appeared as witnesses at the Old Bailey. They could not agree during questioning whether the patient had been conscious, semi-conscious or comatose during the final days of her life.[27] The nursing notes, however, show that far from Mrs Morrell being comatose during the last days of her life, she was in fact sitting up and out of bed to eat her meals. Where a patient in a coma would have a reduced respiratory rate, she had an accelerated respiratory rate;[28] none of this reflected a pattern of overdose, as claimed by the prosecution. Again, the press failed to capture the enormity of this evidence, which cast considerable doubt on the presumption of guilt which was conveyed to the public. Dr Bodkin Adams did not give evidence at his own trial, but a specialist from Harley Street – a London address renowned for its private, reputable medical consultants – gave evidence for the defence, stating that, although it had been unprofessional not to keep records about the drugs administered to patients, he could not say that the doses given to Morrell were the cause of her death.[29]

In summing up for the jury, the judge said:

> a man who, on the known facts, was guilty of folly or perhaps worse might never in his own mind have thought of murder . . . I do not feel I should hesitate to tell you here that the case for the defence seemed a manifestly strong one.[30]

Unsurprisingly, the jury took just 46 minutes to reach their verdict of 'not guilty' at the Old Bailey, following a trial which lasted 17 days. There had been sufficient doubt created about the intention of Bodkin Adams that his defence under the DDE was successful. Had Bodkin Adams been found guilty of murder, the sentence would have been death by hanging.[31] Prior to deliberations, Judge Patrick Devlin directed the jury:

> If the first purpose of medicine, the restoration of health, can no longer be achieved there is still much for a doctor to do, and he is entitled to do all that is proper and necessary to relieve pain and suffering, even if the measures he takes may incidentally shorten life.[32]

While we could debate what Devlin meant by the terms 'proper and necessary', he seemed to indicate to the jury that the incidental shortening of life may not be unlawful. Even if Bodkin Adams had taken a course of action which incidentally shortened life, providing his intention was merely to relieve pain and suffering, he had a clear defence. Thus, the way was open for the DDE to be used as a successful defence for a physician whom the press was vilifying as an unscrupulous murderer of rich old ladies.

2 Dr John Carr (1986)

The next case of a doctor using the DDE as a defence did not occur until 1986. On 1 August 1985, Ronald Mawson returned home to Leeds, Yorkshire, after hospice care for terminal lung cancer. According to his widow, Dr John Carr arrived at their home at 11.15 p.m. for an unrequested home visit. He gave Mawson an injection of phenobarbitone, from a pre-prepared syringe, into his thigh. Mawson became unconscious and died three days later in a hospice. The legal case against Carr centred on the dose of the phenobarbitone and the intention with which it was administered. According to his evidence at trial, Carr had intended to give 150 mg to ease Mawson's suffering but had realised that he had, in fact, made a 'terrible and tragic mistake', administering 1,000 mg instead.

The prosecution alleged that Carr knowingly and intentionally delivered the overdose in order to kill Mawson. The court was told that the physician had admitted administering the phenobarbitone to let Mawson die with dignity.[33] He was acquitted of attempted murder because it could not be proven whether Mawson died of the overdose or of his terminal illness.[34] Carr's intention may have been honourable, and lawful, but the issue of proportionality was left unresolved. Giving a drug known to be lethal in large quantities would have invalidated the DDE were it not for the fact that his evidence was apparently believed by the jury: the amount of the drug he used was indeed a 'terrible and tragic mistake'. In this case, the DDE provided a defence because arguments about errors in drug calculations were used to show that the doctor did not intend the death of his patient.

3 Dr Thomas Lodwig (1990)

While the case of Dr Carr centred on the dose of a legitimate drug used in end-of-life care, Dr Thomas Lodwig's is quite different. Roy Spratley had pancreatic cancer and was in extreme distress. His relatives begged Lodwig, a junior doctor at Battle Hospital in Hampshire, to do something to ease his suffering. Lodwig administered a large dose of lignocaine and potassium chloride, and Spratley died within minutes. Lodwig was charged with murder. The medical evidence presented at trial indeed showed that Spratley had been in extreme pain, despite being treated with morphine, and was in the last days of a terminal cancer. The case centred on the choice of drug used to treat the patient's pain. Lignocaine is a local anaesthetic, used to numb the skin prior to insertion of sharp instruments. Potassium chloride is a mineral compound used to treat low blood levels of potassium, which is necessary to maintain many of the body's natural functions: most importantly, a regular heartbeat. Potassium supplements are administered carefully in very small quantities in recognition that overdose is fatal. Lodwig did not record how much of either drug he gave. At trial, the defence claimed the physician had trained at St Bartholomew's Hospital, London, where the exploratory use of lignocaine and potassium chloride in combination had been introduced for terminal pain control. The prosecution decided to present no evidence against Lodwig because it could not prove the patient had died from the administration of lignocaine and potassium chloride rather than the extremely high levels of morphine recorded in his blood, or from the natural course of the terminal disease. Lodwig was acquitted after the prosecution offered no further evidence at his trial.[35] Two factors seemed to influence the prosecution's withdrawal: the lack of proof of causation and the possible justification for Lodwig's clinical choice if St Bartholomew's exploratory use of drugs had established their combination in extreme cases. Interestingly, this research is not part of standard palliative care and does not appear to have been published, though this may reflect the medical culture not to publish negative research results. So, in this case, the defence using the DDE was never tested.

4 Dr Nigel Cox (1992)[36]

Lilian Boyes was experiencing unbearable suffering from rheumatoid arthritis. Dr Nigel Cox had been Boyes' consultant for 10 years at the Royal Hampshire County Hospital. She was now terminally ill and was on high-dose morphine for pain relief, but, despite increases in dosage, her excruciating pain continued. After pressure from both the patient and her relatives, Cox eventually gave her an undiluted dose of two ampoules of potassium chloride, which he recorded in her medical records, and she died minutes later.[37] The ward sister read the entry about the administration of potassium chloride and reported it to the hospital authorities. Boyes was cremated, which meant that the charge of murder had to be reduced to attempted murder as there was no direct evidence that she had died from the potassium chloride overdose rather than from the natural course of her terminal illness. Cox claimed that he never intended to kill his patient, just to relieve her suffering, but also admitted being emotionally involved in her case because he hated seeing her in such untreatable pain. Much was made of Cox's unblemished reputation and character during the trial. The judge directed the jury as they were sent out to deliberate the verdict: if Cox's prime purpose was to alleviate pain and suffering, he was innocent, but if it was to hasten her death, he was guilty. The judge appears to have ignored the fact that Cox chose a drug which could not relieve pain without killing the patient. Surprisingly, the jury found Cox guilty of attempted murder: they had understood what the judge failed to convey. Once the verdict was delivered, the judge said that Cox's conduct was not only criminal, but a total betrayal of his unequivocal duty as a physician.[38] Cox was given a 12-month jail sentence, suspended for one year.[39] While the doctor failed to establish his defence using the DDE in court, two months later he then faced a disciplinary hearing at the GMC to establish whether he was fit to continue his clinical practice. During this time, he was suspended from his hospital post on full pay. Despite the guilty verdict in court, the GMC found that Cox could continue practising. They decided to 'temper justice with mercy', believing that he had acted in the best interests of Boyes.[40] While the DDE had proven his guilt in law, it was set aside with regard to his professional behaviour.

5 Dr Michael Munro (2007)

The final case is that of Dr Michael Munro, a consultant neonatologist accused of killing two premature babies under his care at Aberdeen Maternity Hospital, Scotland. Both babies were terminally ill, and undergoing what is known as agonal gasping, an involuntary respiratory response to low oxygen levels seen in babies who have had artificial ventilation withdrawn as part of their palliative care. The baby is unaware of the condition because he or she is unconscious, but it is undoubtedly a difficult experience for parents to witness. In the two cases in question, the parents were indeed upset at what they saw, and in both cases Munro gave 23 times the normal dose of pancuronium, a muscle relaxant used in general anaesthetic.[41] This drug stops respiratory effort by paralysing the muscles which control breathing. The babies died within minutes. The first surprising thing to note about this case is that it did not even get to court. Instead, it was heard exclusively by the GMC Fitness to Practise Committee. The GMC said that Munro's actions were tantamount to euthanasia, but found that his fitness to practise was not impaired, accepting his account that he had administered the drug to ease suffering rather than to cause death, with the best interests of each baby in mind at all times.[42] The GMC seemed to have overlooked the fact that the quantity of the drug given on each occasion betrayed the intention – suffering could have been eased with a normal dose of the muscle relaxant. The fact that 23 times the normal dosage was administered suggests that Munro *ought not* to have had a successful defence based on the DDE. Arguably, the only way this quantity of drug could alleviate suffering was by causing death by chemical suffocation. After the hearing, Munro said

> I hope that today's decision will promote further consideration of the treatment of neonates and the end-of-life decision-making and that this, in turn, will lead to clearer professional guidance for doctors, better patient care and greater support for parents.[43]

Textual analysis

To begin a textual analysis of the reportage surrounding the cases of the five doctors, two sets of data were collected from *The Times* and the *Guardian*. Data post-1985 came from the respective newspapers' archives of electronic text, which were relatively straightforward to format for electronic searching. Data from 1985 and before consisted of digitised photographs of the newspaper pages, which made them difficult to analyse electronically. Search terms consisted of the surnames of the five physicians, with false positives subsequently removed. For Bodkin Adams and Lodwig, all of the results referred specifically to their cases and the persons under scrutiny, but as the other three doctors had more common surnames, the majority of text retrieved was unrelated to the events and discarded. Combining the pre-1985 and post-1985 data, the number of relevant articles to appear in *The Times* and the *Guardian* were as shown in Table 11.1.

Once data was collected we were able to categorise the corpus into types of entries, as shown in Table 11.2.

Table 11.1 Number of articles about named doctors in *The Times* and the *Guardian*, 1957–2010

Name	*Number*
Bodkin Adams	113
Carr	4
Lodwig	11
Cox	42
Munro	7

Table 11.2 Categories within media corpus

	Pre-1985	*Post-1985*
Case reports	23	16
Obituaries	8	18
GMC hearings	6	15
Post-case analysis	9	4
Legal analysis	4	12
Pre-case reports	6	5
Shipman	0	8
TV reviews	0	7
Book reviews	3	5

In the collection of post-1985 text, when the most common 'grammar' type items were removed – such as determiners (a, the), pronouns (s/he, it), and auxiliary verbs – in terms of frequency the next 10 most commonly used words were as shown in Table 11.3.

The most frequent items referred to the names of the protagonists; after these, terms that suggested emotional affect emerged, in particular terms around

Table 11.3 Word frequency in post-1985 press reports

Position	*Rank*	*Frequency*	*Item*
1	25	459	Dr
2	39	257	D/doctor(s)
3	42	241	Cox
4	44	237	L/life
5	52	195	D/death(s)
6	53	191	P/patient(s)
7	64	161	M/murder(s) *nominal form*
8	70	152	S/suffering
9	71	149	P/pain
10	73	142	L/law

suffering and pain. Examining words either side of the node word 'pain' produced the following list of occurrences:

- relief/relieve (appearing 17 times); kill/killing/killer (10); ease (five); extreme, terrible, constant (each three times); great, control, physical, severe, abolish (two); begged, agonising, alleviate, considerable, bad, fear, intense, intolerable, intractable, manage, reduce, terminal, unimaginable, unmanageable, unremitting, relentless (one each).

These clusters of words seemed to provide justifications of actions. No ordinary pain was being described. The patients were reported as suffering from 'extreme pain', 'agonising pain', 'intolerable pain', arguably the sort of pain which might justify the act of giving drugs to alleviate anguish with the unfortunate side effect of killing the patient. We then considered whether these clusters were related to one particular category over another, for example as part of a statement from a newspaper article, but here there was no clear pattern. References to 'relieving pain', for example, were found both in case reports and in more analytical, reflective or polemical pieces.

The node word 'suffering' also revealed a similar pattern, though to a lesser extent:

- relief (10); endure (three); ease, patient, ill, great, alleviate, unbearable (two each); prevent, pain, limit, excruciating, intolerable (one each).

What became clear from both items was that those emotive adjectives connected with pain are more frequent in later articles. It can be suggested that emotive words are often used to provoke attitudinal alignment between writer and reader.

As four out of the five doctors stood accused of murder, one would expect the word 'murder' to have emerged as the key theme of the corpus. This, however, was not the case. Out of the 11 key themes identified, euthanasia (mentioned 132 times in its varying forms) is three times more likely to be mentioned than murder (mentioned 47 times). From this, it appears that the press may have emphasised compassionate reasons for killing more than the facts of the cases before them. Other key themes to have emerged out of the corpus include:

- suffer (used 152 times), pain (149), profession (80) – including the phrases 'medical profession' (20) and 'professional guidance' (eight); mercy (55), murder (47), care (40), duty (39), intention (20), suicide (10), abuse (five).

Words that preceded 'mercy' are also interesting, as they suggest a continued pattern of emphasising the motive for killing, providing the reader with grounds for sympathy for the situation in which the physicians found themselves:

- killing (was used 39 times), death (four), tempered with (three), killer (two), act of (two).

What emerged from the linguistic analysis was the number of times Bodkin Adams was referred to in later cases involving doctors on trial. This led us to perform further analysis of the references to Bodkin Adams in popular newspapers (the *Daily* and *Sunday Mirror*, the *Daily* and *Sunday Mail*, the *Daily* and *Sunday Express*, the *(Manchester) Guardian*) and transfer data from photographic images into text. This corpus, specific to Bodkin Adams, contains 402 articles, with 257 articles coming from the 1955–56 period of the trial and acquittal. The articles vary in length from 27 words to 2,011 words. Articles over 1,000 words often contain extensive quotation or reported speech from the trial; hence, many of the articles appear to have very similar content despite being from different newspapers. The tabloids frequently focused on personal interest stories coupled with photographs, which relayed more information through reported speech, and, with the important exception of the *Express*, tended to have articles of shorter length than those found in the broadsheets. The *Mail* and the *Mirror* displayed a tendency to discuss medical matters in dramatic ways, with 'poison(ing)' and its associated lexical items more frequently seen than in the other sources.

The trial was notable for two prominent crime reporters publishing memoirs after Bodkin Adams' 1983 death, safe from the threat of libel. The *Mail* and the *Express*'s principal respective reporters on the case, Rodney Hallworth and Percy Hoskins, took different paths in their reporting of the proceedings, which influenced their papers' evaluative stance. Hallworth's reportage, while avoiding labelling Bodkin Adams as guilty in the months prior to the verdict, certainly might be termed hostile. In 1983, he published *Where There's a Will: The Sensational Life of Dr John Bodkin Adams*, maintaining his belief that the doctor was motivated by the desire to benefit from the estates of his deceased patients.[44] In 1984, the *Express* reporter, Hoskins, published his memoir, *Two Men were Acquitted: The Trial and Acquittal of Dr John Bodkin Adams*, outlining the reasons for his belief in Bodkin Adams' innocence. He recounted how the proprietor, Lord Beaverbrook, threatened to sack him for not following the lead of the *Mail* and the *Mirror*.[45] While Hoskins, perhaps with hindsight, might have portrayed his career to be in more jeopardy than it actually was in order to sell his book, the *Express*'s corpus is unusual in that its articles are often lengthier than those in the broadsheets, and its reporting produced more verbatim quotation from the court proceedings than did the *Guardian*, *The Times* or the *Telegraph*. The *Express* made a clear attempt to describe, in some depth, what the medical experts said, what the verdict meant, and in lay terms what the doctrine of double effect actually meant in practice, with some discussion of the implications to be carried forward.

The approach by Hoskins and the *Express* paid dividends when Bodkin Adams was acquitted, as they were able to pay £10,000 for the exclusive rights to his diaries and photographs. In his later reminiscences, Hoskins suggests that something approaching a friendship developed between Bodkin Adams and himself during the trial. Hoskins visited Bodkin Adams in prison, resolutely maintaining the physician's innocence. It is fascinating to see how these interpersonal relationships affected journalistic stance and subsequent reportage, particularly at a time when newspapers were widely read, highly influential and an important, if not the principal, source of news for most people in the country.[46]

The number of articles published decreased rather rapidly after the Bodkin Adams verdict, showing perhaps that such outcries are short-lived. But the number of press articles issued show two further distinct spikes in terms of frequency: first, following Bodkin Adams' death, and second, coinciding with the 1999–2000 Shipman trial. In the two years following Bodkin Adams' death, Hoskins, Hallworth and the trial judge, Justice Patrick Devlin, all published their memoirs, safe from possible libel action. In their various attempts to facilitate public understanding, it is clear that this trial and its place in the public imagination affected them greatly. Several authors of the true crime genre have since taken an almost salacious interest in the case.[47]

Outside of these two clusters, the 1957 case is mentioned in a wide range of seemingly irrelevant stories. The case took on a life of its own and, like Harold Shipman's, it became part of the social fabric and relational signposts of Britain. In 1992, the famous British comedian Peter Cook was described as going to a prep school in a house next door to one of Bodkin Adams' victims.[48] The 1999 obituary of Jean Burca, a hotelier in Madeira, provided an opportunity to mention that one of his guests had been Bodkin Adams.[49] In 1989, a joke was made in the House of Commons by Ian Gow MP that the former Prime Minister Edward Heath looked like Bodkin Adams.[50]

Conclusion

The use of the doctrine of double effect was intended to demonstrate why the killings in question were wrong, but it has, on occasion, been used as a defence for doctors even though the facts of their cases indicate that they ought to have failed the DDE. From the facts of the 2007 Munro case, it is unclear why he was not referred for police investigation; under extant law, his conduct was indicative of criminal activity. His case bears striking similarities to the 1992 case of Cox, who was found guilty. The GMC finding that the fitness to practise of neither physician had been impaired sends a signal that the DDE is increasingly redundant when a doctor's behaviour is called into question. So long as a practitioner had good intentions and acted in the best interests of the patient, the fact that he performed an unlawful action seems, in these two instances, to have been taken as irrelevant to judgments about fitness to practise. Moreover, the reportage describing the deaths of patients from the actions of the five cases in this chapter also seemed to recognise how complicated end-of-life care can be. The results of the textual analysis suggest that the language around DDE and inferences of intentional killing has shaped public discussions of the limits of medical assistance and of human suffering.

The crime of murder is normally accomplished by a bullet, a knife or a poison, so it is most unusual for a doctor to be charged with murder; however, due to the nature of the drugs they use and the types of patients they treat, they are not immune from such charges. Devlin reflected on the motive for performing a termination prior to the 1967 Abortion Act, which made the procedure legal in England and Wales. One might perform it for compassion: to save the woman from shame or overburden or the child from distress or poverty. At the other end of the spectrum, one might perform it for large fees, as a way of earning a good income. Somewhere in the middle was the back-street abortionist who begins by helping one friend out of compassion and becomes the person in the neighbourhood to whom all 'girls in trouble' are referred. Devlin claims that the actions of Bodkin Adams fall somewhere in the middle of a similar spectrum in terms of 'easing the passing' of elderly patients.[51]

We stand at the threshold of the legalisation of euthanasia or assisted dying in England and Wales. The actions of the doctors reviewed in this chapter might one day be the actions of any physician, providing that they conform to legal regulations. The Director of Public Prosecutions has issued guidelines on when he is more likely to recommend prosecution for assisted suicide. Two things are clear. First, healthcare professionals have less of a defence than relatives – they are meant to be less emotionally involved and to act more professionally.[52] Second, no one performing the assisted suicide should gain from the death of the patient, financially or otherwise.[53] If assisted dying legislation was framed with the same set of concerns as assisted suicide, even acts like those of Bodkin Adams and Cox might become lawful, providing that the defendant could convince a criminal court that they were not so emotionally involved as to permit their clinical judgement to be clouded and were not gaining anything from the estate of a patient. Thus the ultimate complaint about a doctor, that of murder, or at least intentional killing, could become legalised and part of accepted medical practice.

Notes

1 T. Aquinas, *Summa Theologica* (Notre Dame, IN, 2000), Q64. Art 7.
2 J. McHale and M. Fox, *Health Care Law: Texts and Materials* (London, 2007), p. 137.
3 McHale and Fox, *Health Care Law*, p. 269.
4 General Medical Council, 'The Medical Practitioners Tribunal Service (MPTS) a year on', www.gmc-uk.org/about/23047.asp, accessed 22 November 2013.
5 J. Skelton and F. D. R. Hobbs, 'Concordancing: The Use of Language-based Research in Medical Communication', *Lancet*, 353 (1999), pp. 108–111.

6 S. Adolphs, B. Brown, R. Carter, P. Crawford and O. Sahota, 'Applying Corpus Linguistics in a Health Care Context', *Journal of Applied Linguistics*, 1, 1 (2004), pp. 9–28.
7 J. Skelton, A. M. Wearn and F. D. R. Hobbs, '"I" and "we": a Concordancing Analysis of Doctors' and Patients' use of First Person Pronouns in Primary Care Consultations', *Family Practice*, 19, 5 (2002), pp. 484–488.
8 P. Baker, C. Gabrielatos and T. McEnery, *Discourse Analysis and Media Attitudes* (Cambridge, 2013), p. 9.
9 G. Geis, 'Preliminary Hearings and the Press', *UCLA Law Review*, 397 (1961), pp. 397–414.
10 For a full case report, see *Medical Law Review*, 1, 2 (1993), pp. 232–281.
11 A. Mold, *Heroin: The Treatment of Addiction in Twentieth Century Britain* (DeKalb, IL, 2008).
12 *The Times* (14 January 1957).
13 *The Times* (21 August 1956).
14 *The Times* (21 January 1957).
15 *The Times* (21 January 1957).
16 *The Times* (20 December 1956).
17 *The Times* (17 January 1957).
18 *The Times* (23 January 1957).
19 S. Bedford, *The Best We Can Do: An Account of the Trial of John Bodkin Adams* (Harmondsworth, 1958), p. 180.
20 Bedford, *The Best We Can Do*, p. 100.
21 P. Devlin, *Easing the Passing: The Trial of Dr John Bodkin Adams* (London, 1985), p. 81.
22 *The Times* (24 January 1957).
23 *The Times* (19 March 1957).
24 Devlin, *Easing the Passing*, p. 96.
25 Devlin, *Easing the Passing*, p. 97.
26 *The Times* (22 March 1957).
27 *The Times* (22 March 1957).
28 Devlin, *Easing the Passing*, Chapters 8–10.
29 *The Times* (22 January 1957).
30 *The Times* (10 April 1957).
31 The death penalty for murder in England was abolished only in 1965.
32 Devlin, *Easing the Passing*, p. 171.
33 *The Times* (13 November 1986).
34 *The Times* (1 December 1986).
35 *The Times* (16 March 1990).
36 For a full case report, see *Medical Law Review*, 1, 2 (1993), pp. 232–281.
37 *The Times* (11 September 1992).
38 *Guardian* (22 September 1992).
39 *The Times* (22 September 1992).
40 *The Times* (18 November 1992).
41 *The Times* (6 July 2007).
42 *The Times* (11 July 2007).
43 *The Times* (12 July 2007).
44 R. Hallworth, *Where There's a Will: The Sensational Life of Dr John Bodkin Adams* (London, 1983).
45 P. Hoskins, *Two Men Were Acquitted: The Trial and Acquittal of Dr John Bodkin Adams* (London, 1984).

46 K. Williams, *Read All About It! A History of the British Newspaper* (Abingdon, 2010), pp. 173–220.
47 J. Robins, *The Curious Habits of Dr Adam:. A 1950s Murder Mystery* (London, 2013).
48 *The Times* (11 July 1992).
49 *The Times* (9 January 1999).
50 *The Times* (22 November 1989).
51 Devlin, *Easing the Passing*, p. 200.
52 Director of Public Prosecutions, 'Policy for Prosecutors in Respect of Cases of Encouraging or Assisting Suicide' (February 2010), Section 43.14: www.cps.gov.uk/publications/prosecution/assisted_suicide_policy.html, accessed 4 April 2014.
53 Director of Public Prosecutions 'Policy for Prosecutors in Respect of Cases of Encouraging or Assisting Suicide', Section 43.6.

12 Looking back to Bolitho and on to Bristol

Lessons from the 1990s

Jean McHale

The steady rise in civil litigation against healthcare professionals in the UK during the latter half of the twentieth century led to claims that there was a 'malpractice crisis' and that the trends in the UK were following those in the USA.[1] Lawyers were increasingly seen as 'ambulance chasers'. The growth of litigation arising from complaints, it was suggested, was likely to encourage 'defensive medicine'. While there remains dispute as to the extent to which in the USA and in the UK practitioners truly practiced 'defensively' in changing clinical procedures (such as increased use of caesarean sections), the discussion and controversy around this was indicative of changing attitudes and fears among clinicians;[2] indeed, this was a similar phenomena to that which Kim Price describes in the late 1800s.

The twentieth-century hostility caused by the rise in clinical negligence litigation was exemplified by the comment of a Secretary of State for Health, Frank Dobson. In an interview on the BBC television programme *Newsnight* in 1997, he said that 'The best place for a lawyer is on the operating table. Lawyers are milking the NHS of millions of pounds a year – money that would be better spent on patient care'.[3] However, closer examination reveals a much more complex picture. There was certainly a rise in the total number of compensation claims being processed by the NHS and latterly by a dedicated body, the NHS Litigation Authority.[4] Even so, the number of *successful* claims during that time did not radically increase at all. That did not mean the judiciary did not seek to reframe the responsibilities of clinician and patient – a tendency suggested through a number of the chapters in this volume. Nonetheless, as we shall see, the rhetoric of legal scrutiny did not necessarily translate to change in the consequences of litigation. Part of the greatest impetus to change came not from judicial decisions as such. The parameters of professional accountability were being determined instead by events outside the courtroom, resulting in greater scrutiny of the clinical professions – notably the rise of the use of the independent inquiry as mechanism of accountability. The development, too, of professional guidelines and standards and their impact upon structures of care should not be underestimated. In the 1990s, these flowed from professional organisations but also from the Department of Health and the National Health Service themselves.

This chapter begins by exploring the evolution of clinical negligence litigation in the UK in the 1990s, picking up on the wider developments suggested by Rosemary Wall and Alex Mold's chapters, from the perception that 'doctor knows best' to the tendency for judges to be more willing to engage with questions of clinical accountability and to question the professionals. The chapter explores the shifting approach of the courts to medical negligence cases during the 1990s in the area of information disclosure – the so-called 'informed consent' cases – and how the apparent increase in clinical scrutiny of the professional practice standard was, in fact, something much more nuanced and complex. The second part of the chapter examines the increasing use of the inquiry as a means of public scrutiny of clinical practice. It charts the establishment and operation of two notable inquiries into events at the children's pediatric heart unit at Bristol Royal Infirmary (1984–2005) and into the unauthorised retention of organs and tissue at Alder Hey Hospital, Liverpool (1999–2001).[5] It suggests that these inquiries in their disparate ways may have provided a much more effective mechanism of 'complaining about medicine' – at least in terms of raising complaints and concerns – than was afforded by clinical negligence litigation during this period. Finally, it considers how the lessons of history may inform future developments in relation to the legal regulation of clinical practice.

Developing clinical negligence: the movement to Bolitho

The starting point for reviewing the law in this area is inevitably the civil law action in the tort of negligence.[6] In order to establish liability in the tort of negligence, a litigant must demonstrate that the healthcare professional owed them a duty of care, that there was breach of that duty and that consequent harm arose from that breach. The burden of proof is placed on the patient to establish this on the balance of probabilities, i.e. that it was more likely than not. Establishing a duty of care in the context of the standard clinician–patient relationship will generally be straightforward, as it will be assumed that where a patient seeks treatment from a clinician in a professional capacity, such a duty is owed.[7] The second stage is, however, more problematic and concerns whether a breach of duty has arisen. In determining this, the court will assess what standard of care the health professional should be measured against. The standard of a responsible healthcare practitioner is an objective benchmark and it relates to the function that the health professional is performing.[8] So, for example, a junior doctor who purports to be a fully-qualified consultant will be judged by the standard of the fully-qualified consultant; a young nurse on her first day in her post is deemed to be a fully-qualified nurse.

In determining what constitutes the appropriate standard of care in the context of medical negligence law, the starting point is of *Bolam* v. *Friern Hospital Management Committee* by Judge McNair.[9] The facts of this 1957 case concerned a patient with mental illness who was advised to undertake electro-convulsive therapy (ECT). He was not, however, advised of a small risk of a fracture if ECT was administered without a muscle relaxant. He was not subject to physical restraint either, and he subsequently suffered a hip fracture. An action was brought against the hospital in the tort of negligence. McNair commented,

> The test is the standard of the ordinary skilled man exercising and professing to have that special skill. A man need not possess the highest expert skill, it is well established law that it is sufficient if he exercises the ordinary skill of an ordinary competent man exercising that particular art.

He went onto say that:

> A doctor is not guilty of negligence if he has acted in accordance with a practice accepted as proper by a responsible body of medical men skilled in that particular art. . . . Putting it the other way round, a doctor is not negligent, if he is acting in accordance with such a practice, merely because there is a body of opinion that takes the contrary view.[10]

The meaning of these statements has led to considerable debate and discussion during the ensuing years. What is clear is that a doctor cannot simply assert that he acted carefully. S/he needs to provide evidence that the actions were in accordance with a responsible body of clinical practice. What constitutes such a body of clinical practice is to be determined by reference to evidence. Critically it does not need to constitute a large number of clinicians; so, for example, a few members of a very small specialty may be sufficient.[11] It seemed, then, that *Bolam* had the effect that as long as some support from relevant practitioners was provided, this would be enough, and that the court would not then challenge and scrutinise what constituted a responsible body of professional practice.

While in some cases there was evidence of less judicial deference,[12] in others the courts interpreted the *Bolam* test very restrictively indeed. For instance, in *Maynard* v. *West Midlands Regional Health Authority*, a 1985 case decided in the House of Lords, Lord Scarman emphasised that 'a judge's preference for one body of opinion to another is not sufficient to establish negligence in a practitioner whose opinions have received approval, truthfully expressed, honestly held'.[13] In other words, judges could not 'cherry pick' the clinical expert evidence they preferred. However, in relation to consent to treatment, as the House of Lords made clear, that was not to say the clinician would not be subject to external scrutiny.

The evolution of the cases concerning information disclosure illustrate a gradual movement towards recognition of patient autonomy, rather than deference to clinical practice. In *Sidaway* v. *Bethlem Royal Hospital Governors* (1984), the House of Lords were divided in their appraisal of what information should be given to a patient to enable them to make a decision concerning whether to go ahead with a particular course of treatment.[14] The case concerned a patient, Mrs Sidaway, who underwent an operation after having suffered from a recurring pain in her neck, right shoulder and right arm. Even if the operation was performed with appropriate care and skill, it carried a 1–2 per cent risk of damage to the nerve root and the spinal column, with the former carrying a greater probability and severity of damage. Unfortunately, Mrs Sidaway was left severely disabled after the operation. She brought an action in negligence, claiming that she had not been given adequate warning. While the surgeon had informed her of the risks of damage to the nerve root, he had not told her of the risks associated with the spinal column. By acting in this way, he was conforming to what in 1974 would have been accepted as standard medical practice by a responsible and skilled body of neurosurgeons.

Mrs Sidaway's claim in negligence was unsuccessful, but the rulings in this case presented a very influential approach to the law in subsequent years. At one extreme, and in a dissenting judgment, Lord Scarman suggested that the test should not be rooted in what a responsible body of medical practice considered right for disclosure, but rather what a 'prudent patient' wanted to know. This was a judicial reframing of the standard of a professional practice – informed by the approach taken in by the courts in some US states to such issues.[15] At the other extreme was the judgement of Lord Diplock, who defined the issue in terms of the *Bolam* test. As he said,

> no convincing reason has in my view been advanced . . . that would justify treating the Bolam test as doing anything less than laying down a principle of English law that is comprehensive and applicable to every aspect of the duty of care owed by the doctor to his patient.[16]

There was, however, a 'middle way' approach taken by Lords Bridge and Keith in the case. While they accepted that the *Bolam* test was the starting point, at the same time they thought the courts should not automatically accept the approach taken by clinical decision-making. In essence, clinicians would be expected to disclose certain material risks with serious consequences: that an operation might carry a 10 per cent risk of stroke, for instance, or a 50 per cent risk of blindness. Moreover, Lord Templeman, while taking the approach that ultimately the level of disclosure was for the doctor to decide, went onto say that there was a case for disclosing some specific risks such as a 10 per cent risk of stroke. *Sidaway* left some things uncertain. Yes, clinical judgement still played an important part – but how much? The leading healthcare lawyer, Ian Kennedy, stated that 'The message of *Sidaway* is clear. Those who advise doctors already know it. Medical paternalism has had its day'.[17] In cases directly following *Sidaway* in relation to consent to treatment (*Blyth*[18] and *Gold*[19]), Diplock's conservative judgement in Sidaway was followed and it seemed very much a return to 'doctor knows best'.

However, in the 1990s there began to be a significant rattling of the cages. In *Smith* v. *Tunbridge Wells Health Authority* (1994), medical expertise was rejected and it was held that a patient should have been told of the risks of impotence and bladder dysfunction from an operation to repair a rectal prolapse.[20] A further instance, just over a decade later, which was considered a landmark decision, was that of the House of Lords in the negligence case of *Bolitho.*[21] Here, a two-year-old child was taken into hospital with breathing difficulties. At 12.40 p.m. the following day, his condition deteriorated. The nurse rang for the doctor, who failed to appear. The child recovered, but at 2 p.m. the child's condition again deteriorated. The nurse reported this to the doctor over the phone. Again the child recovered, but still the doctor did not attend. At 2.30 p.m., the child collapsed due to respiratory failure and suffered a heart attack. While heart function and breathing were eventually restored, the child was found to have suffered major brain damage. An action was brought in negligence. The issue here concerned the question: if the doctor had attended the patient, would they have initiated treatment that would have avoided the heart attack and later brain damage? Here, Lord Brown-Wilkinson stated that,

> if in a rare case, it can be demonstrated that the professional opinion is not capable of withstanding logical analysis, the judge is entitled to hold that the body of opinion is not reasonable or responsible. I emphasise that in my view it will be very seldom right for a judge to reach the conclusion that views genuinely held by a competent medical expert are unreasonable. The assessment of medical risks and benefits is a matter of clinical judgement which a judge would not normally be able to make without expert evidence . . . it would be wrong to allow such an assessment to deteriorate into seeking to persuade the judge to prefer one of two views both of which are capable of being logically supported. It is only where a judge can be satisfied that the body of professional opinion cannot be logically supported at all that such an opinion will not provide the benchmark by reference to which the defendant's conduct falls to be assessed.[22]

Initially, there was suggestion by legal commentators such as Foster that *Bolitho* represented a 'new Dawn' in clinical negligence litigation.[23] Brazier and Miola also saw that *Bolitho* could be put in context of shifting developments upon clinical practice, such as clinical guidelines and other professional changes (explored later in this chapter).[24] Writing after *Bolitho*, Lord Woolf, a Law Lord, suggested that the position of the courts showing undue deference to doctors had definitely changed;[25] he identified a raft of reasons for this. There was a more general tendency toward less deference to authority, due, for example, to the rise of litigation against public authorities through the procedure known as judicial review. The courts had become increasingly aware of how low the success rates in litigation were (around 16 per cent). There was a greater awareness of patients' rights, in part through the provisions of the European Convention of Human Rights coming into English law, in what came to be the Human Rights Act 1998. There was also a diminution in the 'automatic presumption of beneficence' (that doctors were acting for the benefit of their patients).[26] The courts were aware that other Commonwealth jurisdictions were subjecting doctors to much greater critical scrutiny. Medical negligence was being regarded as 'a disaster' with unproductive litigation. Moreover, the courts were exposed to new challenges concerning medical ethical decisions through, for example, the rise of new health technologies, and were more willing to engage in what Woolf saw as 'more traditional medical issues'.[27]

Other commentators were, however, considerably more cautious as to whether the approach of the court system would radically change and indeed suggested that reports of the death of *Bolam* were greatly exaggerated.[28] For example, Brazier and Miola, writing in 2000, commented:

> While the medical experts are to be required in rare cases to justify their opinions on logical grounds there still appears to be a prima facie presumption that non-doctors will not be able fully to comprehend the evidence. This leads inexorably to a conclusion that the evidence cannot after all be critically evaluated by a judge.[29]

What seemed clear was that while the starting point would be, as before, that of the responsible body of medical practice, this did not mean that such a body of opinion would be automatically accepted. Experts would be required to justify their statements. In addition, reports would need to be clearly reasoned and referenced. But actually succeeding in an action, real scrutiny with 'teeth', was much more problematic. In the *Bolitho* case, however, the litigant failed. Expert evidence supported the view that even if the doctor had gone to see the patient they would not have started active treatment by intubating the patient, so there was no causation, no proof that 'but for' the actions of the defendant the harm would not have occurred. Causation remains a major problem in relation to medical negligence actions, even when breach of duty has been established.

The comments in *Bolitho* concerned diagnosis and treatment but not disclosure of risk. In relation to the latter point, the next major judicial step was that of *Pearce* v. *United Bristol NHS Trust* (1999), concerning an obstetrics case.[30] Here, Lord Woolf took the test for disclosure in relation to consent to treatment and reframed it with a *Bolitho*-type approach. He suggested that,

> if there is a significant risk which would affect the judgement of a reasonable patient then in the normal course it is the responsibility of a doctor to inform the patient of that significant risk, if the information is needed so that the patient can determine for him or herself as to what course she should adopt.[31]

It should be noted, however, that while the test may have been recast, the consequences of the decision remained the same: the litigant in this case lost. It was held that failure to disclose the 0.1–0.2 per cent risk of stillbirth did not amount to negligence. Moreover, the precise significance of this case remains under dispute. Some, such as Jones, have suggested that it can be seen as moving us towards an informed consent doctrine.[32] Brazier and Miola commented that *Pearce* signalled 'that announcements of the stillbirth of "informed consent" in Britain were premature'.[33] In contrast, others (such as MacLean) have been far more cautious and suggest that 'the courts would still rely on the experts to determine the significance of a particular risk'.[34]

The subsequent impact of *Bolitho* in the courtroom proved far less than some commentators initially thought. Yes, there were some cases in which there was clearly enhanced judicial scrutiny, but these were limited and overall judicial reaction was mixed.[35] Was this surprising? Perhaps not, for while the courts had some greater room for manoeuvre, there was still considerable deference to clinical judgement, and an unwillingness or an inhibition when it came to overriding expert evidence. Where the courts were happier to intervene was when there was clear evidence that clinicians had not followed requisite guidelines and protocols. The impact of *Bolitho* outside the courtroom is difficult to ascertain. As Harpwood comments, we simply do not know what the impact of the litigation might have been in influencing cases being settled by the parties pre-trial.[36]

The rise and rise of clinical guidelines

Yet while the judges remained circumspect when it came to curbing clinical discretion within the courtroom, outside developments were moving to do precisely that. Clinicians were increasingly faced by professional guidelines informing their conduct.[37] The proliferation of such guidance inevitably came as a challenge to those in practice and to clinicians' own decision-making autonomy. Guidelines might come from professional practice organisations, such as the myriad of royal medical colleges. These were met with degrees of criticism, but nonetheless they still amounted to regulation being rooted within the professional structures. Through the 1990s, however, guidelines and codes of practice were increasingly emanating from government and from governmental bodies. In two specific areas of clinical practice, statute mandated the production of codes of practice. In the first area of mental health, this arose from the Mental Health Act (1983), which required the production of a code of practice.[38] In the second, the Human Fertilisation and Embryology Authority – a statutory body created to regulate modern fertility treatments under the Human Fertilisation and Embryology Act (1990) – was required to produce a code of practice which provided guidance for clinicians, clinics and patients.[39] A change also arose through the greater use of specific guidelines concerning the legitimacy and safety of particular forms of treatment being promulgated through the National Institute for Clinical Excellence (NICE), a body established by the government in the late 1990s with the aim of reviewing the effectiveness and safety of treatments.

If it was the case that there was a specific set of guidelines for professionals, then in a negligence action this could be evidenced in the courtroom. Moreover, it could also ultimately constrain clinical judgement. As Brazier and Miola have also noted, 'The judge confronted by individual experts who disagree about good practice will in certain cases be able to refer to something approaching a "gold standard"'.[40] It could be argued that a responsible body of professional practice would follow such guidelines and thus that a practitioner would be negligent if they did not follow them.[41] Indeed, as Teff has commented, it could become a case of 'guidelines know best'.[42]

If a health professional has not followed established guidelines in a case in which it was alleged that harm had resulted, this could make it more difficult for them to effectively resist a negligence action.[43] Conversely, if such guidelines existed and the health professional had followed them, it was less likely that they would be held to be negligent. Guidelines could constrain professional autonomy while reducing the risk of liability. One possible consequence of an increase in malpractice litigation, which worried the clinicians, was that of the rise of 'defensive medicine'. However, as noted above, even though the UK courts appeared to accept that defensive medicine was an issue, as Michael Jones noted, there is little empirical evidence that clinical practice changed.[44]

The decade of the inquiry: public vindication of complaints?

While negligence litigation, despite the rhetoric, proved problematic in practice in relation to resolving complaints and reframing professional responsibility, the 1990s were marked by the sustained use of the inquiry as a means of holding the medical profession to account. The use of inquiries in relation to specific areas of health provision had occurred in the past, as discussed in the Introduction to this volume and in Mold's chapter.[45] Yet in the 1990s, major, public and high-profile inquiries established by government as a means of addressing perceived wrongs in healthcare provision marked a sea change in terms of leading to legal reform.[46] There are two particular inquiries which mark out the 1990s, although their reports were not published until 2000 and 2001. It was these reports in particular which marked out changing attitudes and perhaps a sea change in reduced deference to the medical profession, both as clinicians and as researchers. First, there was the Bristol Royal Infirmary Inquiry, triggered by reports of an abnormally high rate of paediatric cardiac deaths, which began in 2008 and finally reported in 2001.[47] There had been rumblings for some time that something was wrong at the cardiology department. The first article about the unit appeared in the satirical journal *Private Eye* in February 1992, but it took almost a decade for events to unravel and the inquiry's report to be published.[48] After a whistleblower emerged – Dr Stephen Bosin, a consultant anaesthetist, who raised concerns about the operation of the unit – the Bristol Children's Heart Action group was established to campaign for an inquiry and action. The inquiry chair appointed by the government was an interesting choice: Professor Ian Kennedy of King's College London. He was the editor, with his colleague Professor Andrew Grubb, of the *Medical Law Review*, the leading academic journal in the area, and he had established the Centre for Medicine Ethics and Law at King's College London. Kennedy was noted for his combativeness and his willingness to challenge clinical orthodoxy.[49] Kennedy's appointment as the inquiry chair was very far indeed from a 'safe' establishment choice. The conclusions and the ramifications of the report can be clearly foreshadowed in that initial appointment. Supporting Kennedy was another eminent academic lawyer, Mavis McClean. The inquiry was held in public, and the hearings themselves attracted a considerable degree of publicity and adverse media coverage for the medical profession.[50]

The recommendations of the Kennedy report, when they finally came in 2001, were extensive. It represented a damning critique of the 'club culture' of the medical profession. Care at Bristol was seen as fundamentally flawed. There had been 'too much power in too few hands'.[51] Moreover, the whole process was problematic, from patient referral through to intensive care. Surgeons were located in one hospital, while the paediatric cardiologists were in another, a few hundred metres away. Although a raft of recommendations was made, here the focus is upon those most closely related to complaining about medicine.

First, the report was highly critical of the manner in which standards were controlled within the NHS. It recommended the establishment of a new body, a Commission for Health Care Improvement. The Government accepted this recommendation and established the body, later named the Commission for Healthcare Audit and Inspection but generally known as the Healthcare Commission, which had the task of independently inspecting health services from the patient's perspective.[52] The Healthcare Commission was itself, in a neat twist of fate, chaired by the now Professor Sir Ian Kennedy. (The Health Care Commission was ultimately in the late 2000s replaced by the Care Quality Commission, an independent regulator which also replaced the Mental Health Act Commission and the Care Standards Commission – and has since its establishment been dogged by criticism.)[53]

Second, the Bristol inquiry report provided a major critique of the processes and procedures concerning consent to treatment. It advocated a more patient-centred approach. It emphasised the need for 'respect and honesty' in healthcare and for the relationship between healthcare professional and patient to be seen as one of partnership. [54] Consent was also to be seen as a process:

> Trust can be only sustained by openness. Secondly, openness means that information be given freely, honestly and regularly. Thirdly, it is of fundamental importance to be honest about the twin concerns of risk and uncertainty. Lastly, informing patients, and in the case of young children, their parents, must be regarded as a process and not as a one-off event.[55]

The report recommended that 'Patients must be given such information as enables them to participate in their care.'[56] It suggested processes for improving the conveyance of information, such as ensuring that information is evidence-based, and that, importantly, 'information should be tailored to the needs, circumstances and wishes of the individual'.[57] It suggested radical new approaches, such as taping the doctor–patient consultation concerning treatment, so that the patient could take this home with them to reflect upon in their own time.[58]

The Kennedy report saw dangers in the existing culture of blame for health mistakes. It also recommended a review of the system of clinical negligence itself. The system then in place was seen as fundamentally flawed. This was followed by a report by the Chief Medical Officer in 2003, which also proposed the introduction of a duty of candour alongside exemptions from disciplinary actions when reporting incidents concerned with patient safety.[59] There needed to be clarity in standards, the Kennedy report argued, and the standards issued by the National Institute for Clinical Excellence needed to be directly enforceable. There needed to be an environment in which errors could be reported safely and acted upon. There should be a national database of sentinel events operated by a government body, the National Patient Safety Agency. Moreover, concerns were voiced as to the problems of bringing litigation, and it was recommended that the current system should be abolished.

> Ultimately, we take the view that it will not be possible to achieve an environment of full, open reporting within the NHS when, outside it, there exists a litigation system the incentives of which press in the opposite direction. We believe that the way forward lies in the abolition of clinical negligence litigation.[60]

The report advised that a further government review of clinical negligence systems should be undertaken. Systems and structures should be designed for safety; this should be led by the Patient Safety Agency. Clinical care standards were to be centrally established and made public to avoid the confusion that had resulted in the past from a range of disparate standards and guidelines produced by different bodies. There needed also, the report said, to be greater involvement of the public via patient forums and patient councils, bodies discussed further in Alex Mold's chapter in this volume. Moreover, services should be designed in the light of the specific needs of children and in consultation with their parents.

Besides arguing for overarching regulation through a Council for the Regulation of Health Care Professions, Kennedy was particularly critical of the regulatory systems which existed for healthcare professionals, which needed reform and the implementation of post-validation training and updating of skills. This approach was subsequently adopted by the medical professional regulatory body the General Medical Council (GMC). The authors of the report further recommended that managers, too, should be subject to similar responsibilities as health professionals and to a regulatory code. In this respect, the lessons of Kennedy took longer to learn. While there had been criticism for many years as to how the system of self-regulation for health professionals actually operated, change came slowly.[61] It was not until a much later inquiry report – the Shipman Inquiry report into GP Dr Harold Shipman, who murdered numerous patients in Cheshire – that radical change to the GMC was finally introduced.[62] The Bristol Report also recommended that patients should be able to obtain information on the performance of consultants and of units within hospitals, something which was subsequently taken up by government with the production of comparative evaluations ('league tables') of surgeons. Ultimately, of course, an inquiry can make recommendations, but it does not have 'teeth': the ability to actually impose sanctions. Indeed, over a decade later, the Francis Report into the events at Mid Staffordshire NHS Trust sadly illustrated that some of the lessons of Kennedy had not been learnt.[63] Events at that hospital led to the unnecessary death of hundreds of patients, many elderly. Some of the Francis recommendations, including those of a duty of candour in relation to NHS staff, echo those of Kennedy. It is interesting to note that Robert Francis QC was one of the lawyers at the Bristol inquiry. The emphasis here, too, was on systems failure. However, as Oliver Quick noted, the former president of the GMC, Sir Donald Irvine, rightly cautioned against undue emphasis on the failure of the system, which may only serve to mask the failings of individuals.[64] This raises the question of whether complaining about medicine is fundamentally concerned with complaints about the professional or the system of provision and, indeed, whether it is possible to effectively disentangle these elements.

The Redfern inquiry

Patient complaints triggered the second major malpractice inquiry of the 1990s, the Redfern inquiry into the retention of organs. The history of this inquiry is itself intertwined with that of Bristol. In May 1996, Helen Rickard sat down to watch a Channel 4 programme from the UK documentary series *Dispatches*, which concerned the events at Bristol Royal Infirmary, where her daughter had died after receiving treatment.[65] After watching the programme, which was a damning critique of events at Bristol, she contacted the hospital and requested her daughter's medical records. It was only on receiving those records that she discovered that her daughter's body had not been buried intact, and that the hospital had retained her organs. This case was then reported to the Bristol Children's Heart Action Group, which raised questions at the Bristol inquiry into the retention of organs. Memorably, in responding to questions at that inquiry, Professor Robert Alderson, a leading authority in paediatric medicine, stated that the 'biggest and best' collection of children's hearts was to be found at Alder Hey in Liverpool.[66] This declaration opened the floodgates. Other parents began to ask questions, and gradually the nature and extent of the retention of human material emerged. Unlike Bristol, this inquiry was triggered not by the actions of a whistleblower but by patients' relatives. The Government Health Secretary, Alan Milburn, commissioned a senior lawyer, Michael Redfern QC, to chair the inquiry into the events at Alder Hey. Nor was this the only investigation into retention concerning human material in the 1990s. It was preceded by a report into organ retention at Bristol by the Bristol inquiry team. As this report illustrated, the issue of organ retention, far from being a 'Liverpool problem', proved in fact to be a national scandal.

The practice of retaining organs and tissue without having obtained consent – from the individual concerned in the case of the living, or from relatives in the case of the dead or concerning adults lacking mental capacity – had been universal until a few years before the Bristol inquiry. Clinical practice had already started to evolve, and the Royal College of Pathologists had themselves begun to produce guidance on the issue.[67] Some of the retentions were, as uncovered subsequently, undoubtedly due to gross ignorance, or to unthinking assumptions of the legitimacy of the use of 'spare' material for treatment and for research purposes. This is still somewhat surprising, particularly given international sensitivities to ethical research practices after the Nuremberg trials of the 1940s and the production of internal guidelines of research by the World Health Organisation in the form of the Declaration of Helsinki (first adopted in 1964); it was not until the 1990s that there was a real attempt at the national level to 'sweep the stables clean'.

The legacy of Alder Hey

These inquiry reports were followed by a census undertaken in 2001 by the Chief Medical Officer, Professor Liam Donaldson, which revealed the full extent of the retention of human material.[68] Donaldson found that there were over 105,000 body parts, stillbirths and fetuses stored in English hospitals and medical schools.

Of these, the census revealed that around 88 per cent of the collections were concentrated in 25 NHS Trusts and medical schools. Nearly half comprised brains, while one-sixth were eyes.[69] In Alder Hey, 2,128 hearts were stored at the Institute of Child Health; 1,564 stillbirths or fetuses were kept which had been collected before 1973, with a further 445 fetuses at a separate collection in Liverpool.[70] In addition, there were 147 brains. Moreover, as Redfern QC commented, 'perhaps the most disturbing specimen [was] the head of an 11-year-old boy'.[71] The legacies of these inquiries were, first, the establishment of the Retained Organs Commission, which placed a moratorium upon the handing back of organs until the full scale of the retention had been realised; second, the uncovering of new incidents and new inquiries in Northern Ireland,[72] Scotland,[73] Manchester,[74] and by Her Majesty's Inspector of Anatomy, the latter revealing the extensive non-consensual retention of brains;[75] and third, after a further three years, the passing of the Human Tissue Act in 2004.[76]

The ultimate legacy was, perhaps, the reinforcing of the idea that public inquiries were the solution to malpractice and misdeeds in medicine.[77] Handing the issue over to a high-profile, independent person can be seen as enabling detachment and transparency, much more than any in-house or governmental investigation could have achieved. However, inquiries can also be regarded as serving a very different purpose. Such inquiries can be seen as a means for the government of the day to detach itself from the specific incident in question, it becoming characterised as a matter of 'localised' concern, albeit with national implications. The government also have the ability to determine the terms of reference of the inquiry and, indeed, to circumscribe its operation. This is, of course, something which is particularly controversial in relation to healthcare decision making. Until the recent NHS reforms contained in the Health and Social Care Act (2012), the Secretary of State for Health under the National Health Service Act (2006) – an act consolidating previous legislation – had various obligations under the law in relation to the establishment and operation of the NHS.[78] While, at a day-to-day level, many of these functions were delegated, nonetheless the overriding responsibility for its operation lay at the very heart of government. Such events are seen as things from which lessons can be learnt. It is interesting that no government minister fell as a consequence of any of these high-profile inquiries into the health service in England and Wales.

Learning the lessons of the 1990s

Despite the media rhetoric about ambulance-chasing lawyers, in practice the 1990s did not lead to a radical change in clinical negligence litigation.[79] Ultimately, the professional practice test remained. Greater scrutiny was possible, but the difficulty of ultimately proving causation, even if there was a more fluid approach to the standard of care, meant that the number of successful claims remained low. Moreover, and as Price has also argued in his chapter in this volume, behind the rhetoric lie other realities of litigation. It is costly, time-consuming and frequently emotionally draining. Litigation requires stamina, drive and confidence; moreover, while it is going on, the litigant cannot move on from the adverse event and indeed is constantly reminded about it. As the NHS Litigation Authority highlighted in the mid-2000s, some 60–70 per cent of claims are not taken forward after an initial contract with a lawyer, and of those taken forward some 30 per cent are abandoned by the person pursuing them.[80] Even where cases are taken forward, the vast majority are settled, usually in favour of the NHS, and only a tiny fraction proceed to trial.[81]

Negligence litigation concerning informed consent is one area which has, at least in procedural terms, moved on since the decisions in *Sidaway*, *Pearce* and the context of Bristol. Not only has there been subsequent guidance in relation to informed consent, judicial statements have also framed information disclosure in terms of autonomy and dignity. Indeed, in *Chester* v. *Afshar* Lord Steyn went further and stated that

> In modern law medical paternalism no longer rules and a patient has a prima facie right to be informed by a surgeon of a small, but well established, risk of serious injury as a result of surgery.[82]

On the face of this, as Devaney commented, 'Autonomy Rules OK!'[83] Yet in the 2000s, Miola countered 'Autonomy Rued OK' when subsequent litigation illustrated that respect for autonomy and patient rights in consent to treatment cases clearly had its limits.[84] In practice, however, the actual process of bringing any negligence action, whether in relation to informed consent or any other form of harm, remains challenging due to the need to *prove* that negligence caused the harm in question. Causation can be particularly problematic in health negligence litigation cases, given that there may be myriad factors which contributed to the resultant harm.[85] Even though the courts are prepared to recognise this – and at times take a more generous approach in relation to consent to treatment – it remains challenging to prove that the action which fell below the standard of professional practice caused the harm suffered. While negligence is of course problematic in civil law, the criminal law presents even more of a problem in bringing successful actions, as Jones and Shanks' chapter suggests. This challenge is evident despite the movement towards enhanced judicial scrutiny of patients' complaints.

Perhaps, then, it was the inquiries which provided the real means of complaining about medicine in the sense of voicing outrage and allowing voices to be heard. The impact of the inquiries was not simply that of multiple cases being heard simultaneously in public, a consequence of collective action with the ability to address the polycentric nature of such decisions. The inquiries – as was the case in many of the instances of complaining about medicine discussed in this collection – were conducted under the heat of huge publicity and with rising professional stakes. They needed to succeed. Did they work? To some extent, it was not only the findings of the inquiries but also their very existence which provided a catalyst for change, at times in unexpected ways. Take the GMC, which, while the Bristol inquiry was underway, decided to publish a code of practice on consent to treatment that placed a far higher duty on a clinician, one much more stringent than anything recommended by the courts.[86] Lord Scarman, in his dissenting judgement in *Sidaway*, talked of what the prudent patient wanted to know; what the GMC was doing here was profoundly more radical – it was what this very patient in front of the doctor would want to know at that time.

What is striking when we reflect upon the findings of those 1990s inquiries is what succeeded and what did not, and, ultimately, what health service failures subsequently emerged. The Alder Hey Inquiry Report did lead to legislation in the 2000s in the form of the Human Tissue Act 2004. The structure of the regulation of human material was radically overhauled and a series of detailed codes of practice were put in place.[87] This is itself was not uncontroversial, leading to major debates in the scientific community and intense lobbying which limited the scope of the legislation in parts. Kennedy's inquiry recommended that there needed to be a reconsideration of the law concerning medical negligence. The government took forward this recommendation, which led to yet a further report by the Chief Medical Officer setting out the alternatives in relation to healthcare negligence redress.[88]

While this report ultimately led to legislation in the form of a new dispute-resolution process for low-level medical complaints under the NHS Redress Act (2006), this has still not been implemented.[89] It was the inquiry established in 2000 following the conviction of the mass murderer Dr Harold Shipman that led to really radical change in relation to the professional regulation of the medical profession.[90] In the late 2000s and early 2010s, the uncovering of high levels of patient deaths and appalling standards of medical care at Mid Staffordshire Hospital led to new inquiries and, eventually, to recommendations for the closure of the hospital itself. Kennedy's words damning the 'club culture' and arrogance of the medical profession can be set alongside another inquiry report which was damning of managers, nurses and regulators. What is striking when these two reports are put alongside each other is what has been lost in the interim. Why is it in the space of less than a decade that another morass of appalling professional practice, unsafe care and bad treatment should emerge in this way? One further tragic twist in the saga was revealed in February 2014 when Chief Medical Officer Sir Bruce Keogh announced yet another inquiry into Bristol Royal Infirmary – this time into six recent deaths of children at that hospital.[91] Perhaps this grim series of events alone should let us reflect that, in healthcare practice, as well as other aspects of the delivery of public service, it is critical that not only professionals but managers and policy-makers alike learn the lessons of history and learn from those complaining about medicine before it is too late.

Notes

1 From 1989 to 1998 the Medical Protection Society reported that claims brought against general practitioners had increased thirteen-fold; C. Dyer, *British Medical Journal*, 318 (1999), p. 820. For further discussions on the 'malpractice crisis', see C. Ham, R. Dingwall, P. Fenn and D. Harris, *Medical Negligence, Compensation and Accountability* (London, 1988); P. Hoyte, 'Unsound Practice: The Epidemiology of Medical Negligence', *Medical Law Review*, 3 (1995), pp. 53–73.
2 See T. Baker, *The Medical Malpractice Myth* (Chicago, 2005); V. Harpwood, *Medicine, Malpractice and Misapprehensions* (Abingdon, 2007), pp. 154–159.
3 Harpwood, *Medicine, Malpractice and Misapprehensions*, p. 23.
4 See discussion below.
5 'The Report of the Public Inquiry into Children's Heart Surgery at the Bristol Royal Infirmary 1984–1995: Learning from Bristol' (Cmnd. 5207 (I) 2001); *Report of the Inquiry into the Royal Liverpool Children's Hospital* [Alder Hey] (London, 2001).
6 See generally M. Jones, *Medical Negligence*, fourth edition (London, 2008).
7 *Barnett v Chelsea & Kensington Hospital Management Committee* [1969] 1 QB 428.
8 *Wilsher v Essex Area Health Authority* [1988] 3 AC 1074.
9 [1957] 2 All ER 118.
10 [1957] 2 All ER 118.
11 *De Freitas v O'Brien* (1995).
12 See *Clarke v Adams* (1950) 94 Sol J 599; *Hucks v Cole* (1960) [1994] 4 Med LR 393.
13 [1985] 1 All ER 635.
14 [1985] 1 All ER 635 at p. 643.
15 See, for example, *Canterbury v Spence* 464 F 2d 772 (DC Cir 1972).
16 [1985] 1 All ER 635.
17 I. Kennedy 'The Patient on the Clapham Omnibus', *Treat Me Right: Essays in Medical Law and Ethics* (Oxford, 1988), pp. 175–212.
18 [1993] 4 Med LR 151.
19 [1988] 1 QB 481.
20 [1994] 5 Med LR 334.
21 See further R. Mulheron, 'Trumping Bolam: A Critical Legal Analysis of Bolitho's Gloss', *Cambridge Law Journal*, 69 (2010), pp. 609–631.
22 [1997] 4 All ER, 771.
23 [1997] 4 All ER 771 at p. 779.
24 M. R. Brazier and J. Miola, 'Bye-bye Bolam: A Medical Revolution?', *Medical Law Review*, 8 (2000), pp. 85–144.
25 Lord Woolf, 'Are the Courts Excessively Deferential to the Medical Profession?' *Medical Law Review*, 9 (2001), pp. 1–16.
26 Woolf, 'Are the Courts Excessively Deferential?'.
27 Ibid., p. 4.
28 H. Teff, 'The Standard of Care in Medical Negligence – Moving on from *Bolam*?' *Oxford Journal of Legal Studies*, 18 (1998), pp. 473–484.
29 Brazier and Miola, 'Bye-bye Bolam'.

30 [1999] PIQR 53.
31 [1999] PIQR 53.
32 M. Jones, 'Informed Consent and Other Fairy Stories', *Medical Law Review*, 7 (2), 1999, pp. 103–134.
33 Brazier and Miola, 'Bye-bye Bolam', p. 119.
34 A. McLean, *Autonomy, Informed Consent and Medical Law* (Cambridge, 2009), p. 176.
35 See Mulheron, 'Trumping Bolam'.
36 See Harpwood, *Medicine, Malpractice and Misapprehensions.*
37 B. Hurwitz, *Clinical Guidelines and the Law: Negligence, Disclosure, Judgement* (Oxford,1998).
38 Mental Health Act 1983, 31 and 32 Eliz. II c.20, s.118.
39 *Human Fertilisation and Embryology Authority Code of Practice*, 8th edn (London, 2012).
40 Brazier and Miola, 'Bye-bye Bolam'.
41 A. Samanta, N. M. Mello, C. Foster, J. Tingle and J. Samanta, 'The Role of Clinical Guidelines in Medical Negligence Litigation: A Shift from the *Bolam* standard', *Medical Law Review*, 14 (3), 2006, pp. 321–366.
42 See also H. Teff, 'Clinical Guidelines, Negligence and Medical Practice', in M. Freeman and A. Lewis (eds), *Current Legal Issues: Law and Medicine* (Oxford, 2000), pp. 67–80, p. 79.
43 See, for example, *Richards* v. *Swansea NHS Trust* [2007] EWHC 487(QB).
44 See M. Jones, 'Breach of Duty', in I. Kennedy and A. Grubb (eds), *Principles of Medical Law*, second edition (Oxford, 2004), p. 369.
45 See further K. Walsh, *Inquiries: Learning from Failure in the NHS* (London, 2002).
46 Though of course inquiries themselves had been utilised in other contexts before in many instances, such as in the context of mental healthcare (see generally Walsh Inquiries).
47 'The Report of the Public Inquiry into Children's Heart Surgery at the Bristol Royal Infirmary 1984–1995: Learning from Bristol' (Cmnd. 5207 (I) 2001).
48 See Harpwood, *Medicine, Malpractice and Misapprehensions*, p. 113.
49 See, for example, Kennedy's Reith Lectures and his subsequent book, *Treat Me Right* (Oxford, 1981).
50 See 'Chaos Reigned at Bristol Heart Centre', *Guardian* (17 March 1999), www.theguardian.com/uk/1999/mar/17/sarahboseley, accessed 10 May 2014.
51 See 'The Report of the Public Inquiry into Children's Heart Surgery at the Bristol Royal Infirmary 1984–1995'.
52 Health and Social Care (Community Health and Standards) Act 2003; and see discussion by C. Newdick, 'The Organisation of the NHS' in A. Grubb and J. Laing (eds), *Principles of Medical Law*, second edition (Oxford, 2004), paras 1.136–1.139.
53 Section 1 of the Health and Social Care Act, 2008.
54 'The Report of the Public Inquiry into Children's Heart Surgery at the Bristol Royal Infirmary 1984–1995'.
55 Ibid.
56 Ibid.
57 Ibid.
58 Ibid.
59 Chief Medical Officer, *Making Amends* (London, 2003), recommendation 12.
60 'The Report of the Public Inquiry into Children's Heart Surgery at the Bristol Royal Infirmary 1984–1995'.
61 See, e.g. M. Stacey, *Regulating British Medicine: The General Medical Council* (Chichester, 1992).

62 The Fifth Shipman Inquiry Report, 'Safeguarding Patients: Lessons from the Past, Proposals for the Future', 9 December 2004, Cm 6394.
63 Mid Staffordshire NHS Foundation Trust: Public Enquiry HC 898–1 (2013).
64 O. Quick, 'Outing Medical Errors: Questions of Trust and Responsibility', *Medical Law Review*, 13 (2000), pp. 22–43, pp. 41–42.
65 See discussion in Bristol Inquiry Interim Report 'Removal and Retention of Human Material' (2000) and see, generally, K. Liddell and A. Hall, 'Beyond Bristol and Alder Hey: The Future Regulation of Human Tissue', *Medical Law Review*, 13 (2005), pp. 170–223.
66 See *Report of the Inquiry into the Royal Liverpool Children's Hospital* [Alder Hey].
67 See, generally, D. Price, *Human Tissue in Transplantation and Research* (Cambridge, 2009).
68 *The Investigation into Retained Organs, Chief Medical Officer's Report on Organ Retention* (London, 2001).
69 Ibid.
70 Ibid.
71 Ibid, paragraph 20.5.
72 *Report of the Human Organ Inquiry* (2002), www.dhsspsni.gov.uk/index/hss/hoi-home/hoi-report.htm, accessed 13 May 2014. Organ retention has also provoked controversy in other jurisdictions; see, for example, G. D. Jones, *Speaking for the Dead* (Aldershot, 2000), for the New Zealand position.
73 Scottish Executive, *Final Report of the Independent Review on the Retention of Organs at Post Mortem* (Edinburgh, 2002).
74 Retained Organs Commission Organ, *Retention at Central Manchester and Manchester Children's University Hospitals Trust* (July 2002), www.nhs.uk/retainedorgans/index.htm, accessed 10 May 2014.
75 *The Investigation of the Events that Followed the Death of Cyril Mark Issacs*, TSO (2003).
76 S. Pinnock, 'Human Tissue Bill could Jeopardise Research: Scientists Warn', *British Medical Journal*, 328 (2004), 1034; and see K. Liddell and A. Hall, 'The Future Regulation of Human Tissue', *Medical Law Review*, 13 (2005), pp. 170–223, pp. 172–173.
77 There is a long history of use of public inquiries as a means of scrutiny; see, for example, R. E. Wraith and P. G. Lamb, *Public Inquiries* (London, 1971).
78 See NHS Act 1976, s.1 and s.3.
79 A. Maclean, 'Beyond *Bolam* and *Bolitho*', *Medical Law International*, 5 (2002), pp. 205–230.
80 See further *Department of Health Full Regulatory Assessment of the NHS Redress Act* (London, 2006).
81 *Department of Health Full Regulatory Assessment.*
82 *Chester v Afshar*, [2004] UKHL 41, para. 16.
83 S. Devaney, 'Autonomy Rules OK!', *Medical Law Review*, 13 (2005), pp. 103–115.
84 J. Miola, 'Autonomy Rued OK', *Medical Law Review*, 14 (2006), 108–114.
85 For a famous illustration of the problems of bringing an action in medical negligence where there may be multiple causes, see *Wilsher v Essex AHA* [1988] 1 AC 1074.
86 General Medical Council, *Seeking Patients' Consent* (London, 2008).
87 See further Human Tissue Authority Codes of Practice 2009–2013, www.hta.gov.uk/legislationpoliciesandcodesofpractice/codesofpractice.cfm, accessed 13 May 2014.
88 *Making Amends: A Consultation Paper Setting Out the Proposals for Reforming the Approach to Clinical Negligence in the NHS* (London, 2003).

89 See further A. M. Farell and S. Devaney, 'Making Amends or Making Things Worse?', *Legal Studies*, 27 (2007), pp. 630–648.
90 The fifth Shipman Inquiry Report: 'Safeguarding Patients: Lessons from the Past; Proposals for the Future', 9 December 2004, Cm 6394.
91 'Inquiry into Bristol Children's Hospital After Deaths', *The Times* (16 February 2014).

Afterword

Going public: the act of complaining

John Clarke

> The culture of delay and denial over NHS complaints in England must come to an end.
>
> (*Clwyd-Hart Review*, October 2013)

Complaints are, once again, at the centre of debates about, and proposals for, the reform of the NHS. As the editors demonstrated in the Introduction to this volume, complaints are a continuous thread woven into the organisations – and re-organisations – of medicine. Nevertheless, we should be wary of assuming that this sense of continuity means that nothing has changed, that complaints are ineffective or that complaints are all just the same. Indeed, the chapters that stand between the Introduction and this Afterword demonstrate the opposite. They point to the variety of settings, practices and forms of complaint – and the diversity of complainants. They testify to the uneven, and sometimes unexpected, impact of complaints. They also reveal the changing contexts and practices of doing medicine that have become the focus of complaints, to which we must add the contemporary concern with medical 'cultures', including the 'culture of delay and denial' named in the quote above. In this brief Afterword, I will draw out four themes from these chapters that fix on connections to questions of culture, power and authority that are my own recurrent concerns in the study of contemporary welfare, public services and their management. First, I am intrigued by the ways in which complaints suggest something profoundly ambivalent about people's relationships to the social institution of medicine. Second, I want to explore how complaining involves the negotiation of difficult boundaries between the public institutions of medicine and the realms of the private and the personal. Third, these studies of complaints raise important issues about the repertoire of resources, techniques and technologies that are in play in the practices of complaining. Finally, I want to pose some questions about the politics of complaint, centred on what seems a perverse paradox of people making modest demands that institutions cannot meet.

Complaints about medicine reveal individual and collective ambivalence about institutions that are ostensibly there to provide care and promote well-being: medicine itself; hospitals, asylums, and other institutional manifestations; and the doctors, nurses and administrators who people them. This ambivalence – in which need and fear are complexly entwined – is visible in the anxieties that other cultural forms and practices reveal. For example, I am struck by the less than positive view of doctors in popular culture: they haunt the pages of crime fiction in the distinctive combination of respectability and threat of being dangerous, whether as the elite and exploitative Harley Street specialist or the genteelly tweedy country doctor in 'Golden Age' stories by Agatha Christie and others. UK television dramas and sitcoms (from *Casualty* to *Getting On*) and their US equivalents (from *ER* to *House*) portray medical staff of all kinds – and medical managers – as flawed heroes and villains. In such cultural forms, there is a persistent ambivalence that unsettles assumptions of popular deference towards doctors, such that scepticism appears to coexist with deference in unpredictable combinations.

What goes on alongside the official world of managed encounters between people and medicine in which roles, positions and exchanges are densely scripted? My own experiences, and those of others, are full of sceptical reflections that recur below the level of public audibility, but in which the professional competence, personal qualities and social skills of particular doctors – and sometimes the entire profession – are called into question. In part, this scepticism reflects, and indeed reflects on, the ways in which forms of authority have been bundled together in medicine – the authority deriving from professional expertise, the authority serving from position in an organised institution (the hospital or the health system), and – in many places – the social authority or prestige claimed by, and granted to, medical professionals. I carry around with me a collection of phrases used by family and friends about medical encounters: 'What do they teach them in medical school?'; 'She just wanted to get me out of there'; 'He couldn't care less'; 'Who does he think he is?'; 'They talked about me as if I wasn't there'. Such phrases speak to a sense of disaffection in the daily experience of institutionalised medicine – focused on feelings of being alienated in medical encounters. So, too, do widely circulating tales of medical incompetence about wrong legs being amputated or incorrect drug doses, patients left lying on trolleys in hospital corridors, or, in the US, wrangles about insurance. Such sceptical views of medical authority may also take more public and collective forms, as Thompson's chapter on the South Wales Coalfield, for example, demonstrates.

For me, this points to a sort of hinterland of complaints in which anxieties, doubts and frustrations may both foreshadow and enable the act of complaining. I am not very sure how to map this landscape, but it might start with the unheard mumble, the muttered deprecation, or the under-the-breath, not quite audible, exhalation of frustration or despair. Then there are all those ways of thinking and speaking that are not exactly complaints: the gripes and grumbles, often ironically cross-referenced by the phrases 'can't complain' and 'mustn't grumble'.[1] This resembles Klein's visible 'iceberg' of complaint that marks the 'submerged' field of potential complaints (composed of grumbles and frictions): an image referred to several times in this volume.[2] I confess to preferring the metaphor of the hinterland to that of the iceberg, because it marks a field of diverse orientations and utterances (or 'mutterances'?). The iceberg seems to be composed of a similarity and a unity – only differentiated by degrees of visibility. Instead, gripes, grumbles, discontented muttering and head-shaking sighs of frustration or disappointment exist below and beyond the act of complaining in the formalised sense. They might, perhaps, be understood as subcultural practices, drawing on languages of grumbling that are widely used and imply the existence of sympathetic audiences ('Oh, I know').

Nevertheless, both metaphors – the iceberg and the hinterland – point to two important issues. First, in cultural terms, complaints do not come out of nowhere. They are underpinned by what we might call vocabularies of grievance – ways of talking about discomforts and disaffections that circulate widely, especially but not only about the institutions of medicine. They imply varieties of what E. P. Thompson once called 'moral economies': the collectively held expectations about relationships, conduct and obligation that animate senses of justice and injustice (in this volume, see the chapter by King).[3] The second consequence of thinking about such cultural hinterlands is that they point to the act of complaining as a moment of transition or translation into a formalised world of public action, in which different vocabularies may be required in order to be heard or recognised. What causes that transition (the act of complaining) and what enables it are critical issues that are illuminated by several of the chapters contained here, not least the questions of the languages or vocabularies through which one might complain, as in the chapters by Léon-Sanz and Mold. But for me, making these hinterlands visible is an important product of the study of complaints, with the process of transition or translation to the act of complaining involving a sort of boundary crossing.

Complaining involves going public, moving from the informal realm of gripes and grumbles into the formal realm of processes and procedures and their associated modes, media and languages of complaint. I will have something more to say about them, but first I want to concentrate on boundaries and boundary crossing. The act of complaining is a decisive step: it makes a grievance public. This is a central theme of the volume, established in the Introduction and richly articulated in many of the chapters, including those by Cook, Scull and Wall. So the act of complaining marks a transition from the private, informal or subcultural worlds in which the grievance is felt and may be first articulated to families, friends or fellow sufferers. In such settings, grievances (or gripes or grumbles) are likely to be articulated conversationally and expressively, attempting to summon an audience that is sympathetic or possibly seeking to move them to action on one's behalf. But the mode is typically informal and conversational; the medium is likely to be speech, although occasionally written in letter form – though the new social media blur the boundaries between personal and public in significant way.[4] The language is also likely to be informal and affect-laden (evoking the *sense* of grievance and the physical or emotional misery associated with it). The transition to making a felt grievance public is often equated with the act of complaining, but it is important to remember that 'voice' (complaining) might co-exist with 'exit' in its different forms.[5] A recent study by Dowding and John of voice and exit in public services has traced different types of exit: 'internal exit' (from one provider to another in the public sector), 'private exit' (to a private sector provider) and 'geographical exit' (moving elsewhere for better services).[6] To these we might add 'service exit', where people absent themselves from the field as a whole, giving up on the possibility of a medical solution to their needs.

As Léon-Sanz's chapter indicates, the transition from the spoken to the written form makes going public with a complaint a very particular sort of transition. The written submission (by letter or by completing a form) changes the medium (from talk to text, in the process creating a permanent public record); it changes the mode to a more formal, distanced address to an authority – and in the process there are complicated calculations to be made about the balance of facticity and affect. What is the correct repertoire through which grievance and suffering is to be conveyed? Such transitions and translations are, of course, likely to be context-specific, as are the boundaries between the public and the domains of the personal or private. The chapters contained here point to a rich variety of forms and languages for complaining – from Wall's and Newsom Kerr's explorations of the types of vocabularies available to complainants, to Cook and to Reinarz and Wynter on different types of public mediation (and the shifting languages of critique and scandal). Medicine operates in a complex way on these boundaries – and might even be said to be one of the fields of institutional practices that helps to constitute them. Medicine largely functions as a public institution (whether or not it is a publicly funded and provided service) and acts on the person (in physical and psychological ways). It enters the private, domestic worlds of families and households, with a variety of public authorisations that range from health visitors scrutinising child development and parental performance to the forced removal of children at risk, or of adults who are deemed to represent a danger to themselves or others (see, for example, Scull's chapter). It also summons – more or less forcibly – individuals to submit themselves to the publicly backed authority of the medical professions. As Illich pointed out, the authoritative reach of medicine is extensive and extending as different experiences and conditions become medicalised, even if, for much of the time, people submit themselves willingly to its judgements and interventions. But such submission is always – as the chapters collected here demonstrate – contingent rather than absolute.

But the boundary between the public and the personal or private is more blurred and shifting than the basic distinction would imply. Conventionally, medical practitioners take considerable steps to guarantee the 'privacy' of the person, or at least, they perform the privacy of the patient in public settings (the ritual of drawing curtains around the hospital bed). The institutional practices and interventions of medicine are often transgressive of the public–private boundary – whether it involves putting things into the body, collecting personal data, or probing the 'invisible wounds' of psychological trauma.[7] Indeed, much of the codification of professional practice, standards and ethics is directed to managing the problematic quality of these transgressive practices. Many of the chapters in this collection point to the amount of effort that the professions and institutions expend on establishing the notion of consent – and the maintenance of legitimacy in the face of dissent. Of course, in Western societies, the trangressive possibilities of medicine have most often surfaced around questions of sexual intrusion, invasion and exploitation; but their range of 'dangerous' possibilities extends much wider – from shifting and contested understandings of what behaviour is deemed 'inappropriate' to the threat of murderous interventions, as addressed by McHale and by Jones and Shanks. These fears reflect in part the ways in which medicine works on the person, but also the perverse effect of conducting a public purpose (medical intervention) in relatively private or enclosed (unsurveilled) spaces.

My point here is that forms of publicness and the personal are both entangled and blurred in the organisation and practice of medicine, and this forces those who initiate an act of complaining to negotiate a blurred and problematic boundary. To what sort of 'public authority' is the complaint addressed? How is the personal experience of the complainant to be made knowable and recognisable to this authority? How is the experience to be moved beyond 'mere anecdote' to become an objectified event? Finally, there is the question that haunts appeal to public authorities: how independent is this authority; does this authority collude with the object(s) of the complaint (an issue that has unusual power so soon after the Care Quality Commission has been accused of covering up knowledge of health service failings in Britain)? The chapters in the book by Price and Ingram offer rich explorations of the problem of who judges complaints – and how.

Going public is a difficult and risky step, and its accomplishment requires a set of capacities and resources. There are important issues about how this move is made. They concern the triggers that make people shift register from private to public; the routes to complaining; and the cultural repertoires through which complaints can come to voice. Let me take the second of these points first: in what *vocabularies* can complaining be effectively communicated? There is a long-running sociological interest in how people use particular 'vocabularies of account' and varieties of 'justification' that might be productive here.[8] If people have a grievance, how do they learn and use the 'proper' language through which to frame and lodge their complaint? Such languages are – we might conclude from the chapters by King, Wall and Léon-Sanz – historically and socially specific, but are probably not clear-cut in any particular moment because of what has to be negotiated in the act of complaining. The personal suffering, the experience of becoming disaffected, the identification of institutional or professional failures, and the languages of formalised demands for attention (and/or justice) have to be articulated into a clear, compelling and persuasive (yet not too emotional) message. In particular, I am intrigued by the problem of how languages of emotion and affect act in these settings. What is the right balance of emotional/experiential and quasi-judicial style? What cultural–political repertoires can be drawn upon to make the case compelling? During the workshop from which this book flows, we discussed a range of such resources – from the models provided by religious parables to the imagery of rights and entitlements, referencing (more or less consciously and explicitly) the foundational French Declaration of the Rights of Man and of the Citizen.

The issue of different routes to complaining is identified in Léon-Sanz's discussion of the change from an oral to a written process of complaining. In the contemporary world of British public (and indeed private) service provision, there has been a proliferation of possible routes to complaining. For example, my own local hospital in Milton Keynes has a 'Patient Experience Team' that acts as a point of connection for the expression of complaints, compliments and concerns (a pleasant alliteration). It solicits comments from patients (and other users) as part of creating what managerial and organisational development experts refer to as a 'customer-centred culture'. This contemporary organisational enthusiasm for complaints is an interesting puzzle, given that it now appears to be an intrinsic feature of organisational design (as outlined in the Introduction to this volume), rather than merely a bolted-on mechanism. Complaints then become an element of the performance management of the organisation, with systematic reporting on the numbers of complaints and their outcomes. So, in Milton Keynes Hospital Trust, complaints are part of the business of the Quality Committee which also provides the Board with assurance about the actions taken by the Trust in response to serious incidents and complaints, including individual issues and analysis of trends and learning. The Board also receives a monthly report on the number of serious incidents and complaints through the regular 'Monthly Board dashboard'.[9]

The proliferation of complaining possibilities arises at the intersection of a number of different changes, including the rise of the 'customer satisfaction survey' as a device to be applied to almost all encounters and transactions in the effort to create the imagined 'self-regulating organisation' or, at least, to create the impression of giving attention to the 'customer experience'. Notably, new technologies have enabled organisations to provide (relatively) accessible routes to address the organisation with complaints and the capacity to store, analyse and respond to comments and complaints. They also enable new practices of complaining and digital activism. Such technologies emerged alongside the 'decline of deference' among service users in the emergence of what Giddens called 'reflexive modernity':

> The development of social reflexivity is the key influence on a diversity of changes that otherwise seem to have little in common. Thus the emergence of 'post-Fordism' in industrial enterprises is usually analysed in terms of technological change – particularly the influence of information technology. But the underlying reason for the growth of 'flexible production' and 'bottom-up decision-making' is that a universe of high reflexivity leads to greater autonomy of action, which the enterprise must recognise and draw on.
>
> The same applies to bureaucracy and to the sphere of politics. Bureaucratic authority, as Max Weber made clear, used to be a condition for organizational effectiveness. In a more reflexively ordered society, operating in the context of manufactured uncertainty, this is no longer the case. The old bureaucratic systems start to disappear, the dinosaurs of the post-traditional age. In the domain of politics, states can no longer so readily treat their citizens as 'subjects'.[10]

I am not wholly convinced by this narrative of modernisation – not least because the chapters collected here (notably those by King, Price and Scull) suggest that deference to forms of social authority was always more conditional and contingent than this story implies. Indeed, it might be that the supposed deference of the past would be better understood as calculated compliance, or even performed deference. Nevertheless, the narrative of modernisation has had substantial popular and political impact in the UK, not least in New Labour's enthusiasm for imagining the users of public services as consumers (an enthusiasm both predating the 1990s and sustained by the Coalition government of the early 2010s, and discussed in some detail by Mold in this volume). For me, this was perfectly expressed in a distinction made by Harry Cayton (at the time, 2003, Director for Patients and the Public at the Department of Health):

> So often in state provision of services universal provision meant the equity of the mediocre. That might have been acceptable to those lying down patients of the past but it will not do for the standing up consumers of the future. What we aspire to is the equity of excellence and choice is a necessary, though not sufficient, part of that transformation.[11]

This is not the place to pursue the question of this consumerist shift.[12] Rather, I want to concentrate on the problem of maintaining institutional control of the complaining process in the face of emerging social media. A governmental enthusiasm for performance data across all public services, and the associated exposure of providers to judgements on the 'patient experience', is intended to promise continuous service improvement (and to devolve responsibility for performance to the service and individual units within it). But this is also 'Trip Advisor World' in which user and consumer routes to voice are proliferating in non-official settings, enabling a demotic culture of comment and complaint.[13] Some public services attempt to combine the two modes: for example, Ofsted (the UK Office for Standards in Education) samples parental views in the process of school inspection and also has a 'Parent View' section of its website in which parents are invited to comment (through a 12-point survey) on individual schools. So, what pressures do official routes to complaining confront in the emerging field of new media; and how do those possibilities change which voices get to be heard?

Of course, the question of which voices get heard – and responded to – involves a much wider set of processes than the available forms of media. Such processes range from wider political arrangements (identifying which citizens, users and publics are entitled to come to voice through to more localised institutional, professional and organisational conditions and their capacity to filter, disallow and ignore certain complaints) and among certain types of complainant. Complaining is a complex relational practice – in at least two senses. As several of the chapters here show, complaints often address infractions of what is perceived to be the normal or proper relationship between professionals and patients (and between various professionals). Such normative understandings of how relationships should be ordered remain significant for public engagement with public services, including healthcare. Indeed, in our study of 'citizen-consumers', respondents often emphasised the importance of the 'relational' aspect of healthcare, contrasting it sharply with the 'consumer' experience, arguing that it was 'not like going shopping'; for example, as a user of health services put it in an interview:

> I am a patient and that's the word I understand . . . I don't feel I'm a customer of the National Health Service, or any health service for that matter. I feel I am a patient and I would like to develop my relationship with my healthcare professional. Because the way I view it is, being a diabetic, and any other problem I may have health wise, I'm the one whose got it and I have to lead it. The people who are around me are my team who are helping me get there. And a healthcare professional is part of my team. But I am his patient or her patient . . . I think customer is a very distant relationship. I don't think it is a relationship because I can walk into a shop over the road and be a customer, but not necessarily know the person who is serving me. But I think it's important that you know the person who is dealing with you as a patient.[14]

But complaining is relational in a second sense – the complaint enters a field of relationship after it is launched. It enters institutional settings, becomes an object to be managed and processed. It evokes other real and imagined relationships as it is assessed and evaluated. The judgement of the complaint carries relational implications – confirming or changing positions and identities. It may be this quality that locates the act of complaining in a series of actions that I have been thinking about under the idea of 'modest demands'. I am interested in these modest demands because they are often small in their apparent scope and significance. They are also often voiced modestly, if not apologetically. Yet they often prove difficult for institutions to manage effectively – indeed, the act of complaining already marks the failure to recognise or address a grievance at an earlier stage. I am not sure how many of these 'modest demands' there might be. For me, they include the recurrently expressed desire in our study of citizen-consumers to be recognised and treated 'as a person'. This has a long history (in medicine, but in other services, too) and is closely linked to desires for 'respect'. As my colleagues and I argued in our study of public service users, the desire to be treated with respect, or to be viewed as a 'partner' in the processes of healthcare, has strong affinities with Richard Sennett's subtle conception of 'respect' in welfare provision as the condition that would allow people to be treated as 'competent to participate in the terms of their own dependency'.[15]

This complicated usage (like that of being a partner) has found echoes in government discourse and policy (New Labour had a particular enthusiasm for both terms), but such echoes bent these ideas towards a more governmentalised and 'top down' insistence on respect and partnership as public obligations (rather than the obligations of public institutions). Both of these terms feed into the drive towards 'personalisation' in social and public policy, although that policy narrative is also shaped by other governmental and political forces.[16]

This model of 'modest demands' also came to my attention in a paper by Helen Graham that explored interactions between a museum and people who had contributed oral histories to the museum.[17] When the exhibits changed, the museum staff found themselves being contacted by these members of the public (with whom they had conducted formal legal copyright processes about the rights to use the recorded material) saying that it would be nice if the museum told them when the exhibit was changing and what was happening to their story. This is not even a complaint, just a polite request. But it carries with it a weight of political, cultural and affective resonances about the person's story and its movement between the personal and the public. Complaints have this quality, too. Although they may focus on specific mishaps and misfortunes, personal grievances and disasters, they address an imagined order of how relationships should be conducted – evoking modest norms of respect, dignity and recognition, the proper conduct of relationships and how the person should be dealt with in institutional/public spaces. As the chapters by King and Scull suggest, it is precisely in the relational spaces in which people encounter institutions such as medicine that desires and demands such as these emerge and form the basis of how people hope to be treated. They are profoundly effective in underpinning senses of grievance and injustice. I am intrigued by these modest demands because of the ways in which they jump scales, being highly individual and personal, yet evoking norms of social and organisational conduct that organisations find it difficult to engage with, much less deliver in practice.

Although they are modest, they call into question the implicit structuring of professional and institutional orders. In particular, they appear in the midst of relations of power and threaten to interrupt them. In that respect, it is not surprising that modest demands are rarely fulfilled: institutions (and occupations) have invested much in acting as they do – in being professional, in being effective and efficient, in being high-performance organisations, and so on. Modest demands may appear singular, personal and particular – but they evoke a world of relationships (real and imagined). These are the micro-politics of complaint, which need to be set alongside the broader political questions of the right to complain, to be heard and to be treated – with respect – as a person, as a citizen, as a patient. During the French Revolution, the Abbé Gregoire addressed the members of the Constituent Assembly on the right to complain. In the contemporary context, where all citizens are urged to be 'active', and those who are not are viewed with suspicion, his starting point is particularly interesting:

> I know in Paris citizens who are not active, who live in a sixth floor attic and are for all that able to give enlightenment and useful opinion (applause from the benches). Would you reject these citizens? . . . They will address themselves to you in order to claim their rights when they have been slighted, as the Declaration of Rights is after all common to all men. Will you refuse to hear their demands? Will you regard their sighs as acts of rebellion, their complaints as an attack against the laws? And whom would we prohibit non-active citizens from addressing? Administrators, municipal officials, those who should be the defenders of the people, the guardians and fathers of the poor. Is complaint not a natural right? And should a citizen not have, precisely because he is poor, the right of soliciting protection from the public authority? . . . If you deprive the poor citizen of the right to present petitions, you detach him from public affairs, you even make him their enemy. Unable to complain in legal ways, he will resort to tumultuous movements and replace reason by despair.[18]

Notes

1 On gripes, see J.-C. Kaufmann, *Gripes: The Little Quarrels of Couples* (Cambridge, 2009, translated by H. Morrison).
2 R. Klein, *Complaints Against Doctors: A Case Study in Professional Accountability* (London, 1973).
3 E. P. Thompson, 'The Moral Economy of the English Crowd in the Eighteenth Century', *Past and Present*, 50 (1971), pp. 76–136.
4 See, for example, R. Gambles, 'Going Public? Articulations of the Personal and the Public on Mumsnet.com', in N. Mahony, J. Newman and C. Barnett (eds), *Rethinking the Public: Innovations in Research, Theory and Politics* (Bristol, 2010), pp. 29–42.
5 A. Hirschman, *Exit, Voice and Loyalty: Responses to Decline in Firms, Organisations and States* (Cambridge, MA, 1970).
6 K. Dowding and P. John, *Exits, Voices and Social Investment: Citizens' Reactions to Public Services* (Cambridge, 2012).
7 See, for example, M. Allsopp, *Emotional Abuse and Other Psychic Harms: Invisible Wounds and their Histories* (Basingstoke, 2012).
8 On accounts, see M. Scott and S. Lyman, 'Accounts', *American Sociological Review*, 33, 1 (1968), pp. 46–62. For a recent approach to justification, see L. Boltanski and L. Thévenot, *On Justification: Economies of Worth* (Princeton, NJ, 2006, translated by C. Porter).
9 www.mkhospital.nhs.uk/board-of-directors/trust-committees, accessed 29 June 2013.
10 A. Giddens, *Beyond Left and Right: The Future of Radical Politics* (Cambridge, 1994), p. 7.
11 H. Cayton, *Trust Me, I'm A Patient: Can Healthcare Afford the Informed Consumer?*, speech delivered to the Royal College of Physicians, BUPA Health Debate, 2 September 2003, London.
12 The issue is discussed at length in J. Clarke, J. Newman, N. Smith, E. Vidler and L. Westmarland, *Creating Citizen-Consumers: Changing Publics and Changing Public Services* (London, 2007).
13 On the distinction between demotic and democratic arrangements, see G. Turner, *Ordinary People and the Media: The Demotic Turn* (London, 2010); and J. Clarke, 'Enrolling Ordinary People: Governmental Strategies and the Avoidance of Politics?', *Citizenship Studies*, 14, 6 (2010), pp. 637–650.
14 Clarke *et al.*, *Creating Citizen-Consumers*, p. 132.
15 Clarke *et al.*, *Creating Citizen-Consumers*; R. Sennett, *Respect: The Formation of Character in an Age of Inequality* (London, 2003), p. 178.
16 C. Needham, *Personalising Public Services: Understanding the Personalisation Narrative* (Bristol, 2011).
17 H. Graham, 'Open to the Public and on Behalf of the Public: Museums and their Democratic Deficit', paper presented to the 'Creating Publics, Creating Democracies' workshop, organised by the Centre for Citizenship, Identities and Governance, The Open University, Goldsmiths' College and the University of Westminster (18–19 June 2012).
18 Abbé Gregoire: *Le Moniteur universel*, vol. 8, p. 354. Quoted in S. Wahnich, *In Defence of the Terror* (London, 2012, translated by D. Fernbach), p. 84.

Index